Oettgen

Gangliosides and Cancer

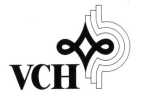

© VCH Verlagsgesellschaft mbH, D-6940 Weinheim (Federal Republic of Germany), 1989

Distribution:

VCH Verlagsgesellschaft, P. O. Box 10 11 61, D-6940 Weinheim (Federal Republic of Germany)

Switzerland: VCH Verlags-AG, P. O.-Box, CH-4020 Basel (Switzerland)

Great Britain and Ireland: VCH Publishers (UK) Ltd., 8 Wellington Court, Wellington Street, Cambridge CB1 1HW (Great Britain)

USA and Canada: VCH Publishers, Suite 909, 220 East 23rd Street, New York, NY 10010-4606 (USA)

ISBN 3-527-27835-4 (VCH Verlagsgesellschaft)   ISBN 0-89573-877-5 (VCH Publishers)

Gangliosides and Cancer

Edited by H. F. Oettgen

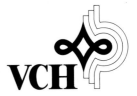

Herbert F. Oettgen, M. D.
Memorial Sloan-Kettering Cancer Center
1275 York Avenue
New York, N.Y. 10021, USA

1st edition 1989

Published jointly by
VCH Verlagsgesellschaft, Weinheim (Federal Republic of Germany)
VCH Publishers, New York, NY (USA)

Editorial Director: Dr. Michael G. Weller
Production Manager: Dipl.-Wirt.-Ing. (FH) Bernd Riedel
Production Director: Maximilian Montkowski
Composition: Hagedorn GmbH, D-6806 Viernheim
Printing: Colordruck Kurt Weber GmbH, D-6906 Leimen
Bookbinding: Georg Kränkl, D-6148 Heppenheim

British Library Cataloguing-in-Publication Data:
Gangliosides and cancer
  1. Man. Cancer. Role of gangliosides. Man.
Neurons. Gangliosides. Role in cancer
  I. Oettgen, Herbert F.
616.99'4079

ISBN 3-527-27835-4

Deutsche Bibliothek Cataloguing-in-Publication Data:
Gangliosides and cancer / ed. by H. F. Oettgen. – 1. ed. –
Weinheim ; Basel (Switzerland) ; Cambridge ; New York, NY :
VCH, 1989
  ISBN 3-527-27835-4 (Weinheim ...) Gb.
  ISBN 0-89573-877-5 (Cambridge ...) Gb.
NE: Oettgen, Herbert F. [Hrsg.]

Table of Contents

Symposium held at the European Academy, Nonnweiler/Trier,
June 17–19, 1988.

List of Contributors

D. Bajorin
Memorial Sloan-Kettering Cancer Center,
1275 York Avenue,
New York, NY 10021, USA

B. L. Bauer
Institute of Neurosurgery,
Universität von Marburg,
3550 Marburg/Lahn,
Federal Republic of Germany

B. Bechtel
Wistar Institute of Anatomy and Biology,
3601 Spruce Street,
Philadelphia, PA 19104-4268, USA

H. Bernhard
Medizinische Klinik,
Johannes Gutenberg-Universität Mainz,
6500 Mainz, Federal Republic of Germany

J. Biedler
Memorial Sloan-Kettering Cancer Center,
1275 York Avenue,
New York, NY 10021, USA

E. Boosfeld
Memorial Sloan-Kettering Cancer Center,
1275 York Avenue,
New York, NY 10021, USA

K. Bosslet
Research Laboratories of Behringwerke AG,
3550 Marburg/Lahn,
Federal Republic of Germany

S. Canevari
Division of Experimental Oncology E,
Instituto Nationale Tumori,
Via Venezian 1,
20133 Milano, Italy

C. Cardon-Cardo
Memorial Sloan-Kettering Cancer Center,
1275 York Avenue,
New York, NY 10021, USA

P. J. Chandler
John Wayne Cancer Clinic and
Armand Hammer Research Laboratories,
University of California,
School of Medicine,
Louis Factor # 9-267,
Los Angeles, California 90024, USA

P. B. Chapman
Memorial Sloan Kettering Cancer Center,
1275 York Avenue,
New York, NY 10021, USA

N. K.V. Cheung
Memorial Sloan-Kettering Cancer Center,
1275 York Avenue,
New York, NY 10021, USA

M. J. Colnaghi
Instituto Nationale Tumori,
Via Venezian 1,
20133 Milano, Italy

J. Di Maggio
Memorial Sloan-Kettering Cancer Center,
1275 York Avenue,
New York, NY 10021, USA

W. Dippold
First Department of Internal Medicine,
Universität von Mainz,
Langenbeck-Str. 1, 6500 Mainz,
Federal Republik of Germany

T. Feizi
Clinical Research Center,
Watford Road,
Harrow, Middlesex HA 1 3 UJ, England

P. Fredmann
Department of Psychiatry and
Neurochemistry,
Göteburg Universität,
St. Jørgen's Hospital,
42203 Hisings Bacha, Sweden

T. Fujimori
Department of Pathology,
Tokai University School of Medicine,
Isehara, Kamagawa 250-11, Japan

S.-I. Hakomori
The Biomembrane Institute,
201 Elliott Ave. West,
Seattle, WA 98119, USA

Y. Harada
Center for Neurobiology
and Molecular Immunology,
School of Medicine,
Chiba University,
Chiba 280, Japan

A. N. Houghton
Memorial Sloan-Kettering Cancer Center,
1275 York Avenue,
New York, NY 10021, USA

R. F. Irie
Department of Surgery,
UCLA School of Medicine,
10833 Le Conte Avenue,
Los Angles, CA 90024, USA

K. Ishii
Department of Biochemistry,
Shizuoka College of Pharmacy,
2-2-1 Oshika, Shizuoka 422, Japan

J. D. Johnson
Department of Physiological Chemistry,
The Ohio State University,
473 West 12th Avenue,
Columbus, Ohio 43210, USA

J. P. Johnson
Institute for Immunology,
Goethestraße 31, 8000 München 2,
Federal Republic of Germany

J. Kawashima
Department of Oncology,
Tokyo Metropolitan Institute
of Medical Science, Honkomagome,
Bunkyo-ku, Tokyo 113, Japan

R.V. Kleist
Gesellschaft für
Biotechnologische Forschung, GBF,
Mascheroder Weg 1, 3000 Braunschweig,
Federal Republic of Germany

R. Klingel
First Department of Internal Medicine,
Universität von Mainz, 6500 Mainz,
Federal Republic of Germany

B. H. Kushner
Memorial Sloan-Kettering Cancer Center,
1275 York Avenue,
New York, NY 10021, USA

S. Ladisch
Division of Hematology/Oncology,
Department of Pediatrics,
UCLA School of Medicine,
Los Angles, CA 90024, USA

F. Leoni
Division of Experimental Oncology E,
Instituto Nationale Tumori,
Via Venezian 1,
20133 Milano, Italy

P. O. Livingston
Memorial Sloan-Kettering Cancer Center,
1275 York Avenue,
New York, NY 10021, USA

K. O. Lloyd
Memorial Sloan-Kettering Cancer Center,
1275 York Avenue,
New York, NY 10021, USA

B. K. Mc Illroy
Department of Physiological Chemistry,
The Ohio State University,
473 West 12th Avenue,
Columbus, Ohio 43210, USA

H. D. Mennel
Institute of Neuropathology,
Universität von Marburg,
3550 Marburg/Lahn,
Federal Republic of Germany

W. D. Merritt
Children's Hospital
National Medical Center
III Michigan Avenue, N.W.
Washington, D.C. 20010, USA

K. H. Meyer zum Büschenfelde
First Department of Internal Medicine,
Universität von Mainz, 6500 Mainz,
Federal Republic of Germany

S. Miotti
Division of Experimental Oncology E,
Instituto Nationale Tumori,
Via Venezian 1, 20133 Milano, Italy

P. Mühlradt
Gesellschaft für
Biotechnologische Forschung,
Mascheroder Weg 1, 3300 Braunschweig,
Federal Republic of Germany

J. Müthing
Gesellschaft für
Biotechnologische Forschung,
Mascheroder Weg 1,
3300 Braunschweig,
Federal Republic of Germany

D. H. Munn
Memorial Sloam-Kettering Cancer Center,
1275 York Avenue,
New York, NY 10021, USA

A. Myoga
Department of Biochemistry,
Shizuoka College of Pharmacy 2-2-1,
Oshika, Shizuoka 422, Japan

Y. Nagai
Department of Biochemistry,
Faculty of Medicine,
University of Tokyo, Hongo,
Bunkyo-ku, Tokyo, Japan

H. F. Oettgen
Memorial Sloan-Kettering Cancer Center,
1275 York Avenue,
New York, NY 10021, USA

L. J. Old
Memorial Sloan-Kettering Cancer Center,
1275 York Avenue,
New York, NY 10021, USA

J. Portoukalian
Laboratory of Immunology,
Center Léon Bérnard,
69373 Lyon, CX 08, France

M. H. Ravindranath
John Wayne Cancer Clinic and
Armand Hammer Research Laboratories,
University of California,
School of Medicine,
Los Angeles, California 90024, USA

G. H. Reaman
Children's Hospital,
National Medical Center,
III Michigan Avenue, N.W.,
Washington, D.C. 20010, USA

S. L. Ren
Department of Pharmacology,
Yale University
School of Medicin,
333 Cedar Street,
New Haven, CT 06510, USA

G. Riethmüller
Department of Immunology,
University of München,
Goethestr. 31, 8000 München,
Federal Republic of Germany

G. Ritter
Memorial Sloan-Kettering Cancer Center,
1275 York Avenue,
New York, NY 10021, USA

F. Rodden
Institute of Neurosurgery,
Universität von Marburg,
3550 Marburg/Lahn,
Federal Republic of Germany

M. Sakatsume
Division of Molecular Immunology,
Center for Neurobiology and
Molekular Immunology,
School of Medicine, Chiba University,
Chiba 280, Japan

Y. Sanai
Department of Biochemistry,
Faculty of Medicine,
University of Tokyo,
Bunkyo-ku, Tokyo 113, Japan

A. C. Sartorelli
Department of Pharmacology,
Yale University
School of Medicine,
333 Cedar Street,
New Haven, CT 06510, USA

H. H. Sedlacek
Research Laboratories of
Behringwerke AG,
3550 Marburg/Lahn,
Federal Republic of Germany

S. Sonnino
Department of Biochemistry,
University of Milano,
Medical School, Via Saldini 50,
20133 Milano, Italy

S. Spiegel
Department of Biochemistry,
Georgetown University
School of Medicine,
3900 Reservoir Road N.W.,
Washington DC 20007, USA

S. M. Stock
Division of Neuropathology,
The Ohio State University,
473 West 12th Avenue,
Columbus, Ohio 43210, USA

M. B. Sztein
Department of Medicine,
The George Washington University
School of Medicine and Health Sciences,
Washington DC 20037, USA

N. Tada
Department of Pathology,
Tokai University School of Medicine,
Isehara, Kanagawa 250-11, Japan

T. Tai
The Tokyo Metropolitan Institute
of Medical Science, 18–22,
Honkomagone, 3-Chome, Bunkyo-ku,
Tokyo 113, Japan

T. Taki
Department of Biochemistry,
Shizuoka College of Pharmacy,
2-2-1 Oshika, Shizuoka 422, Japan

M. Taniguchi
Department of Immunology,
Chiba University School of Medicine,
1-8-1 Inohana, Chiba 280, Japan

J. Thurin
The Wistar Institute,
Thirty-Sixth-Street at Spruce,
Philadelphia, PA 19104-4268, USA

T. Tsuchida
John Wayne Cancer Clinic and
Armand Hammer Research Laboratories,
University of California,
School of Medicine,
Los Angeles, California 90024, USA

S. Tsuji
Department of Biochemistry,
Faculty of Medicine,
University of Tokyo, Hongo,
Bunkyo-ku, Tokyo 113, Japan

N. Usmani
Departments of Pediatrics,
Pathology, Medicine, and
Sloan Kettering Institute,
Memorial Sloan-Kettering Cancer Center,
New York, NY 10021, USA

F. Wagner
Institute of Pathology,
Universität von Gießen, 6300 Gießen,
Federal Republic of Germany

J. D. Walters
College of Medicine,
and College of Dentistry,
The Ohio State University,
473 West 12th Avenue Columbus,
Ohio 43210, USA

K. Welte
Memorial Sloan-Kettering Cancer Center,
1275 York Avenue,
New York, NY 10021, USA

H. Wiegandt
Physiologisch-Chemisches Institut,
Universität von Marburg,
Lahnberge, 3550 Marburg,
Federal Republic of Germany

X. J. Xia
Department of Pharmacology,
Yale University
School of Medicin,
333 Cedar Street,
New Haven, CT 06510, USA

A. J. Yates
Ohio State University,
Division of Neuropathology,
Room 111 Upham Hall,
473 West 12th Avenue, Columbus,
Ohio 43210, USA

S. D. Yeh
Memorial Sloan-Kettering Cancer Center,
1275 York Avenue,
New York, NY 10021, USA

R. Yu
Department of Biochemistry,
Medical College of Virginia,
Box 614,
Richmond, VA 23298, USA

H. Yuasa
Memorial Sloan-Kettering Cancer Center,
1275 York Avenue,
New York, NY 10021, USA

1. Gangliosides and Cancer: Introduction

H. F. Oettgen

The term ganglioside was coined in 1942 in reference to lipids of the central nervous system that contained neuraminic acid, to signify their prime location in ganglion cells and their glycosidic nature (1).

Until 1979, many years later, ganglioside research was centered mainly on nervous tissue. In that year, however, a ganglioside identified by thin-layer chromatography and carbohydrate analysis, called GD3, was found to be a prominent constituent of a human cancer, malignant melanoma, that did not arise from the nervous system (2). In the following year, a glycolipid antigen on cultured human melanoma cells was identified by mouse monoclonal antibody (3) and later shown to belong to the ganglioside GD3 (4). Further, therapy with the IgG3 monoclonal antibody R24, which recognizes GD3, was found to be associated with partial regression of melanoma metastases in a small proportion of cases (5), raising expectations for gangliosides as points of therapeutic attack. Other gangliosides identified with mouse monoclonal antibodies as prominent human cancer cell surface antigens include GD2 and GM2 in malignant melanoma (6, 7), GD2 in neuroblastoma (8), and sialylated lacto-series gangliosides in epithelial cancers (9).

It was later established that melanoma gangliosides can also be recognized by the human immune system (10–12), and active immunization of patients became a second mode of therapy to be explored. In fact patients have been shown to produce antibodies against GM2 in response to immunization with a purified GM2 vaccine (13). Retrospective analysis suggests that production of GM2 antibodies was associated with delay in recurrence of melanoma, and this is now being tested in a prospective study.

With rising clinical interest in gangliosides came a pressing need to promote and facilitate communication not only among those concerned in the study and treatment of cancer but also with investigators engaged in research on other aspects of the gangliosides. This symposium was designed to serve that very purpose.

In addition to substantiating, extending and detailing our knowledge of ganglioside and glycolipid expression in cancer and consequent approaches to therapy, we discussed a wide range of topics, including the molecular structure and three-dimensional conformation of gangliosides and other glycolipids, the role of gangliosides in cellular signal transmission, the effects of gangliosides on immunological functions and other cellular interactions and, again with a view toward therapy, ways to augment the immunogenicity of gangliosides. This book is an account of the information we shared.

It remains for me to thank those who have contributed so generously – Sen-itiroh Hakomori, Herbert Wiegandt, and Kenneth Lloyd for their invaluable help in developing and formulating the program, all participants for sharing results of their most recent work freely, and Dr. Thomas Stiefel and Dr. Harald Porcher of Biosyn for their excellent logistic support and assistance in arranging timely publication.

References

1. Klenk, E. Über die ganglioside, eine neue Gruppe von zuckerhaltigen Gehirnlipoiden. Hoppe-Seyler's Z. Physiol. Chem. 273, 76–86, 1942.
2. Portoukalian, J., Zwingelstein, G., and Dorre, J. Lipid composition of human malignant melanoma tumors at various levels of malignant growth. Eur. J. Biochem. 94, 19–23, 1979.
3. Dippold, W. G., Lloyd, K. O., Li, L.T. C., Ikeda, H., Oettgen, H. F., and Old, L. J. Cell surface antigens of human malignant melanoma: Definition of six antigenic systems with monoclonal antibodies. Proc. Natl. Acad. Sci. USA 77, 6114–6118, 1980.
4. Pukel, C. S., Lloyd, K. O., Travassos, L. R., Dippold, W. G., Oettgen, H. F., and Old, L. J. GD3, a prominent ganglioside of human melanoma. Detection and characterization by mouse monoclonal antibody. J. Exp. Med. 155, 1133–1147, 1982.
5. Houghton, A. N., Mintzer, D., Cordon-Cardo, C., Welt, S., Fliegel, B., Vadhan, S., Carswell, E., Melamed, M. R., Oettgen, H. F., and Old, L. J. Mouse monoclonal IgG3 antibody detecting GD3 ganglioside: a phase I trial in patients with malignant melanoma. Proc. Natl. Acad. Sci. USA 82, 1242–1246, 1985.
6. Watanabe, T., Pukel, C. S., Takeyama, H., Lloyd, K. O., Shiku, H., Li, L.T. C., Travassos, L. R., Oettgen, H. F., and Old, L. J. Human melanoma antigen AH is an autoantigenic ganglioside related to GD2. J. Exp. Med. 156, 1884–1889, 1982.
7. Natoli, E. J., Livingston, P. O., Pukel, C. S., Lloyd, K. O., Wiegandt, H., Szalay, J., Oettgen, H. F., and Old, L. J. A murine monoclonal antibody detecting N-acetyl and N-glycolyd-GM2. Cancer Res. 46, 4116–4120, 1986.
8. Cheung, N-K.V., Saarinen, U. M., Neely, J. E., Landmeier, B., Donovan, D., and Coccia, P. F. Monoclonal antibodies to a glycolipid antigen on human neuroblastoma cells. Cancer Res. 45, 2642–2649, 1985.
9. Hakomori, S. Tumor associated carbohydrate antigens. Ann. Rev. Immunol. 2, 103–126, 1984.
10. Cahan, L. D., Irie, R. F., Singh, R., Cassidenti, R., and Paulson, J. C. Identification of a human neuroectodermal tumor antigen (OFA-1-2) as ganglioside GD2. Proc. Natl. Acad. Sci. USA 79, 7629–7633, 1982.
11. Tai, T., Paulson, J. C., Cahan, L. D., and Irie, R. F. Ganglioside GM2 as a human tumor antigen (OFA-1-1). Proc. Natl. Acad. Sci. USA 280, 5392–5396, 1983.
12. Yamaguchi, H., Furukawa, K., Fortunato, S. R., Livingston, P. O., Lloyd, K. O., Oettgen, H. F., and Old, L. J. Cell-surface antigens of melanoma recognized by human monoclonal antibodies. Proc. Natl. Acad. Sci. USA 84, 2416–2420, 1987.
13. Livingston, P. O., Natoli, E. J., Jones-Calves, M., Stockert, E., Oettgen, H. F., and Old, L. J. Vaccines containing purified GM2 ganglioside elicit GM2 antibodies in melanoma patients. Proc. Natl. Acad. Sci. USA 84, 2911–2915, 1987.

2. The Chemical Structure of Gangliosides

H. Wiegandt

Gangliosides are lipid constituents of the cellular plasma membrane. Their lipophilic residue, composed of an amide-linked long chain sphingoid base and a fatty acid, the ceramide, is believed to participate in the formation of the outer leaflet of the cell membrane lipid bilayer. The carbohydrate portion of the ganglioside molecule is oriented towards the outer environment. In this strategic position, gangliosides contribute to the very special surface features that characterize cells according to animal species and cell types. The component profile of the gangliosides also varies greatly with the developmental stage of the cells and their mode of growth. Cellular differentiation or dedifferentiation due to oncogenic transformation correlate with changes in ganglioside distribution. No "tumour-associated" ganglioside species appear to exist that cannot also be found at some other location in normal tissue.

Analysis of the tumour-associated ganglioside component profile, however, may aid in the characterization of tumour cells and their degree of malignant transformation. Furthermore, gangliosides that become prominently exposed on tumour cells during oncogenic dedifferentiation may be used as targets for specific immuno-histological identification and possible therapeutic approaches.

The aim of this chapter is to enumerate the chemical structures of all gangliosides known today. This should provide a basis for the discussion of "Gangliosides and Cancer" (see Appendix).

As do other glycosphingolipids, gangliosides differ from one another by their carbohydrate moieties. They are distinguished from other glycosphingolipids by the presence of one or more residues of sialic acid*.

In animals, sialic acid is present only in phyla of the deuterostomia. D-glucuronic acid may take a similar position as sialic acid in glycosphingolipids from animals of the protostomia.

Glycosphingolipids may be biologically related to one another through the stepwise addition or removal of single monosaccharides. Such glycolipids can therefore be arranged in series. Sialic acid containing glycolipids, i.e. gangliosides, occur within all these carbohydrate series (see Appendix).

Commencing the buildup of the carbohydrate moiety with lactose from glucose and galactose, further extension by N-acetylglucosamine, galactose or N-acetylgalactosamine leads to the formation of oligosaccharides of the "lacto"-, "globo"- or the "ganglio"-series, respectively (Figure 1).

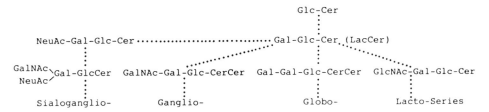

Figure 1. Arrangement of Glycosphingolipids according to Carbohydrate Series.

---

* The generic name for variously substituted neuraminic acids, the sialic acid, is derived from the sialic acid rich mucins of saliva (greek, τὸ σίαλον).

There appears to be a tendency for glycolipids of the ganglio-, globo- or the lacto-series to occur preferentially in cells derived from the ekto-, meso-, or entodermal germ layer, respectively.

Some related glycolipids lack glucose as the first sugar. Instead, they commence their oligosaccharide chain with galactose attached to the ceramide. Such glycolipids occur substituted by sialic acid or sulfate, or they are extended by neutral sugars much in the same way as other compounds of the ganglio- or the globo-series.

If, as is the case with the classical major brain gangliosides, the transfer of N-acetyl-galactosamine to the lactose is preceded by substitution with sialic acid, members of the "sialoganglio"-series are formed (Figure 1). As a consequence, cell types that carry glycolipids of the sialoganglio-series, frequently have gangliosides as their most prominent glycolipid constituents. Conspicuously, such cells appear in many cases to be of a neuroektodermal origin.

Tumours that result from dedifferentiation of neuroectodermal cells, such as gliomas, neuroblastomas, melanomas or small cell lung carcinomas, therefore, can be characterized by altered patterns of their sialoganglio-series gangliosides. As a more general phenomenon, these neuroectodermal tumours contain gangliosides of a lesser degree of structural complexity, such as mono- and disialogangliotriaosylceramide and mono- and disialolactosylceramide.

The identification of the chemical structure of gangliosides on a small scale is greatly aided by the use of monoclonal antibodies. Such antibodies that recognize sialic acid containing immune-epitopes have been described for some gangliosides of all carbohydrate series (see Appendix). In many instances, the sialo-immune-epitopes are composed of a three sugar unit, or in the case one member carries a monosaccharide substitution a four sugar unit. Good examples for this are provided by the antibodies that were raised against epitopes specific for the mono-, bis-, and trissialoganglio-series gangliosides, but also against gangliosides of other carbohydrate series (see Appendix).

The puzzling question posed by the intricate wealth of systematic chemical structures among the ganglioside-sialooligosaccharides indeed has not been answered satisfactorily. It remains to be seen whether the many carbohydrates of varying constitution provide a rich matrix of information for biological processes, or whether they exert their influences by the creation of special physico-chemical environments necessary for biological functions at the cell membrane.

Appendix

The structures of gangliosides are enumerated following the chemical constitution of their respective sialooligosaccharide moieties. The gangliosides are arranged according to the oligosaccharide series, i.e.
I.   Ganglio-series
II. Monosialoganglio-series
III. Bis(a)- and Tris(c)-sialoganglio-series
IV. Globo- and isoGlobo-series
V.   Lacto-series
VI. neoLacto-series
In order to facilitate a quick one glance view of the known ganglioside structures, their oligosaccharides, as well as some structurally related milk sugars, are depicted in schematic presentations (Figure 2).

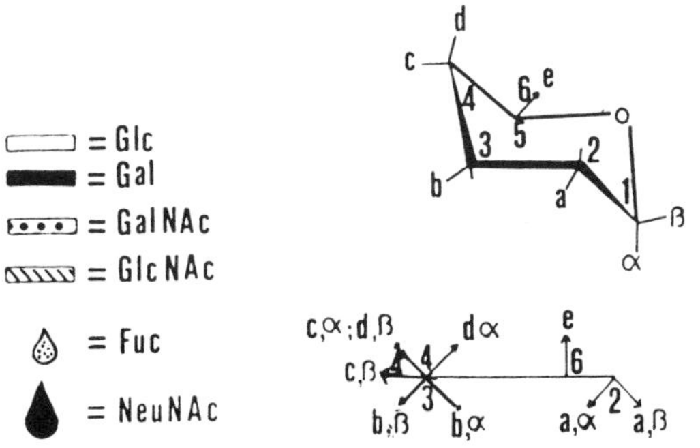

Figure 2. System of the schematic presentation of ganglioside-derived oligosaccharides. The sugar structures are given from right to left, their reducing end at the right. Substitution positions are indicated by angles that also depend on the equatorial or axial position of the aglycosidic hydroxyl, respectively.

The schematic presentations are complemented by a list of proposed minimal ganglioside- and milk sugar designations for computer usage. As a reference, the first report on the chemical constitution of the respective gangliosides is cited from the literature. Footnote quotations refer to publications of ganglioside – directed monoclonal antibodies.

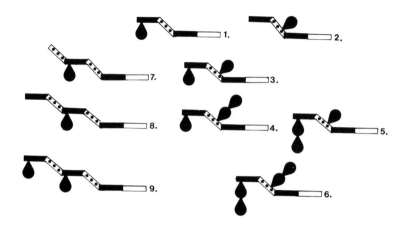

Gangliosides of the Ganglio-Series

I. Ganglio-series gangliosides (ω-series)

Nr.	Ganglioside structure	Computer designation* References
1.	IV^{3}NeuAc-Cg$_4$Cer	4433SxBDBA Hirabayashi, Y., & al. (1979) FEBS Lett. 100, 153-7; Watanabe, K., & al. (1979) JBC 254, 8223-9
1a.	NeuAcα2, 3Galβ1, 3GalNacβ1, 4GalCer	433SxBDB Watanabe, K., & al. (1979) Biochem. 18, 5502-4
2.	III^{6}NeuAc-Gg$_4$Cer	443B6SxDBA not yet reported
3.	IV^{3}NeuAc-, III^{6}NeuAc-Gg$_4$Cer	4433SxB6SxDBA Ohashi, M. (1981) Glycoconjugates, Proc. VI. Int. Symp. Tokyo, pp 33-4
4.	IV^{3}NeuAc-, III^6(NeuAc)$_2$-Gg$_4$Cer	4433SxB68SxSxDBA Ohashi, M. (1981) Glycoconjugates, Proc. VI. Int. Symp. Tokyo, pp 33-4
5.	IV^3(NeuAc)$_2$-, III^{6}NeuAc-Gg$_4$Cer	44338SxSxB6SxDBA Ohashi, M. (1981) Glycoconjugates, Proc. VI. Int. Symp. Tokyo, pp 33-4
6.	IV^3(NeuAc)$_2$-, III^6(NeuAc)$_2$-Gg$_4$Cer	44338SxSxB68SxSxDBA Ohashi, M. (1981) Glycoconjugates, Proc. VI. Int. Symp. Tokyo, pp 33-4
7.	IV^{3}NeuAc-Gg$_5$Cer	4434D3SxBDBA Ilyas, A., & al. (1988) J. Biol. Chem. 263, 4369-73
8.	IV^{3}NeuAc-Gg$_6$Cer	44343BD3SxBDBA not yet reported
9.	VI^{3}NeuAc-, IV^{3}NeuAc-Gg$_6$Cer	443433SxBD3SxBDBA not yet reported

*Computer Designations (C.D.) for oligosaccharides: Monosaccharide constituents, A = βDGlcp; B = βDGalp; C = βDGlcNAcp; D = βDGalNacp; F = βLFucp; S = βSialp. The core oligosaccharide chain is read in two directions, first, from the reducing end the glycosidic substitution positions. These numbers are written in the C.D. beginning from left to right; second, from the non-reducing terminal the monosaccharide constituents from left to right, also written in the C.D. from left to right, e. g. gangliotriaose, i. e. GalNAcβ1, 4Galβ1, 4Glc, 44DBA. x-anomeric glycopyranosides are indicated by an x (l. c.), e. g. globotriaose, i. e. Galx1, 4Galβ1, 4Glc, 44BxBA. In the case of branching oligosaccharides, the longest chain, except for substitutions in the 6-position, is considered as the core sequence. Substituents in branching positions are then placed within the straight core oligosaccharide chain designation with the corresponding positional numberings, e. g. ganglioside II^3(NeuAc)$_2$-Gg$_4$Cer, 443BD3SSxSxBA. If two ligands ccould be read as in terminal position, except for fucose and sialic acid, the one with the lower glycosidic positional number will be considered as in branching position.

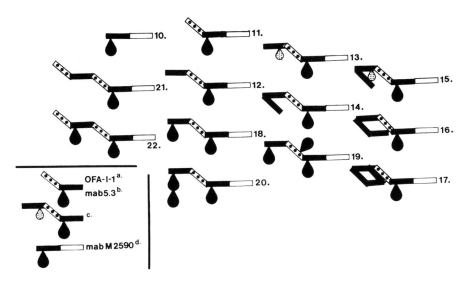

Gangliosides of the Monosialo-Ganglio-Series

II. Monosialoganglio-series Gangliosides (a-series)

Nr.	Ganglioside structure	Computer designation* References
10.	II^3NeuAc-LacCer	43SxBA Kuhn, R., & al. (1964) Zschr. Naturforsch. 19b, 256-7
11.	II^3NeuAc-Gg$_3$Cer	44D3SxBA Kuhn, R., & al. (1963) Chem. Ber. 96, 866-80
12.	II^3NeuAc-Gg$_4$Cer	443BD3SxBA Kuhn, R., & al. (1963) Chem. Ber. 96, 866-80
13.	IV^2Fuc-, II^3NeuAc-Gg$_4$Cer	4432FxBD3SxBA Wiegandt, H. (1973) H.-S. Zschr. Physiol. Chem. 354, 1049-56
14.	IV^3Galx-, II^3NeuAc-Gg$_4$Cer	4433BxBD3SxBA Ohashi, M. (1982) Lipids 14, 52-7
15.	IV^3Galx-, IV^2Fuc-, II^3NeuAc-Gg$_4$Cer	4433Bx2FxBD3SxBA Holmes, E. H., & al. (1982) J. Biol. Chem. 257, 7698-703
16.	IV^3Galβ-3Galx-, II^3NeuAc-Gg$_4$Cer	44333BBxBD3SxBA Ohashi, M. (1982) Lipids 14, 52-7
17.	IV^3Galx-3Galβ-Galx-, II^3NeuAc-Gg$_4$Cer	443333BxbBxBD3SxBA Ohashi, M. (1982) Lipids 14, 52-7
18.	IV^3NeuAc-, II^3NeuAc-Gg$_4$Cer	4433SxBD3SxBA Kuhn, R., & al. (1963) Zschr. Naturf. 18b, 541-3
19.	IV^3NeuAc-, III^6NeuAc-, II^3NeuAc-Gg$_4$Cer	4433SxB6SxD3SxBA Nakamura, K., & al. (1988) Proc. Jap. Germ. Symp. Sial. Acids, Berlin, Schauer, Yamakawa, eds, Kieler Verlag Wissenschaft, pp 86-7
20.	IV^3(NeuAc)$_2$-, II^3NeuAc-Gg$_4$Cer	44338SxSxBD3SxBA Ando, S., & al. (1977) J. Bio. Chem. 252, 6247-59
21.	II^3NeuAc-Gg$_5$Cer	4434DBD3SxBA Iwamori, M., & al. (1978) J. Biochem. 84, 1601-8
22.	IV^3NeuAc-, II^3NeuAcc-Gg$_5$Cer	4434D3SxBD3SxBA Svennerholm, L., & al. (1973) J. Biol. Chem. 248, 740-2

a. Tai, T., & al. (1983) Proc. Natl. Acad. Sci. (USA) 80, 5392-6
b. Natoli, E. J., & al. (1986) Cancer. Res. 46, 4116-20
c. Fredman, P., & al. (1986) Biochi. Biophys. Acta 875, 316-23
d. Hirabayashi, Y., & al. (1985) J. Biol. Chem. 260, 13328-33 (Lactone: Nores, G., & al. (1987) J. Immunol 139, 3171-6)

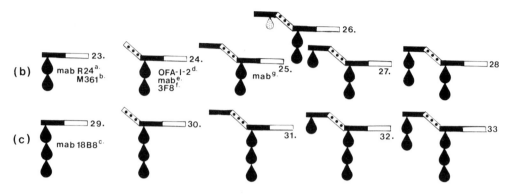

Gangliosides of the Bis-(b), and Tris-(c)sialo-ganglio-Series

III. Bissialoganglio-series gangliosides (b-series)

Nr.	Ganglioside structure	Computer designation* References
23.	$II^3(NeuAc)_2Lac$	438SxSxBA Kuhn, R., & al. (1964) Zschr. Naturf. 19b, 256-7
24.	$II^3(NeuAc)_2\text{-}Gg_3Cer$	44D38SxSxBA Klenk, E., & al. (1968) H.-. Zschr. Physiol. Chem. 349, 288-92
25.	$II^3(NeuAc)_2\text{-}Gg_4Cer$	443BD38SxSxBA Kuhn, R., & al. (1964) Zschr. Naturf. 18b, 541-3
26.	$IV^2Fuc\text{-}, II^3(NeuAc)_2\text{-}Gg_4Cer$	4432FxBD38SxSxBA Sonnino, S., & al. (1978) J. Neurochem. 31, 947-56
27.	$IV^3NeuAc\text{-}, II^3(NeuAc)_2\text{-}Gg_4Cer$	4433SxB38SxSxBA Kuhn, R., & al. (1963) Zschr. Naturf. 18b, 541-3
28.	$IV^3(NeuAc)_2\text{-}, II^3(NeuAc)_2\text{-}Gg_4Cer$	44338SxSxBD38SxSxBA Ishizuka, I., & al. (1972) Biochi. Biophys. Acta 260, 279-85

Trissialoganglio-series gangliosides (c-series)

Nr.	Ganglioside structure	Computer designation References
29.	$II^3(NeuAc)_3\text{-}LacCer$	4388SxSxSxBA Yu, R. K. (1980) Adv. Exptl. Med. Biol. 125, 33
30.	$II^3(NeuAc)_3\text{-}Gg_3Cer$	44D388SxSxSxBA Ohashi, M., & al. (1977) J. Biochem. 81, 1675-90
31.	$II^3(NeuAc)_3\text{-}Gg_4Cer$	443BD388SxSxSxBA Ishizuka, I., & al. (1972) Biochi. Biophys. Acta 260, 279-85
32.	$IV^3(NeuAc)_2\text{-}, II^3(NeuAc)_3\text{-}Gg_4Cer$	4433SxBD388SxSxSxBA Ishizuka, I., & al. (1972) Biochi. Biophys. Acta 260, 279-85
33.	$IV^3(NeuAc)_2\text{-}, II^3(NeuAc)_3\text{-}Gg_4Cer$	44338SxSxBD388SxSxSxBA Ishizuka, I., & al. (1972) Biochi. Biophys. Acta 260, 279-85

a. Pukel, C., & al. (1982) J. exptl. Canc. Res. 155, 1133-47
b. Thurin, J., & al. (1987) Canc. Res. 47, 1229-33
c. Dubois, C., & al. (1986) J. Biol. Chem. 261, 3826-30
d. Cahan, L. D., & al. (1982) Proc. Natl. Acad. Sci. (USA) 79, 7629-33
e. BW 625, BW 704, Boslet, K., & al. (1988), see present volume.
f. Cheung, N. K.V., & al. (1987) J. Clin. Oncol. 5, 1430-40
g. Fredman, P., & al. (1985) FEBS Lett. 189, 23-6

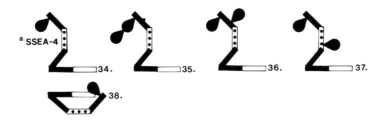

a. SSEA-4

Gangliosides of the Globo-Series

IV. Globo-series gangliosides

Nr.	Ganglioside structure	Computer designation* References
34.	V^3NeuAc-Gb$_5$Cer	4433SxBDBxBA Hogan, E. L., & al. (1981) Glycoconjugates, Proc. 6. Int. Symp. Tokyo, pp 74-5
35.	V^3(NeuAc)$_2$-Gb$_5$Cer	44338SxSxBDBxBA Hogan, E. L., & al. (1981) Glycoconjugates, Proc. 6. Int. Symp. Tokyo, pp 75-5
36.	V^3NeuAc-, V^6NeuAc-Gb$_5$Cer	4433Sx6SxBDBxBA Kundu, S. K., & al. (1983) J. Biol. Chem. 258, 13857-66
37.	V^3NeuAc-, IV^6NeuAc-Gb$_5$Cer	44333SxSx6SxDBxBA Ishizuka, I. (1987)

isoGlobo-series gangliosides

38.	V^3NeuAc-iGb$_5$Cer	43333SxBDBxBA Breimer, M. E., & al. (1982) J. Biol. Chem. 257, 557-68

a. Kannagi, R., & al. (1983) EMBO J. 2, 2355-61

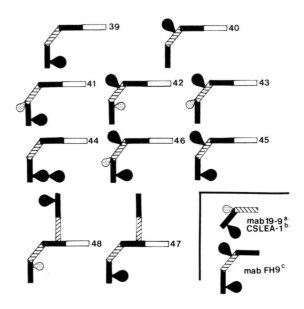

Gangliosides of the Lacto-Series

V. Lacto-series gangliosides

Nr.	Ganglioside structure	Computer designation* References
39.	$IV^3NeuAc\text{-}Lc_4Cer$	4333SxBCBA Nilsson, O., (1985) FEBS Lett. 182, 398-402
40.	$III^6NeuAc\text{-}Lc_4$	433B6SxCBA milk oligosaccharide: Kuhn, R., & al. (1953) Chem. Ber. 86, 827
41.	$IV^3NeuAc\text{-}, III^4Fuc\text{-}Lc_4Cer$	4333SxB4FxCBA Magnani, J. L. (1982) J. Biol. Chem. 257, 14365-9
42.	$IV^2Fuc\text{-}, III^6NeuAc\text{-}Lc_4$	4332FxB6SxCBA milk oligosaccharide: Wieruszeski, & al. (1986) Carb. Res. 137, 127-38
43.	$III^4Fuc\text{-}, III^6NeuAc\text{-}Lc_4Cer$	433B4Fx6SxCBA Nudelman, E., & al. (1986) J. Biol. Chem. 261, 5487-95
44.	$IV^3(NeuAc)_2\text{-}Lc_4Cer$	43338SxSxBCBA Brodin, T., & al. Biochim. Biophys. Acta 837, 349-53
45.	$IV^3NeuAc\text{-}, III^6NeuAc\text{-}Lc_4$	4333SxB6SxCBA milk oligosaccharide: Grimmonprez, L., & al. (1968) C. R. Acad. Sci. Paris 265, 2124
46.	$IV^3NeuAc\text{-}, III^6NeuAc\text{-}Lc_4Cer$	4333SxB4Fx6SxCBA Nudelman, E., & al. (1986) J. Biol. Chem. 261, 5487-95
47.	$IV^3NeuAc\text{-}, II^6LacNAc\text{-}Lc_4$	4333SxBC64BCBA milk oligosaccharide: Yamashita, K., & al. (1976) Arch. Biochem. Biophys. 174, 582-91
48.	$IV^2Fuc\text{-}, II^6(II^3NeuAc\text{-}LacNAc)\text{-}Lc_4$	4332FxBC643SxBCBA milk oligosaccharide: Yamashita, K., (1976) Arch. Biochem. Biophys. 174, 582-91

a. Falk, K.-E., & al. (1983) Biochem. Biophys. Res. Com. 110, 383-91
b. Chia, D., & al. (1985) Canc. Res. 45, 435-7
c. Fukushi, Y., & al. (1986) Biochem. 25, 2859-66

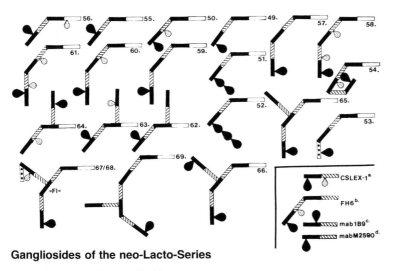

Gangliosides of the neo-Lacto-Series

VI. neoLacto-series gangliosides

Nr.	Ganglioside structure	Computer designation* References
49.	IV³NeuAc-nLc₄Cer	4343SxBCBA Wiegandt, H. (1968) Zschr. Naturf. 24b, 945-6
50.	IV³NeuAc-, III³Fuc-nLc₄Cer	4343SxB3FxCBA Fukushima, J., & al. (1984) Canc. Res. 44, 5279-85
51.	IV³(NeuAc)₂-nLc₄Cer	43438SxSxBCBA Murakami-Murofushi, K., & al. (1983) J. Biochem. 93, 621-9; Kundu, K., & al. (1983) J. Biol. Chem. 258, 13857-66
52.	IV³(NeuAc)₃-nLc₄Cer	434388SxSxSxBCBA Murakami-Murofushi, K., & al. (1983) J. Biochem. 93, 621-9
53.	IV³NeuAc-3Galβ-nLc₄Cer	43433SxDBCBA Watanabe, K., & al. (1979) J. Biol. Chem. 254, 8223-9
54.	IV³(NeuAc-3GalNAcx)-, II²Fuc-nLc₄Cer	434333SxBDx2FxBCBA Clausen, H., & al. (1987) J. Biol. Chem. 262, 14228-34
55.	IV⁶NeuAc-nLc₄Cer	4346SxBCBA Wiegandt, H. (1973) H.-S. Zschr. Physiol. Chem. 354, 1049-56; Watanabe, K., & al. (1979) JBC 254, 8223-9
56.	IV⁶NeuAc-, I³Fuc-nLc₄	4346SxBCB3FxA milk oligosaccharide: Groenberg, 1987
57.	VI³NeuAc-nLc₆Cer	434343SxBCBCBA Wiegandt, H. (1974) Eur. J. Biochem. 45, 367-9
58.	VI³NeuAc-, V³Fuc-, III³Fuc-nLc₆Cer	434343SxB3FxCB3FxBCBA Fukushi, Y., & al. (1984) J. Biol. Chem. 259, 10511-7
59.	VI⁶NeuAc-nLc₆Cer	434346SxBCBCBA Watanaabe, K., & al. (1979) J. Biol. Chem. 254, 8223-9
60.	VI⁶NeuAc-, III³Fuc-nLc₆Cer	434346SxBCB3FxCBA Hakomori, S., & al. (1984) Biochem. Biophys. Res. Com. 113, 791-8
61.	VI⁶NeuAc-, V³Fuc-, III³Fuc-nLc₆Cer	434346SxB3FxCB3FxCBA
62.	IV⁶NeuAc-, II⁶LacNAc-nLc₄	4346SxBC64BCBA milk oligosaccharide: Yamashita, K., & al. (1976) Arch. Biochem. Biophys. 174, 852-91
63.	IV⁶NeuAc-, II⁶(II²Fuc-LacNAc)-nLc₄Cer	4346SxBC642FxBCBA milk oligosaccharide: Yamashita, K., & al. (1976) Arch. Biochem. Biophys. 174, 852-91
64.	III³Fuc-, II⁶(II⁶NeuAc-LaNAc)-nLc₄	434B3FxC646SxBCBA milk oligosaccharide: Lundgren 1987
65.	VI³NeuAc-, IV⁶LacNAc-nLc₆Cer	434343SxBC64BCBCBA Watanabe, K., & al. (1978) J. Biol. Chem. 253, 8962-7
66.	VI³NeuAc-, IV⁶(II²Fuc-LacNac)-nLc₆Cer	434343SxBC642FxBCBCBA Feizi, T. & al. (1979) J. exptl. med. 149, 975
67.	VI³NeuAc-, IV⁶(II³NeuAc-LacNAc)-nLc₆Cer	434343SxBC643SxBCBCBA Kundu, S. K., & al. (1983) J. Biol. Chem. 258, 13857-66
68.	VI³NeuAc-, IV⁶(II²Fuc-, II³Galx-LacNAc)-nLc₆Cer	434343SxBC642Fx3BxBCBCBA Watanabe, K., & al. (1978) J. Biol. Chem. 253, 8962-7
69.	VIII³NeuAc-, VI⁶LacNAc-nLc₈Cer	43434343SxBC64BCBCBCBA

a. Fukushima, K., & al. (1984) Canc. Res. 44, 5279
b. Fukushi, Y., & al. (1985) Canc. Res. 45, 3711
c. Hakomori, S., & al. (1983) J. Biol. Chem. 258, 11819; Nilsson, O., & al. (1985) Biochim. Biophys. Acta 835, 577

3. Bimodal Regulation of Cell Growth by Endogenous Gangliosides

S. Spiegel

Abstract

Gangliosides have long been implicated in cell growth regulation (1). The B subunit of cholera toxin, which is pentavalent and binds exclusively to the oligosaccharide moiety of ganglioside GM1 exposed on the cell surface was used as a ganglioside-specific probe to study the role of endogenous gangliosides in the process of cellular proliferation. The B subunit induced proliferation of resting thymocytes and of quiescent, non-transformed mouse 3T3 fibroblasts. In contrast, the B subunit inhibited the growth of *ras*-transformed 3T3 cells (Ha-, Ki-, and N-*ras)*, rat glioma C6 cells with elevated levels of GM1, as well as normal 3T3 cells during rapid growth phase. The finding that a bimodal response to the B subunit can be observed in the same cells just by varying their state of growth, suggests that endogenous gangliosides may be bimodal regulators of both positive and negative signals for cell growth.

To elucidate the mechanism by which the B subunit stimulates cell growth, its effects on several transmembrane signalling systems which have been suggested to play a vital role in cell growth regulation were examined. The B subunit did not increase cAMP levels nor activate adenylate cyclase. The B subunit induced a rapid and profound increase in intracellular free Ca^{2+}, as measured with the fluorescent Ca^{2+}-sensitive dye quin 2/AM. Removal of external Ca^{2+} completely inhibited the signal, thus suggesting that the B subunit elevates intracellular Ca^{2+} through a net influx of extracellular Ca^{2+} rather than by causing the release of Ca^{2+} from intracellular stores. These findings are consistent with the observations that the B subunit induced reinitiation of DNA synthesis without activation of phospholipase C. There was no increase in the formation of inositol trisphosphate, the second messenger that mediates release of Ca^{2+} from intracellular stores. In addition, the B subunit still stimulated DNA synthesis in Swiss 3T3 cells pretreated with phorbol ester to down regulate protein kinase C. These results suggest that the mitogenic effects of the B subunit are mediated mainly by facilitation of Ca^{2+} influx and that activations of adenylate cyclase, phospholipase C, or protein kinase C are not obligatory steps in the initiation of cell growth by the B subunit. Furthermore, the observation that Ca^{2+} ionophores, such as ionomycin and A23187, are not mitogenic implies that additional undefined growth signaling pathways probably exist which may be regulated through endogenous gangliosides.

Introduction

Gangliosides, sialic acid-containing glycosphingolipids, have long been recognized as characteristic constituents of the plasma membrane of mammalian cells (2) where their only function identified so far is as receptors for bacterial toxins (3) and viruses (4). Interest in these membrane constituents has increased due to the discovery that many monoclonal antibodies raised against tumor cells recognize carbohydrate moieties present on gangliosides which appear to be tumor-specific antigens (reviewed in References 5–7). Furthermore, there are profound changes in ganglioside composi-

tion and biosynthesis during cell development, differentiation and oncogenic transformation (1, 7, 8). The recent observations that exogenously added gangliosides alter
the growth of a variety of cell types (9–14) suggests that gangliosides may play an
important role in the regulation of cell growth. It has been shown that exogenous gangliosides can stimulate the growth of some cell types (reviewed in 15) and inhibit the
growth of others (9, 10, 12, 14). Even slight alterations in ganglioside structure can leas
to opposite effects on cell growth (16). It has usually not been determined whether the
effects of the exogenous gangliosides are the result of insertion into the plasma
membranes in a physiologically relevant fashion. More importantly, the relationship
between these observations and the function of endogenous gangliosides in the
process of cellular proliferation remains unclear (5). To directly examine potential
functions for endogenous gangliosides in the control of cell growth, a new approach
was developed. The B subunit of cholera toxin, which is pentavalent and binds only to
ganglioside GM1, was used as a probe to interact specifically with endogenous GM1
(17, 18).

The B Subunit of Cholera Toxin Stimulates DNA Synthesis and Cell Division in Quiescent Cells

The B subunit was found to be mitogenic for rat thymocytes as measured by
[^{3}H]thymidine incorporation. Mitogenesis was dependent on the direct interaction
between the B subunit and ganglioside GM1 on the cell surface (17). The ability of the
B subunit to stimulate resting cells to divide was not limited only to rat thymocytes, as
the B subunit also stimulated DNA synthesis and cell division in quiescent cultures of
murine 3T3 fibroblasts (NIH 3T3, Balb/C 3T3, and Swiss 3T3). The three non-transformed 3T3 cell lines, arrested in the Go/G1 phase of the cell cycle, exhibited similar
degrees of sensitivity and mitogenic response to the B subunit (18). A major advantage of Swiss 3T3 fibroblasts is that they can be grown in serum-free medium (19).
In chemically defined conditions, the B subunit by itself was as mitogenic for these cells

Table 1. Effects of the B subunit and growth promoting agents on DNA synthesis in quiescent swiss 3T3 cells.

Stimulator		Other Addition [^{3}H]Thymidine Incorporation (cpm x 10^{-3})			
B	I	None	EGF	Bombesin	FCS
−	−	7	25	14	200
+	−	15	53	34	303
−	+	13	204	52	ND
+	+	91	313	107	ND

Quiescent cultures of Swiss 3T3 cells were exposed to the indicated mitogens in the absence (−)
or presence (+) of the B subunit and/or insulin (I) and assayed for [^{3}H]thymidine incorporation.
Data are the means of triplicate determinations. The standard deviation was < 10 %. The concentrations of the agents were as follows: B, 1 µg/ml; I, 2 µg/ml; EGF, 5 ng/ml; Bombesin, 12 nM;
Fetal Bovine Serum (FCS), 10 % (v/v). ND, not determined.

as other known mitogens, such as insulin, bombesin, epidermal growth factor (EGF), and platelet-derived growth factor (PDGF). The mitogenic response to the B subunit was greatly potentiated in the presence of insulin which also enhanced the effects of the other mitogens (Table I). In addition to synergism with insulin, the B subunit also potentiated the effect of optimal stimulatory concentrations of EGF, bombesin, and even unfractionated FCS (Table I). Thus the response of the cells to B plus the growth factors was much greater than the sum of the responses to each of the effectors alone. The synergistic interaction between B and growth factors was observed even when both EGF and insulin or bombesin and insulin were tested together; while the two growth factors synergized with each other, addition of B caused a further potentiation of [^{3}H]thymidine incorporation. This synergistic effect suggests that the B subunit mediates its effects in a fundamentally different way than any of these growth factors, probably through a specific but not yet defined pathway. The B subunit may also enhance the responsiveness of the cells to other mitogens by directly modulating a common effector system crucial for cell proliferation

B subunit effects on transmembrane signalling pathways

The discovery that the interaction of the B subunit with ganglioside GM1 on the surface of resting cells leads to cellular proliferation, suggests a fundamental role for endogenous gangliosides in the regulation of cell growth (18). The signalling pathways used by the cells to transmit information from the outer leaflet of the lipid bilayer of the plasma membrane, where the gangliosides reside, across the cytoplasm to the machinery in the nucleus responsible for replicating DNA need to be identified. The main intracellular second messenger systems that are involved in mitogenic responses are gradually being clarified (reviewed in 19–21). It has been suggested that the two inositol lipid intermediates, diacyl glycerol (DAG) and inositol trisphosphate (IP$_3$), formed by increased degradation of polyphosphoinositides via a receptor-coupled phospholipase C, play a central role in the transduction of growth signals (22). DAG is an endogenous activator of protein kinase C (21) and IP$_3$ causes a release of Ca^{2+} from intracellular stores (22). Recently it has been shown that a proliferative response can occur in the absence of PI breakdown (23) or protein kinase C activation (24). However, an increase in cytosolic free Ca^{2+} appears to be an early and general response to mitogenic stimulation. The classical second messenger, cAMP, has also been implicated in the signal transduction process (19). To elucidate the mechanism by which the B subunit stimulates cell growth, its effects on these transmembrane signalling systems were examined.

The Effect of the B Subunit on Adenylate Cyclase

To determine whether the stimulatory activity of the B subunit was due to contamination of this reagent with the A subunit of CT, which is known to activate adenylate cyclase (3), the ability of the B subunit to cause accumulation of cAMP was measured. The B subunit did not activate adenylate cyclase or increase the cytoplasmic level of cAMP in rat thymocytes, nor in quiescent Swiss 3T3 fibroblasts (Table II). Therefore, the mitogenic effect of the B subunit is clearly independent of an increase in cAMP.

Table 2. Effect of the B subunit on adenylate cyclase and cAMP production.

Cells	Additions	Adenylate Cyclase (pmol/10 min/mg)	cAMP Accumulation (pmol/mg)
Rat thymocytes	None	51 ± 4	48 ± 7
	B	53 ± 3	49 ± 5
	CT	181 ± 15	890 ± 94
Swiss 3T3 fibroblasts	None	22 ± 2	71 ± 11
	B	19 ± 4	103 ± 33
	CT	460 ± 26	5020 ± 230

Rat thymocytes and quiescent Swiss 3T3 fibroblasts were exposed to CT or the B subunit (1 µg/ml). Activation of adenylate cyclase and the cellular content of cAMP was measured (17, 25).

Effect of the B Subunit on Phosphoinositide Breakdown and Phospholipase C

To determine whether the B subunit activates phospholipase C, which catalyzes the breakdown of phosphatidylinositol 4,5-bisphosphate to IP_3 and DAG (22), the B-mediated increase in the production of [^{3}H]-labelled inositol phosphates was measured directly. Addition of bombesin to quiescent Swiss 3T3 fibroblasts and Con A to rat thymocytes induced a large increase in the levels of inositol phosphates, IP_1, IP_2, and IP_3 (Table III). In contrast to the marked stimulation induced by these mitogens, the B subunit did not stimulate the production of inositol phosphates in the same experiment. Even a combination of insulin plus B which was capable of reinitiating DNA synthesis 45 % of that produced by FCS in Swiss 3T3 cells, failed to significantly stimulate levels of IP_1, IP_2, or IP_3 (Table III). Increasing the B concentration to more than 100 times that required to elicit the maximum mitogenic effect was also without effect. These results show that the B subunit induced reinitiation of DNA synthesis in quiescent cells without activation of phospholipase C.

Table 3. Effects of the B subunit on the level of inositol phosphates.

Cells	Addition	Level of [^{3}H]inositol phosphates		
		IP_1	IP_2 (cpm per well)	IP_3
Rat thymocytes	None	1836 ± 178	303 ± 85	258 ± 27
	B	1733 ± 231	360 ± 26	250 ± 25
	Con A	3766 ± 166	740 ± 43	378 ± 11
Swiss fibroblasts	I	2451 ± 416	375 ± 97	193 ± 27
	I + B	1948 ± 570	355 ± 53	285 ± 32
	I + Bombesin	12719 ± 258	1071 ± 730	1031 ± 287

[^{3}H]Inositol-labelled quiescent Swiss 3T3 cells and rat thymocytes were incubated with the indicated agents for 10 min at 37 °C in medium containing 10 mM LiCl and levels of [^{3}H]inositol phosphates were measured (25). The concentrations of the agents were as follows: B, 1 µg/ml; Con A, 2 µg/ml; I, 1 µg/ml; Bombesin, 100 nM.

The Effect of the B Subunit on Protein Kinase C

Since these results suggest that the polyphosphoinositide signalling pathway is not essential for the B subunit-induced mitogenesis, it was expected that protein kinase C, the putative target of DAG, would not be essential for the proliferative response induced by the B subunit. Indeed, the B subunit still stimulated DNA synthesis in Swiss 3T3 fibroblasts made effectively protein kinase C-free by preincubation with a high concentration of TPA (25). In control experiments, TPA no longer induced DNA synthesis in these protein kinase C-deficient cells. In addition, the B subunit had no effect on the distribution of protein kinase C in rat thymocytes, while under the same conditions, both TPA and Con A caused activation of protein kinase C; i.e. a decrease in cytoplasmic kinase C levels and a corresponding increase in membrane-associated kinase activity (26). Thus, these data indicate that the B subunit does not require activation of either phospholipase C or protein kinase C to stimulate DNA synthesis in quiescent cells.

The Effect of the B Subunit on Na^+/H^+ Exchange

It has been suggested that activation of Na^+/H^+ exchange, resulting in cyoplasmic alkalinization, is a key event leading to the initiation of cellular proliferation (27). Using the fluorescent pH-sensitive dye BCECF, it was found that the B subunit did not have any effect on pH_i, both in thymocytes and in 3T3 cells (Table 4). This indicates that the B subunit has no acute effect on Na^+/H^+ exchange or other pH_i modulating systems.

The Effect of the B Subunit on Intracellular Free $[Ca^{2+}]$

An increase in cytosolic free Ca^{2+} appears to be an early and general response to mitogenic stimulation (28). Using the intracellularly trapped fluorescent Ca^{2+} indicator, quin 2, it was found that the B subunit induced a pronounced increase in intracellular Ca^{2+} in lymphocytes as well as in quiescent 3T3 cells (Table 4).

Removal of external Ca^{2+} completely inhibited the B-induced Ca^{2+} signal, while readdition of Ca^{2+} rapidly restored the response. This inhibitory effect is not due to a lack of binding of the B subunit to the cells since the binding of the B subunit to GM1 is a Ca^{2+}-independent process (3, 17). These findings clearly indicate that the increase in $[Ca^{2+}]_i$ induced by the B subunit arises from a net influx of Ca^{2+} from extracellular sources and not from a release of Ca^{2+} from intracellular stores and are consistent with the observation that inositol trisphosphate, the second messenger that mediates release of Ca^{2+} from intracellular stores, was not elevated in response to the B subunit.

In summary, the B subunit induces an increase in intracellular Ca^{2+} levels, but does not affect cAMP accumulation, phosphoinositide hydrolysis, or cytoplasmic pH. Thus, activation of adenylate cyclase, phospholipase C, protein kinase C, or Na^+/H^+ exchange are not obligatory steps in the initiation of cell growth by the B subunit of CT. The regulation of Ca^{2+} permeability by endogenous gangliosides has important implications for their potential function in many other cellular processes.

Table 4. The effect of the B subunit on intracellular pH and intracellular free Ca^{2+}.

Cells	Additions	ΔpH_i	$\Delta[Ca^{2+}]_i$ (nM)
Rat thymocytes	B	0	80
	EGTA + B	ND	0
	Con A	0.1	110
3T3 swiss fibroblasts	B	0	100
	EGTA + B	ND	0
	Bombesin	0.15	230

Cytoplasmic free Ca^{2+} and intracellular pH was monitored fluorimetrically using quin 2 and bis(carboxyethyl)-5,6-carboxyfluorescein (BCECF), respectively (25, 26). The results are expressed as changes resulting from the addition of the agents relative to untreated controls. The concentrations of the agents were as follows: B, 1 μg/ml; Con A, 2 μg/ml; Bombesin, 100 nM; EGTA, 1 mM. ND, not determined.

In order to determine whether the early increase in intracellular $[Ca^{2+}]_i$ was sufficient to induce DNA synthesis, [^{3}H]thymidine incorporation was measured in quiescent 3T3 fibroblasts after exposure to calcium ionophores. Ionomycin and A23187 (100 nM), which cause an increase in $[Ca^{2+}]_i$ similar to that induced by the B subunit, do not stimulate DNA synthesis, even in the presence of insulin (Table 5). To avoid possible cytotoxic effects after prolonged exposure to the ionophores, the cells were incubated with the ionophores or the B subunit for only 5 h, then washed and incubated further in medium containing either insulin or 10% FCS. Short incubation of the fibroblasts with the ionophores, followed by incubation with insulin alone, did not potentiate the response to insulin. Although the ionophores did not induce DNA synthesis, cells treated with the ionophores are still competent to respond to FCS, indicating that the ionophores do not damage the cells irreversibly (Table 5). The increases in intracellular free $[Ca^{2+}]_i$ produced by ionophores are sufficient to produce short term effects, such as the increased expression of c-fos and c-myc genes (29). However, this induction is not sufficient to commit the quiescent cells to DNA syn-

Table 5. Effect of calcium ionophores on DNA synthesis.

Initial addition	[^{3}H]Thymidine Incorporation (cpm x 10^{-3} per well)		
	Without washing	Second incubation plus I	plus FCS
None	14.0 ± 1.2	16.5 ± 0.9	173 ± 21
A23187	10.1 ± 1.9	14.2 ± 1.9	157 ± 21
Ionomycin	16.5 ± 2.1	17.5 ± 1.4	192 ± 33
B	81.6 ± 10.7	98.7 ± 7.3	287 ± 34

Quiescent cultures of Swiss 3T3 cells were incubated in culture medium supplemented with insulin (2 μg/ml) and the various agents. Where indicated, the cultures were washed 5 h later followed by a second incubation in the presence of insulin (2 μg/ml) or 10% FCS for an addditional 15 h. [^{3}H]thymidine incorporation was measured after 20 h (25).

thesis. In contrast, short incubation of the fibroblasts with the B subunit followed by Tab. 5
addition of insulin alone produced a stimulation which was similar to that observed when both the B subunit and insulin were present for the entire incubation period (Table 5). This is due to the tight interaction between the B subunit and ganglioside GM1 ($Kd = 10^{-10}$ M) which makes it impossible to remove the B subunit by washing. Thus, the interaction of the B subunit with endogenous ganglioside GM1 was sufficient to invoke the long term response, that is, progression of the cells into the S phase leading to cellular proliferation. These results could be explained by the existence of another hitherto unknown signalling pathway, in addition to Ca^{2+}, that may also be involved in eliciting cellular proliferation.

The B Subunit Inhibits Growth of Transformed Cell Lines

In contrast to results described above that the B subunit interacts with endogenous gangliosides to induce lymphocyte stimulation and proliferation of confluent, non-dividing fibroblasts, others have found that antibodies, directed to certain gangliosides present on the plasma membranes of tumor cells, inhibit their growth (30, 31). Therefore, it was of interest to study the effect of the B subunit on the proliferation of transformed cells (18). The B subunit inhibited the growth of *ras*-transformed 3T3 fibroblasts (Ha-, Ki-, and N-*ras*). This family of mammalian genes encode highly conserved 21 kD proteins (p21^{ras}) that appear to be intimately involved in the control of cellular growth. Although the three transformed cell lines exhibit different degrees of sensitivity to the B subunit (1 µg/ml B inhibits proliferation of Ha-, Ki-, and N-*ras*, by 60, 51, and 41 %, respectively), all three cell lines were significantly affected by a very low concentration of the B subunit and these inhibitory effects were observed even in the presence of FCS (18). To rule out the possibility that the inhibitory action was specific to *ras*-transformed NIH 3T3 cells, the effect of the B subunit on the growth of C6 cells was explored. The major advantages of the rapidly dividing C6 cell line are that they have no detectable GM1 and can readily take up GM1 from the medium and insert it into the plasma membrane in a physiologically functional manner (3). The B subunit had no effect on the proliferation of control C6 cells which bind only trace amounts of iodinated CT. Prior treatment of C6 cells with GM1, which caused an increase in iodinated CT binding, rendered the cells sensitive to the B subunit (Table 6). The inhibitory effect of the B subunit appeared to be specific, as Con A, a lectin which can bind to cell surface glycoconjugates, had no effect on the growth of the control or GM1-treated C6 cells (Table 6). Furthermore, treatment of the cells with asialo-GM1, which does not does not increase CT binding, did not render the cells responsive to the B subunit (Table 6). The maximum B subunit-dependent inhibition of DNA synthesis increased as the amount of exogenous GM1 added was increased. A maximum inhibition of 25 %, 35 %, and 80 % was found with C6 cells that were treated with 0.2, 1.0, and 5.0 µmolL^{-1} GM1, respectively (32). The dose-dependency for the growth inhibition effect by the B subunit at the three different concentrations of exogenous GM1 correlated closely with the dose-dependence of iodinated CT binding (32). Since butyrate is known to induce ganglioside GM1 biosynthesis in rat glioma C6 cells, the effects of the B subunit were studied on cells in which the endogenous levels of GM1 were elevated by treatment with butyrate. There was an increase in iodinated CT binding with a corresponding inhibition of DNA synthesis by the B subunit in butyrate-treated cells (Table 6). Treatment with acetate, which does not increase GM1 levels, did not render the cells responsive to the B subunit. It is interesting to note that treatment of the cells with 40 nmolL^{-1} exogenous ganglioside GM1, which induces the same increase in iodinated CT binding, also caused a similar B subunit-dependent growth inhibition as did treatment with butyrate (Table 6). Thus, when the levels of GM1 are increased to the same extent, either with exogenous addition or by increasing biosynthesis, there are similar effects on the cells. As shown previously, the ability of the B subunit to inhibit cell growth by interacting with cell surface GM1 was independent of adenylate cyclase activation or increases in intracellular cAMP levels (32). It should be noted that in all the transformed cell lines examined, the anti-proliferative activity of B was not associated with any cytotoxic effects, since the number of viable cells, determined by trypan blue exclusion, was always more than 95 %.

Table 6. Effects of the B subunit of cholera toxin on DNA synthesis and iodinated CT binding in rat glioma C6 cell.

Culture Treatment	[^{3}H]Thymidine Incorporation (cpm x 10^{-4})/well			^{125}I-CT Bound (fmol/mg protein)
	none	Con A	B	
Control	13	13	12	34
Butyrate (5 mM)	9	10	7	412
GM1 (40 nM)	12	13	11	389
GM1 (0.2 µM)	12	12	9	2240
Asialo GM1 (0.2 µM)	13	13	13	35

Cells were cultured without or with GM1 or with asialo-GM1 (16 h), or with butyrate (48 h), washed with medium and incubated in the presence of various additions for 20 h and than [^{3}H]thymidine incorporation was determined (32). Data are means of triplicate determinations. Standard deviations are less than 5 %. Specific iodinated CT binding was assayed on duplicate cultures by incubating the cultures with 20 nM iodinated CT for 1h (32).

Bimodal Effects of the B subunit on Growth of Normal Fibroblasts

The opposite effects of B on resting thymocytes and confluent, quiescent 3T3 cells and on the rapidly dividing transformed cell lines suggested that the difference might be due either to inherent differences in response patterns of normal and transformed cells or to differences between quiescent and proliferating cells. Experiments with growing, normal 3T3 cells demonstrated that a bifunctional response pattern to the B subunit can be observed in the same cell line (Table 7).

Thus, in contrast to the observation that B induced proliferation of quiescent, non-dividing cells, when the cells were exponentially growing, B inhibited their proliferation. Similar to the result shown for the transformed cells, the inhibitory effects of the B subunit were observed regardless of whether EGF or FCS were added to the cells even though these factors by themselves increased [^{3}H]thymidine incorporation. Thus, the B subunit can inhibit the growth of rapidly dividing, normal 3T3 cells as well

Table 7. Inhibition of DNA synthesis in exponentially growing mouse 3T3 cells by the B subunit of cholera toxin.

	[³H]Thymidine incorporated (c.p.m. x 10^{-3})			
	NIH 3T3 Cells		Swiss 3T3 Cells	
B added (1 µg/ml)	−	+	−	+
Other Additions				
None	58	33	62	42
EGF (40 ng/ml)	64	40	79	56
FCS (5%)	120	91	84	61

Exponentially growing mouse 3T3 cells were incubated with the indicated mitogens and incorporation of [³H]thymidine was determined (18). Values are the means of triplicate determinations. Standard deviations are less than 5%.

as transformed cells. Whether the same or different signal transduction mechanisms are involved in the stimulatory and inhibitory responses to the B subunit remain to be determined. The *ras*-transformed 3T3 cells used in these studies have less GM1 than normal NIH 3T3 cells and the levels of cell surface gangliosides increase as normal NIH 3T3 cells reach confluency (1, 7, 33). The bimodal response to B may be related to the amount of surface GM1 being occupied. Although it is unusual for the same effector to both stimulate and inhibit the growth of cells, it is not unprecedented. Transforming growth factor β (TGF-β) is a bifunctional regulator of cell growth (34). TGF-β inhibits the growth of many tumor cells, yet stimulates the growth of non-neoplastic fibroblasts. The response of a cell to a growth factor may depend not only on the growth factor itself but also on the total set of stimulatory and inhibitory agents that are operating on the cell at that time.

The elucidation of the mechanisms of the control of cellular proliferation is one of the fundamental problems in biological science. This knowledge is a crucial prerequisite for the understanding of the cause or causes underlying the unrestrained proliferation of cancer cells. Gangliosides may play an important role in the regulation of cell growth. The discovery that the B subunit of cholera toxin regulates cell growth by interaction with cell surface ganglioside GM1 suggests that endogenous gangliosides may be "biomodulators" of both positive and negative growth control signals.

Acknowledgements – I thank Dr. Sheldon Milstien for reviewing the manuscript. This work was supported in part by NIH grant 1R 29 GM39718-01.

References

1. Hakomori, S. Glycosphingolipids in cellular interaction, differentiation, and oncogenesis. Ann. Rev. Biochem. 50, 733, 1981.
2. Wiegandt, H. The gangliosides. Adv. Neurochem. 4, 149, 1982.
3. Fishman, P. H. Role of membrane gangliosides in the binding and action of bacterial toxins. J. Membrane Biol. 69, 85, 1982.

4. Markwell, M. A. K., L. Svennerholm, and J. C. Paulson. Specific gangliosides function as host cell receptors for Sendai virus. Proc. Natl. Acad. Sci. USA 78, 5406, 1981.
5. Marcus, D. M. A review of the immunogenic and immunomodulatory properties of glycosphingolipids. Molec. Immunol. 21, 1083, 1984.
6. Feizi, T. Demonstration by monoclonal antibodies that carbohydrate structures of glycoproteins and glycolipids are onco-developmental antigens. Nature 314, 53, 1985.
7. Hakomori, S. Aberrant glycosylation in cancer cell membranes as focused on glycolipids: Overview and perspectives. Cancer Res. 45, 2405, 1985.
8. Fishman, P. H., and R. O. Brady. Biosynthesis and function of gangliosides. Science 194, 906, 1976.
9. Bremer, E. G., S. Hakomori, D. F. Bowen-Pope, E. Raines, and R. Ross. Gangliosidemediated modulation of cell growth, growth factor binding, and receptor phosphorylation. J. Biol. Chem. 259, 6818, 1984.
10. Bremer, E. G., J. Schlessinger, and S. Hakomori. Ganglioside-mediated modulation of cell growth. J. Biol. Chem. 261, 2434, 1986.
11. Katoh-Semba, R., L. Facci, S. Skaper, and S. Varon. Gangliosides stimulate astroglial cell proliferation in the absence of serum. J. Cell. Physiol. 126, 147, 1986.
12. Keenan, T. W., E. Schmid, W. W. Franke, and H. Wiegandt. Exogenous glycosphingolipids suppress growth rate of transformed and untransformed 3T3 mouse cells. Exp. Cell Res. 92, 259, 1975.
13. Tsuji, S., M. Arita, and Y. Nagai. GQ1b, a bioactive ganglioside that exhibits novel nerve growth factor (NGF)-like activities in the two neuroblastoma cell lines. J. Biochem. (Tokyo) 94, 303, 1983.
14. Whisler, R. L., and A. J. Yates. Regulation of lymphocyte responses by human gangliosides: Characteristics of inhibitory effects and the induction of impaired activation. J. Immunol. 125, 2106, 1980.
15. Ledeen, R. W. Biology of gangliosides: Neuritogenic and neuronotrophic properties. J. Neurosci. Res. 12, 147, 1984.
16. Hanai, N., T. Dohi, G. A. Nores, and S. Hakomori. A novel ganglioside, de-N-acetyl-GM3 ($II^3NeuNH_2LacCer$), acting as a strong promoter for epidermal growth factor receptor kinase and as a stimulator for cell growth. J. Biol. Chem. 263, 6296, 1988.
17. Spiegel, S., P. H. Fishman, and R. J. Weber. Direct evidence that endogenous ganglioside GM1 can mediate thymocyte proliferation. Science 230, 1283, 1985.
18. Spiegel, S., and P. H. Fishman. Gangliosides as bimodal regulators of cell growth. Proc. Natl. Acad. Sci. USA 84, 141, 1987.
19. Rozengurt, E. Early signals in the mitogenic response. Science 234, 161, 1986.
20. Bell, R. M. Protein kinase C activation by diacylglycerol second messengers. Cell 45, 631, 1986.
21. Nishizuka, Y. Studies and perspectives of protein kinase C. Science 233, 305, 1986.
22. Berridge, M. J. Inositol trisphosphate and diacylglycerol as second messengers. Biochem. J. 220, 345, 1984.
23. Besterman, J. M., S. P. Watson, and P. Cuatrecasas. Lack of association of epidermal growth factor-, insulin-, and serum-induced mitogenesis with stimulation of phosphoinositide degredation in BALB/c 3T3 fibroblasts. J. Biol. Chem. 261, 723, 1986.
24. Tsuda, T., K. Kaibuchi, Y. Kawahara, H. Fukuzaki, and Y. Takai. Induction of protein kinase C activation and Ca^{2+} mobilization by fibroblast growth factor in Swiss 3T3 cells. FEBS Lett. 191, 205, 1985.
25. Spiegel, S., and C. Panagiotopoulos. Mitogenesis in 3T3 fibroblasts induced by endogenous gangliosides is not mediated by cAMP, protein kinase C, or phosphoinositides turnover. Exp. Cell Res. 177, 414, 1988.

26. Dixon, S. J., D. Stewart, S. Grinstein, and S. Spiegel. Transmembrane signalling by the B subunit of cholera toxin: Increased cytoplasmic free calcium in rat lymphocytes. J. Biol. Chem. 105, 1153, 1987.

27. Pouyssegur, J., J. C. Chambard, A. Franchi, G. L'Allemain, S. Paris, and E. Van Obberghen-Schilling. Growth-factor activation of the Na^+/H^+ antiporter controls growth of fibroblasts by regulating intracellular pH. Cancer Cells 3, 409, 1985.

28. Tsien, R. Y., T. Pozzan, and T. J. Rink. Calcium homeostasis in intact lymphocytes: Cytoplasmic free calcium monitored with a new, intracellularly trapped fluorescent indicator. J. Cell Biol. 94, 325, 1982.

29. Tsuda, T., K. Kaibuchi, B. West, and Y. Takai. Involvement of Ca^{2+} in platelet-derived growth factor-induced expression of c-myc oncogenes in Swiss 3T3 fibroblasts. FEBS Lett. 187, 43, 1985.

30. Lingwood, C. A., and S. Hakomori. Selective inhibition of cell growth and associated changes in glycolipid metabolism induced by monovalent antibodies to glycolipids. Exp. Cell Res. 108, 385, 1977.

31. Dippold, W. G., A. Knuth, and K. H. M. Zum Buschenfelde. Inhibition of human melanoma cell growth in vitro by monoclonal anti-GD3-ganglioside antibody. Cancer Res. 44, 806, 1984.

32. Spiegel, S. Insertion of ganglioside GM1 into rat glioma C6 cells renders them susceptible to growth inhibition by the B subunit of cholera toxin. Biochim. Biophys. Acta 969, 249, 1988.

33. Matyas, G. R., S. A. Aaronson, R. O. Brady, and P. H. Fishman. Alteration of gangliosides in ras transfected NIH 3T3 cells. Proc. Natl. Acad. Sci. USA 84, 6065, 1987.

34. Roberts, A. B., M. A. Anzano, L. M. Wakefield, N. S. Roche, D. F. Stern, and M. B. Sporn. Type β transforming growth factor: A bifunctional regulator of cellular growth. Proc. Natl. Acad. Sci. USA 82, 119, 1985.

4. Biological Significance of Ecto Biosignal Transduction: Carbohydrate Recognition Coupled with Cell Surface Protein Phosphorylation

Y. Nagai and S. Tsuji

Introduction

Most of the biosignal transduction mechanisms of cells have been known to be coupled in certain steps with protein phosphorylation. Each of those protein phosphorylations is catalyzed by specific protein kinases as exemplified by cAMP-dependent (kinase A), cGMP-dependent (kinase G), Ca^{2+}/calmodulin-dependent and Ca^{2+}/phospholipid-dependent (kinase C) kinases as well as receptor autophosphorylation. These kinases are known to be localized intracellularly and thus should be categorized as endo protein kinases, while kinases localized on the cell surface may be categorized as ecto protein kinases (1). The biological significance of ecto protein phosphorylation has been discussed by several workers, though its precise molecular mechanism is unclear.

During the course of an investigation of ganglioside effects on neuronal differentiation, particularly on neurite outgrowth (neuritogenesis), we found that addition of a particular tetrasialoganglioside, GQ1b [IV^{3}a(NeuAc)$_2$II^{3}a(NeuAc)$_2$-GgOse$_4$Cer], exerts strong, nerve growth factor (NGF)-like neuritogenic action on neuroblastoma cells, especially two human neuroblastoma cell lines, GOTO and NB-1 (2). A GQ1b concentration of only a few nanomoles, almost equivalent to the required concentration of NGF, was sufficient for the development of neuritogenic activity (2, 3).

Subsequent studies using these two cell lines revealed the interesting facts that the GQ1b biological activity is most probably mediated by the cell surface-localized receptor-like function which rigorously recognizes the oligosaccharide structure of GQ1b (oligo-GQ1b), that exogenous GQ1b enhances protein phosphorylation *in situ* (4) and that the addition of GQ1b together with γ-^{32}P-ATP to intact cells specifically and instantly enhanced phosphorylation of a particular set of cell surface proteins (5, 6). These observations will be discussed with particular emphasis on the cell biological significance of carbohydrate-mediated ecto protein phosphorylation as a novel ecto biosignal transduction system.

Neuritogenic Activity of GQ1b

It must be emphasized that a very minute amount of GQ1b (5 to 10 ng/ml of culture medium) is sufficient for expression of its biological activity, which is in sharp contrast to other exogenous gangliosides so far described with respect to growth factor-dependent cell growth and receptor phosphorylation (7), hematopoietic progenitor cell differentiation (8) and effects on other neuroblastoma cell lines (e. g., mouse Neuro2a) (9).

Abbreviations used
   The abbreviations for glycosphingolipids follow Svennerholm's nomenclature system (17, 18). Oligo-GQ1b; the oligosaccharide portion of GQ1b, Gg; ganglioside, kinase A; cAMP-dependent protein kinase, kinase G; cAMP-dependent protein kinase, kinase C; Ca^{2+}/phospholipid-dependent protein kinase, Gg kinase; ganglioside-dependent protein kinase.

The necessity of the carbohydrate structure for the activity was absolute, and deletion of any of the four sialic acid residues resulted in complete loss of the activity (3) (Figure 1). Furthermore, simultaneous addition of the oligosaccharide portion of GQ1b (oligo-GQ1b) which itself did not have any effect inhibited the biological effect of GQ1b in a dose dependent fashion. All results strongly indicate the involvement of a receptor-like function that rigorously recognizes the GQ1b-oligosaccharide structure on the cell surface.

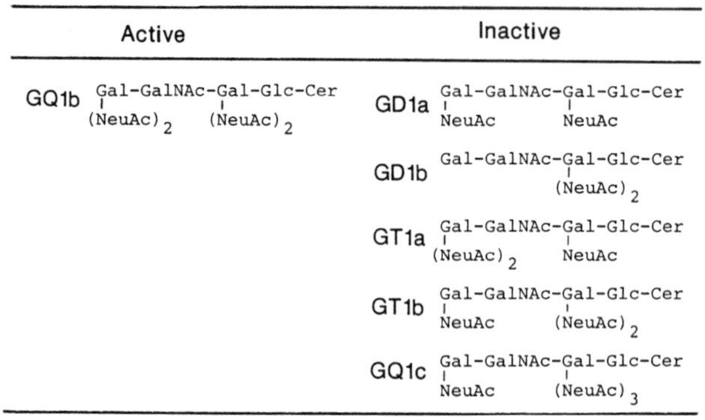

Active	Inactive

GQ1b   Gal-GalNAc-Gal-Glc-Cer
       | |
     (NeuAc)$_2$ (NeuAc)$_2$
	GD1a Gal-GalNAc-Gal-Glc-Cer
	          |
	         NeuAc NeuAc

	GD1b Gal-GalNAc-Gal-Glc-Cer
	                  |
	               (NeuAc)$_2$

	GT1a Gal-GalNAc-Gal-Glc-Cer
	          |
	       (NeuAc)$_2$ NeuAc

	GT1b Gal-GalNAc-Gal-Glc-Cer
	          |
	        NeuAc (NeuAc)$_2$

	GQ1c Gal-GalNAc-Gal-Glc-Cer
	          |
	        NeuAc (NeuAc)$_3$

Figure 1. Active and inactive gangliosides.

Ganglioside-dependent Protein Phosphorylation (4)

Exogenous GQ1b in biologically active concentrations (5–10 ng/ml) also stimulates protein phosphorylation in the above-mentioned GOTO cells (4). Distinct stimulation was observed 30 minutes after addition of GQ1b to the intact cells. This ganglioside-stimulated protein phosphorylation system was found to be solely localized in the plasma membrane fraction of the cells. Not only some *(de novo)* proteins of the membrane but also purified histones (H1) and tubulin were phosphate-accepting. The phosphorylation system depended upon Ca^{2+} (50–100 μM). GQ1b/Ca^{2+}, however, could not directly activate known protein kinases (kinases A, G, C, and Ca^{2+}/calmodulin) and was inhibitory for kinase C. Interestingly, the specificity of GQ1b for this phosphorylation system of plasma membranes was not strict; not only GQ1b but also GT1a, GT1b, GD1a, GD1b, GD3, and GM1 stimulated the system, although the degree of stimulation by the other gangliosides was less than that mediated by GQ1b, and varied among the gangliosides tested. This broad specificity sharply contrasted with the specific action of GQ1b on the intact cells.

GQ1b-dependent Cell Surface Protein Phosphorylation (5, 6)

Very recently we found that cell surface proteins of GOTO cells are strongly phosphorylated after addition of a few nM GQ1b and $1\mu M$ γ-^{32}P-ATP (3.7×10^5Bq/well) to the intact cells. The phosphorylation became distinct within a few minutes

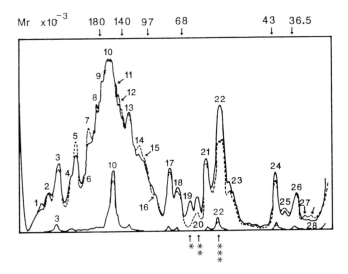

Figure 2. Endogenous protein substrates for the ecto type protein kinase activity in intact GOTO cells.

The ecto-protein kinase assay was performed according to Ehrlich et al. with a slight modification (1). Neuroblastoma cells in the exponential growth phase were distributed into 96-well plates at an inoculum size of 2×10^4 cells, followed by incubation for 2 days. Before the experiment, the cells were rinsed three times in FCS-free medium (RPMI : MEM = 1 : 1) and then incubated in serum-free fresh medium (50 μL) containing ganglioside GQ1b (10 ng/mL) for 1 hour at 37 °C. The reaction was started by adding 1 μmolL^{-1} γ-^{32}P-ATP (3.7×10^5 Bq/well) to the attached cells and terminated by adding the termination buffer (50 μL: 0.5 molL^{-1} Tris-HCl, 10 % SDS, 6.0 M urea, 1 % 2-mercaptoethanol, pH 6.8) after 1 hour incubation with gentle shaking at 30 °C. Samples were resolved on 4–20 % polyacrylamide gel gradients according to Laemmli (16) and then autoradiographed for one or two weeks.

A: the autoradiograph was scanned with a microdensitometer. Solid line: with GQ1b, reaction time; 5 minutes and 1 hour, broken line: with GQ1b, reaction time; 5 minutes and 1 hour, *: 64 KDa, **: 60 KDa, ***: 54 KDa.

The molecular markers were: DNA dependent RNA polymerase B from *Thermus thermophilus* HB8 (a: 43 KDa, X: 97 KDa, b: 140 KDa, and b': 180 KDa), bovine serum albumin (868 KDa) and lactate dehydrogenase from swine muscle (36.5 KDa).

B: time course of protein phosphorylation in intact GOTO cells with γ-^{32}P-ATP.

After the autoradiography, the autoradiogram was traced with a densitometer. The peak areas for the 64 KDa protein were estimated. Open circles: GQ1b (10 ng/mL) added; closed circles: No GQ1b added.

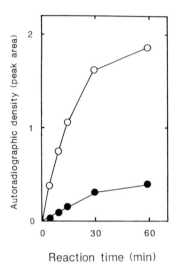

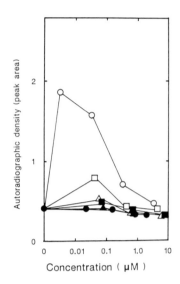

Figure 3. Ganglioside specificity of the stimulation of ecto-type protein phosphorylation (64 KDa phosphorylation).

   The cell surface phosphorylation assay was performed as described in the legend to Figure 2, except for the use of various amounts of purified gangliosides. This figure only shows the results for the 64 KDa protein. The results for the 60 and 54 KDa proteins were almost the same as those for the 64 KDa protein. ○ GQ1b; □ GT1b; △ GD1a; ● GM1; ■ GA1; ▲ oligo-GQ1b.

after addition and linearly increased up to at least 30 min. GQ1b specifically stimulated phosphorylation of three proteins (54, 60 and 64 KDa) among at least 28 cell surface proteins which were phosphorylated by γ-^{32}P-ATP alone (Figure 2). Thr of the 64 KDa protein and Ser/Thr (60 and 54 KDa proteins) but not Tyr were phosphorylated. There was no discernable difference in the protein composition (examination of gels) or in the total protein content between GQ1b-treated cells and cells not exposed to GQ1b. This observation precludes the possibility that certain newly synthesized proteins ready to be phosphorylated appeared during the incubation of the cells with GQ1b. The results strongly indicate the existence of ecto type protein phosphorylation which is catalyzed by a specific, ganglioside-activated, ecto type protein kinase. It is to be noted that the ganglioside specificity of this system is very narrow. Only GQ1b (5 nM) but not GD1a, GM1, GA1, oligo-GQ1b was active and, to a far lesser degree, GT1b at 50 nM concentration (Figure 3).

   The existence of an ecto type protein kinase is also supported by the following evidence: (1) The phosphorylation did not occur after incubation with ortho-32-phosphoric acid (3.7 x 10^5 Bq/well) for 30 minutes. After longer incubation phosphory-lation occurred, but the phosphorylated protein pattern was different from the pattern seen after short term phosphorylation as described above. It is likely that newly syn-thesized ATP from intracellularly incorporated ATP is utilized in the latter phosphory-lations, including intracellular phosphorylation. Exogenous ATP is known to make some cells permeable to small molecular weight compounds (10–13). However, in these cases higher concentrations of ATP in the absence of divalent cations were used in contrast to the conditions used in our experiments, 1 μmolL^{-1} γ-^{32}P-ATP in the presence of divalent cations. (2) 5'-p-Fluorosulfonyl-benzoyl-adenosine (1 μmolL^{-1}) or AMP-PCP (0.1 mmolL^{-1}) inhibited almost all the ecto type phosphorylations. These phosphorylations were also inhibited by a protein kinase inhibitor, k-252a (14). (3) The phosphorylation sites for 54, 60, and 64 KDa proteins were localized on the cell surface as evidenced by their susceptibility to mild and brief trypsin treatment. Based on these facts we proposed to call the ganglioside-stimulated protein kinase of the ecto type ecto Gg protein kinase (5, 6). Up to now, several protein kinases (kinases A, G, and C, and Ca^{2+}/calmodulin kinase) including a partially purified new enzyme (J-kinase) which is stimulated by ganglioside (15) have been known. These kinases reside intracellularly or on the inner surface of the plasma membrane and are therefore categorized as endo protein kinases (5).

Biological Implication of Ecto Gg Kinase

In the previous sections we dealt with two membrane-related phosphorylation systems. One is ecto Gg kinase-catalyzed phosphorylation, the ganglioside specificity of which is very high. It is very likely that only GQ1b is responsible for its stimulation. The other system, on the other hand, resides in the plasma membrane fraction prepared from the same GOTO cells, and its spectrum of ganglioside specificity is relatively broad. It is still too early to draw conclusions as to whether or not we are dealing with the same protein kinase.

With regard to the former we should add the interesting fact that ecto Gg phosphorylation of 54, 60, and 64 KDa proteins or GOTO cells by GQ1b was inhibited by simultaneous addition of oligo-GQ1b in a dose dependent fashion. This finding is in accord with our previous observation that GQ1b-promoted neuritogenesis is inhibited in the same manner by oligo-GQ1b. Both phenomena indicate the participation of a carbohydrate biosignal recognizing receptor molecule in this activation system. At present, however, we do not know whether or how the GQ1b receptor is coupled with ecto Gg kinase. It is interesting to note that the ganglioside specificity of, and the optimal concentration required for, the stimulation of the ecto type phosphorylation in GOTO cells resembled the conditions under which neuritogenic activity was induced in the same cells (3). Photo-affinity labelling of the cell surface with 8-azide-ATP led to complete inhibition of both ecto type phosphorylation and GQ1b-stimulated neuritogenesis. Although the ecto type phosphorylation may be closely associated with the neuritogenic effect of GQ1b, it remains unclear whether or not the molecular mechanisms underlying the neuritogenic effect of GQ1b observed in the presence and absence of exogenous ATP are different from each other. At present we have no data on the function of the ecto proteins that are phosphorylated in GOTO and NB-1 cells and those that are susceptible to ganglioside-dependent ecto type phosphorylation in other types of cells. However, the hypothesis of a receptor-coupled ecto Gg kinase system leads us to propose a *cis* and *trans* carbohydrate recognition model of cells (Figure 4), with *trans* recognition involved in cell biological phenomena including differentiation, development, malignant cell transformation and metastasis of the malignant cells. The model also emphasizes the biological importance of a carbohydrate biosignal recognizing receptor lectin of the cells.

Ganglioside modulating the cellular information process

1. cis−recognition   2. trans−recognition

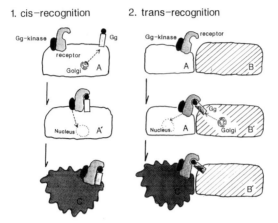

Figure 4. Cis- and trans-carbohydrate recognition model.

Summary

Recently we found that a tetrasialoganglioside GQ1b specifically stimulates phosphorylation of several cell surface proteins of human neuroblastoma cells, when both the ganglioside and ATP are added to the intact cells. The results strongly indicate the possibility that this cell surface protein phosphorylation is carried out by a unique cell surface membrane protein kinase which is specifically activated by a particular ganglioside, and we proposed to call this type of kinase ecto-Gg kinase (ganglioside-dependent ecto protein kinase). We also reported that GQ1b can specifically promote neuritogenesis of the same cell line. A procedure that inhibited the cell surface protein phosphorylation also resulted in inhibition of the GQ1b-dependent promotion of neuritogenesis, strongly suggesting an association between those two cellular events. It is likely that a new type of biosignal transduction exists that is mediated through cell surface carbohydrate recognition (ecto biosignal transduction system).

Acknowledgements

This work was supported in part by a Grant-in-Aid for the Promotion of Science and a Grant-in-Aid for Cancer Research, both from the Ministry of Education, Science and Culture of Japan. The support by a Grant-in-Aid from the Ministry of Health and Welfare of Japan is also gratefully acknowledged.

References

1. Ehrlich, Y. H., Davis, T. B., Bock, E., Kornecki, E., and Lenox, R. H. Ecto-protein kinase activity on the external surface of neural cells. Nature 320, 67–70, 1986.
2. Tsuji, S., Arita, M., and Nagai, Y. GQ1b, a bioactive ganglioside that exhibits novel nerve growth factor (NGF)-like activities in the two neuroblastoma cell lines. J. Biochem. 94, 303–306, 1983.
3. Nakajima, J., Tsuji, S., and Nagai, Y. Bioactive gangliosides: analysis of functional structures of the tetrasialoganglioside GQ1b which promotes neurite outgrowth. Biochim. Biophys. Acta. 876, 65–71, 1986.
4. Tsuji, S., Nakajima, J., Sasaki, T., and Nagai, Y. Bioactive gangliosides IV. Ganglioside GQ1b/Ca^{2+} dependent protein kinase activity exists in the plasma membrane fraction of neuroblastoma cell line, GOTO. J. Biochem. 97, 969–972, 1985.
5. Nagai, Y. and Tsuji, S. Cell biological significance of gangliosides in neuronal differentiation and development: Critique and proposals.; in Ledeen, R.W. (eds.), New Trends in Ganglioside Research: Neurochemical and Neuroregenerative Aspects, in press.
6. Tsuji, S., Yamashita, T., and Nagai, Y. A novel, carbohydrate signal-mediated cell surface protein phosphorylation: Ganglioside GQ1b stimulates ecto-protein kinase activity on the cell surface of human neuroblastoma cell line, GOTO. J. Biochem. 104, in press, 1988.
7. Bremer, E. G., Hakomori, S., Bowen-Pope, D. F., Raines, E., and Ross, R. Ganglioside-mediated modulation of cell growth, growth factor binding, and receptor phosphorylation. J. Biol. Chem. 259, 6818–6825, 1984.
8. Nojiri, H., Takaku, F., Terui, Y., Miura, Y., and Saito, M. Ganglioside GM3: An acidic membrane component that increases during macrophage-like cell differentiation can induce monocytic differentiation of human myeloid and monocytoid leukemic cell lines HL-60 and U937. Proc. Natl. Acad. Sci. USA 83, 782–786, 1986.
9. Tsuji, S., Yamashita, T., Tanaka, M., and Nagai, Y. Synthetic sialyl compounds as well as natural gangliosides induce neuritogenesis in a mouse neuroblastoma cell line (Neuro2a). J. Neurochem. 50, 414–423, 1988.
10. Bennett, J. P., Cockcroft, S., and Gomperts, B. D. Rat mast cells permeabilized with ATP secrete histamine in response to calcium ions buffered in the micromolar range. J. Physiol. 317, 335–345, 1981.
11. Gomperts, B. D. Involvement of guanine nucleotide-binding protein in the gating of Ca^{2+} by receptors. Nature 306, 64–66, 1983.
12. Gomperts, B. D. and Fernandez, J. M. Techniques for membrane permeabilization. TIBS Nov. 1985, 414–417, 1985.
13. Whetton, A. D., Huang, S. J., and Monk, P. N. Adenosine triphosphate can maintain multipotent haemopoietic stem cells in the absence of interleukin 3 via a membrane permeabilization mechanism. Biochem. Biophys. Res. Commun. 152, 1173–1178, 1988.
14. Kase, H., Iwahashi, K., and Matsuda, Y. K-252a, a potent inhibitor of protein kinase C from microbial origin. J. Antibiotics 39, 1059–1065, 1986.
15. Chan, K.-F. J. Ganglioside-modulated protein phosphorylation. Partial purification and characterization of a ganglioside-stimulated protein kinase in brain. J. Biol. Chem. 262, 5248–5255, 1987.
16. Laemmli, U. K. Cleavage of structural proteins during the assembly of the head of the bacteriophage T4. Nature 277, 680–685, 1970.
17. Svennerhol, L. Chromatographic separation of human brain gangliosides. J. Neurochem. 10, 613–623, 1963.
18. IUPAC-IUB Commission on Biochemical Nomenclature (CBN): The nomenclature of lipids. Eur. J. Biochem. 79, 11–21, 1977.

5. Cyclic AMP Dependent Protein Kinase and Cyclic Nucleotide Phosphodiesterase Activities are Modulated by Gangliosides

A. J. Yates, J. D. Walters,
S. M. Stock, B. K. McIlroy, and
J. D. Johnson

Summary

The catalytic subunit of cAMP-dependent protein kinase (cAK) phosphorylates proteins of 180 kDa, 49 kDa, 31 kDa, 21 kDa, and 14 kDa in rabbit sciatic nerve membranes *in vitro*. Gangliosides GT1b[1], GD1a, and GM1 inhibited cAK phosphorylation of these proteins with $I_{50} = 7$ μM, 21 μM, and 25 μM, respectively. Results of studies using several non-ganglioside lipids and sialic acids show that there are three structural determinants of this inhibitory effect: (a) The chemical nature of the lipid component; (b) The oligosaccharide chain length; (c) The number of negative charges per molecule. GM1 inhibits cAK phosphorylation of histone IIA (Ki = 108) in a manner which is competitive with respect to substrate. GM1 also inhibits autophosphorylation of cAK ($I_{50} = 15$ μM) consistent with a direct inhibitory effect of ganglioside on this enzyme. GM1 stimulated cyclic nucleotide phosphodiesterase (PDE) (half maximal = 0.3 μM) to essentially the same degree as calcium and calmodulin by increasing Vmax. These results suggest that ganglioside may modulate the activity of cAK through two distinctly different mechanisms: (a) Reduction of cAMP by activating PDE; (b) Direct inhibition of cAK. The latter mechanism may be responsible for biological events such as the stellation response of astrocytes (2), which are stimulated by cAMP but inhibited by gangliosides without reducing intracellular cAMP levels.

Introduction

Gangliosides have a wide range of biological and biochemical effects when administered both *in vivo* and *in vitro* (3–8), but the specific molecular mechanisms through which they exert these effects are still not known. Goldenring et al. (9) demonstrated that gangliosides affect endogenous phosphorylation of rat brain membranes, suggesting that gangliosides may operate by modulating protein kinase systems. Experimental results from several laboratories have supported this hypothesis. The cAMP-dependent protein kinase (cAK) is of special relevance to the biology of tumors because of the pivotal role of cAMP in regulating cell proliferation

---

[1] Ganglioside nomenclature is that of Svennerholm (1).
Abbreviations:
cAK: cyclic AMP-dependent protein kinase
GA1:   asialo GM1
PDE: cyclic nucleotide phosphodiesterase
SDS: sodium dodecyl sulfate
PAGE: polyacrylamide gel electrophoresis
lysoPS: lysophosphatidylserine
lysoPC: lysophosphatidylcholine
NeuNAc: N-acetylneuraminic acid
NeuNGc: N-glycolylneuraminic acid
GalCer: galactosylceramide
CTH: ceramide trihexoside
PKC: protein kinase C
MBP: myelin basic protein

(10). The observation that gangliosides added exogeneously to culture medium inhibit growth of several types of cells *in vitro* (11–13) makes it a reasonable possibility that gangliosides alter cell growth by altering levels of intracellular cAMP and/or modulating the activity of cAK.

Our laboratories are particularly interested in the biological roles of gangliosides, and the mechanisms through which they may participate in the pathogenesis of gliomas and other diseases of the nervous system. Therefore, we have studied the effects of gangliosides on cAK activity and its phosphorylation of proteins in peripheral nerve membranes. The results indicate that gangliosides in the low micromolar range have a direct inhibitory effect of cAK. Furthermore, in the submicromolar range, gangliosides are potent stimulators of cyclic nucleotide phosphodiesterase (PDE), which catalyzes the breakdown of cAMP. These findings indicate that gangliosides may modulate cAK activity through two different mechanisms at concentrations of gangliosides which differ by over an order of magnitude.

Materials and Methods

Sciatic nerves were dissected from female adult New Zealand white rabbits under deep pentobarbital and diethyl ether anaesthesia. The nerves were immediately placed into an ice cold solution of 0.29 M sucrose in 10 mM Hepes buffer (pH 7.4) with EGTA (1.0 mM), soybean trypsin inhibitor (0.7 µM), phenylmethylsulfonyl fluoride (290 µM), EDTA (500 µM), leupeptin (10 µM), and pepstatin (12 µM). Adherent connective tissues were dissected free, the nerves initially minced and then homogenized in a Thomas tissue grinder. A membrane fraction was isolated which consists of a variety of membranous structures and some myelin (14). Total protein was determined on this fraction using the method of Lowry et al. (15).

Phosphorylation of membrane proteins (750 µg/ml) was carried out for 1 minute at 23 °C in 200 µl of 50 mM sodium phosphate at pH 6.5 containing 2 mM EGTA, 3 mM $MgCl_2$, and 7 nM $[\gamma^{32}P]ATP$ (3000 Ci/mmol). Some reactions contained catalytic subunit of cAK (2.5 µg/ml) and either gangliosides or control lipids (0–200 µM). The reaction was halted by boiling with 40 µl stop solution (160 mM Tris-HCl pH 6.8, 20 % glycerol, 10 % SDS, 1.2 % dithioerythitol, and trace bromphenol blue). SDS-PAGE was performed with 25 µg protein per well (16), the gels stained with Coomassie blue, dried and processed for autoradiography using Kodak XAR-5 film. Protein molecular weights were determined according to mobilities relative to known molecular weight standards. The degree of phosphorylation in bands seen on the autoradiograms was quantitated by scanning densitometry using an LKB Ultroscan XK densitometer.

cAK was isolated from pig heart by the method of Reimann and Beham (17) using DEAE-cellulose and hydroxylapatite column chromatography. The activity of cAK was determined in 0.1 ml 50 mM Tris-HCl (pH 7.5) containing 10 mM $MgCl_2$, 150 µM $[^{32}P]ATP$ (6.7 mCi/mole), histone (200–300 µg/ml), and either ganglioside or control lipid (0–250 µM). Cyclic nucleotide phosphodiesterase was isolated from bovine brain by chromatography on DEAE-cellulose, calmodulin sepharose and Sephadex G-200 as described by Sharma et al. (18).

Phosphodiesterase activity was determined by the method of Johnson et al. (19). The method of Walker and Schmidt (20) was used to determine Vmax and Km of phosphodiesterase.

GM1 was obtained from Fidia Research Laboratories and GA1 was a gift of Dr. Subhash Basu. All other glycolipids and lysophosphatidylserine (lysoPS) were from Supelco. Lysophosphatidylcholine (lysoPC), NeuNAc, NeiNGc, colominic acid, and histone type IIA were all purchased from Sigma Chemical Co., $[\gamma^{32}P]$ATP was from New England Nuclear. Molecular weight standards were from Biorad and 2'methylanthraniloyl-cGMP was from Molecular Probes.

Results

Effects of Ganglioside on Cyclic Nucleotide Phosphodiesterase

Saturating amounts of calmodulin stimulated cyclic nucleotide phosphodiesterase (PDE) activity 40-fold over basal levels. GM1 either in the presence (0.73 mM $CaCl_2$) or absence (2 mM EGTA) of Ca^{2+}, stimulated PDE 32-fold over basal activity. Figure 1a shows that GM1 activation of PDE was dose-dependent with half maximal stimulation at 0.3 µM and maximal at 1 µM. PDE activity was decreased above 1 µM GM1. An analysis of the activation kinetics showed that calmodulin and GM1 both increased Vmax of PDE by 46-fold (Figure 1b). Calmodulin also decreased the Km for cGMP to 2.7 µM, while GM1 had a minimal effect on Km (6.4 µM). The entire ganglioside molecule is required for PDE activation, because neither GA1 nor GalCer had any effect on PDE. Sulfatide, another negatively charged glycosphingolipid, was also incapable of stimulating PDE. These results suggest that GM1 is a potent activator of PDE even in the absence of calcium.

Effects of Gangliosides on cAK Activity

The activity of cAK is calcium-independent, therefore, all phosphorylation reactions were performed in the presence of 2 mM EGTA to inhibit endogenous calcium-dependent kinases. Under these conditions, only two major protein bands (31 and 21 kDa) were phosphorylated by endogenous kinases (Figure 2 lane 1). The addition of cAK increased the phosphorylation of both the 31 kDa (2-fold) and 21 kDa (2.4-fold) proteins and dramatically enhanced phosphorylation of 180 kDa (11-fold), 49 kDa (7.6-fold), and 14 kDa (2.3-fold) (Figure 2 lane 2). The 40 kDa protein represents autophosphorylation of cAK. Figure 2 lanes 3–8 shows the effect of increasing concentrations of GM1 on the phosphorylation of these proteins by cAK. Figure 3 shows the effect of increasing concentrations of GM1 on the cAK phosphorylation of 180 kDa, 49 kDa, and 21 kDa proteins. The phosphorylation of each protein was half maximally inhibited near 25 µM GM1. Gangliosides GD1a and GT1b also inhibited cAK mediated phosphorylation (Table 1). GM1 and GD1a were approximately equal in inhibitory activity (I_{50} = 20–25 µM); GT1b was considerably more potent (I_{50} = 7 µM).

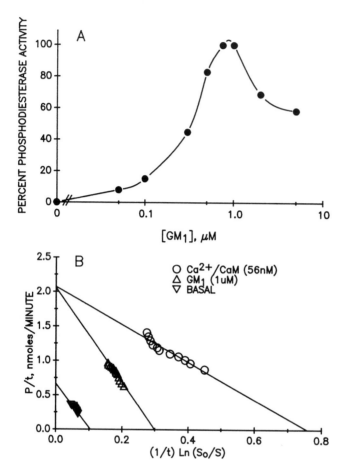

Figure 1a. Dose-response effect of GM1 on cyclic nucleotide phosphodiesterase activity as estimated by the rate of cGMP hydrolysis (19). Phosphodiesterase (3.6 µg/ml) was assayed in 10 mM MOPS, pH 7.0, containing 90 mM KCl, 6 mM $MgCl_2$, 0.73 $CaCl_2$ and 8 µM methylanthraniloyl-cGMP. Enzyme activity corresponding to 100 % is 3.2 nmol cGMP/min.

b. Effects of calcium/calmodulin and GM1 on the Km and Vmax of phosphodiesterase. Calmodulin and ganglioside-stimulated phosphodiesterase (1.3 µg/ml) and unstimulated phosphodiesterase (20 µg/ml) were assayed at 25 °C. The method of Walker and Schmidt (20) was used to estimate Km and Vmax.

Sulfatide, a negatively charged non-ganglioside glycosphingolipid was equally inhibitory to GM1 and GD1a (I_{50} = 25 µM). This suggests that a negatively charged lipid might be a structural requirement for inhibition. However, the negatively charged lysoPS was considerably less inhibitory. LysoPC, which is Zwitterionic, caused 14–22 % inhibition at 100 µM. N-acetylneuraminic acid (NeuNAc), N-glycolylneuraminic acid (NeuNGc), and colominic acid (a polymer of NeuNAc) had no inhibitory effect on cAK phosphorylation of nerve membrane proteins. GA1, globoside and CTH (100 µM) caused only 39–48 % inhibition and GalCer was almost inactive at 100 µM (9–14 % inhibition). These findings indicate that the degree of inhibition is

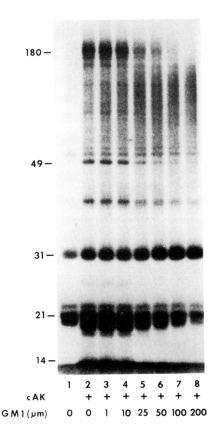

Figure 2. Autoradiograph of SDS-PAGE showing dose-response effect of GM1 on cAK-dependent phosphorylation of rabbit sciatic nerve membrane proteins. Additives to the phosphorylation system are shown below the figure. Numbers at the side are molecular weights determined from the mobility of standards.

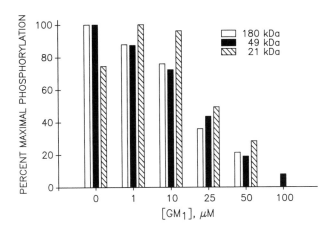

Figure 3. Dose-response effect of GM1 on cAK-catalyzed phosphorylation of 180 kDa, 49 kDa and 21 kDa proteins in rabbit sciatic nerve membranes. Results are expressed as per-cent maximal phosphorylation, correcting for cAK-independent phosphorylation.

Table 1. Inhibition of cAK-Catalyzed. Protein Phosphorylation by Lipids[a].

Glycolipid	Protein (kDa)	I_{50} (μM)
GM1	180, 49, 21	20–25
GD1a	180, 49	21
GT1b	180, 49	7
Sulfatide	180, 49	25

Control Lipid (100 μM)	Substrate Protein (kDa)	Phosphorylation Inhibition %
GA1	180	40
	49	48
Globoside	180	39
	49	44
CTH	180	43
	49	45
GalCer	180	14
	49	9
LysoPS	180	46
	49	40
LysoPC	180	14
	49	22

[a] Phosphorylation was carried out as described in Methods using membranes isolated from rabbit sciatic nerve as substrates. Phosphorylated proteins were separated using 11% SDS-PAGE, visualized with autoradiography, and degree of phosphorylation quantitated by scanning densitometry.

determined by each of the following: (a) Nature of the lipid moiety; (b) Length of oligosaccharide chain; (c) Number of negative charges per molecule.

The inhibitory effects of various lipids on cAK activity was also studied using a more defined system with histone as the substrate protein. Figure 4 shows the effect of increasing concentrations of GM1 on cAK phosphorylation of histone. GM1 was a competitive inhibitor (Figure 5) of cAK phosphorylation of histone (Ki = 108 with respect to substrate). At 250 μM GM1 completely inhibited histone phosphorylation; similar concentrations of other glycolipids were much less inhibitory: sulfatide (24%), GA1 (16%), GalCer (8%). This confirms that the sialic acid containing oligosaccharide is a major structural determinant of the inhibitory activity of gangliosides on cAK.

To determine if GM1 interacts directly with cAK we studies the effects of GM1 on autophosphorylation of cAK. In these studies only purified cAK was added to the phosphorylation system. In the absence of GM1, a 40 kDa protein was visualized with autoradiography, representing autophosphorylation of cAK (21). GM1 inhibited this autophosphorylation of cAK with I_{50} = 15 μM, providing evidence for direct inhibition of cAK by GM1 (Figure 4).

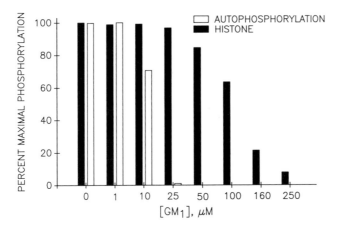

Figure 4. Dose-response effect of GM1 on cAK-catalyzed phosphorylation of histone (solid bars) and cAK autophosphorylation (open bars).

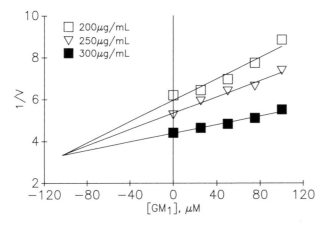

Figure 5. Kinetic analysis of the inhibitory effect of GM1 on cAK-catalyzed phosphorylation of histone is competitive with respect to substrate (Ki = 108 μM).

Discussion

The phosphorylation state of many proteins is a major determinant of their biological functions (22). At least three types of kinases have been shown to be important in regulating cell growth and proliferation. These include growth factor receptor tyrosine kinases (23), protein kinase C (PKC) and cAK. Polypeptide growth factor receptors (platelet derived growth factor, epidermal growth factor, nerve growth factor and insulin like growth factor), and the transforming principle of many retroviruses (oncogenes including erb-B and sis) share many common features including their tyrosine kinase activity and stimulation of cell growth (23–25). Growth factors binding to their receptors activate their tyrosine kinase activities and result in the phosphorylation of specific sets of cellular proteins on their tyrosine residues (23). This phosphorylation alters the activity of these substrate proteins and results in alterations in cell growth and proliferation. Both PKC and cAK have been shown to phosphorylate growth factor receptors and to alter their abilities to bind ligands (growth factors) as well as their tyrosine kinase activity. The phosphorylation events regulated by tyrosine kinases are thought to be of primary importance in regulating cell growth, differentiation and proliferation (23, 25).

Currently it is uncertain if PKC and cAK regulate cell growth and proliferation directly or if they alter ligand binding and tyrosine kinase activity of growth factor receptors via their phosphorylation of these receptors. PKC is known to be involved in the regulation of many biological functions, including gene expression and cell proliferation (26), and cAK has been shown to have dramatic effects on the progression of the cell through its cell cycle (10). Thus alterations in the activity of growth factor receptor tyrosine kinase, PKC and cAK can all have dramatic consequences on cell growth and proliferation.

In a relatively short time, experimental evidence has accumulated which shows that gangliosides can alter the activities of a variety of protein kinases (Table 2; Yu et al. – this volume). The activity of some of these is inhibited, while others are stimulated by gangliosides. Most reports suggest that PKC is inhibited by gangliosides under most conditions studied (see reference 27 for a review). However, gangliosides can also stimulate the initial rate of PKC phosphorylation of myelin basic protein (MBP). There is evidence that some protein kinases are specifically regulated by gangliosides (9, 28, 29), but the *in vivo* relevance of ganglioside modulated activity for any protein kinase is still uncertain.

Cyclic AMP has many effects on the biology of tumors, including growth and a variety of differentiation associated events. In cells cultured from dorsal root ganglia (30a) and some tumors of the nervous system (31, 32), cAMP can induce neuritogenesis. This is considered to be an expression of differentiation in neuronal tumors, and a process related to axonal regeneration *in vivo* which is also stimulated by cAMP (33, 34). Therefore, understanding the molecular mechanisms which regulate intracellular levels of cAMP and the activity of cAMP-dependent kinase should yield insights into important pathogenetic aspects of some neural tumors.

We found that cAK can phosphorylate endogenous proteins in membranes isolated from rabbit sciatic nerve in an *in vitro* phosphorylation assay. The major proteins phosphorylated by endogenous kinase activity in the absence of Ca^{2+} were 21 kDa and 31 kDa, which, based on their molecular weights, are probably the two major proteins (MBP and Po) of peripheral nerve myelin. These two proteins also serve as substrates for exogenously added PKC (35). Exogenous cAK increased the phosphorylation state of these 2 proteins as well as 180 kDa, 49 kDa, and 14 kDa proteins, the identities of which are uncertain. All gangliosides tested (Table 2 and Figure 1) inhibited cAK-catalyzed phosphorylation of 180 kDa, 49 kDa, 21 kDa, and 14 kDa proteins with half maximal inhibition occuring in the low micromolar concentration range. GT1b was the most inhibitory; GD1a, GM1, and sulfatide were about equally effective. Comparing these results with those obtained with other glycolipids and compounds which are components of the ganglioside molecule, it appears that negatively charged lipids are in general inhibitory to cAK. Neutral glycolipid structural analogues of gangliosides and the Zwitterionic lysoPC had much less inhibitory effect; NeuNAc, NeuNGc, and colominic acid, a polymer of NeuNAc, were all ineffective. Therefore, it appears that both the hydrophilic ceramide and the negatively charged oligosaccharide portions of

Table 2. Effects of Gangliosides on Protein Kinase Activities.

Enzyme	Source	Substrate	Effect	Half Maximal Ganglioside Concentration	Reference
PKC	myelin	endogenous MBP	inhi-bition	GM1 – 160 µM, GD1a – 65 µM, GD1b – 65 µM, GT1b – 40 µM	46
	HL-60 leukemia cells	histone IIIS MBP MBP peptide	inhi-bition	Mixed brain gangliosides 30 µM	47
	rat brain	MBP	stimu-lation	GM1 – 241 µM GD1a – 67 µM	28
Ganglioside Kinase	Rat brain membranes	endogenous proteins	stimu-lation	Ca^{2+}-gangliosides complex GD1 – 50 µM	9
	guinea pig myelin	endogenous 62 kDa protein	stimu-lation	GM1, GT1b – 73 µM	28
	guinea pig synaptosome membrane	endogenous proteins	stimu-lation	GT1b – 20 µM GD1b – 36 µM	29
	guinea pig brain membranes	synthetic peptide	inhi-bition	GD1a – 4.8 µM GD1b – 5.2 µM GM1 – 8.4 µM complete at 0.4 µM GT1b	30
PDGF Receptor	Swiss mouse 3T3	autophosphory-lation	inhi-bition	GM1; GM3 10 µM	48
EGF Receptor	epidermoid	autophosphory-lation	inhi-bition	GM1; GM3 2.5 µM	49
cAK	pig heart	rabbit nerve membrane	inhi-bition	GM1 20 – 25 µM GD1a 21 µM	50
		endogeous proteins		GT1b	
		autophosphory-lation	inhi-bition	GM1 15 µM	
		Histone IIA	inhi-bition	GM1 – 108 µM	

the ganglioside molecule are essential for full inhibitory activity. The finding that GT1b, which has 3 negatively charged sialic acids, was slightly more inhibitory than GD1a or GM1 (which have 2 and 1 sialic acid residues per molecule, respectively) suggests that the degree of inhibition is directly related to the number of negative charges on the compound. Similarly, at least up to a tetrasaccharide, the oligosaccharide chain length, which confers a dregee of hydrophilicity to the molecule, is directly related to the degree of inhibition caused by the neutral glycolipids. GalCer, which has only one sugar residue, had almost no inhibitory effect. Neutral glycolipids with 3 (CTH) or 4 (GA1, globoside) sugars were all more inhibitory than GalCer.

There are two forms of cAMP-dependent protein kinases in mammalian tissues, referred to as Types I and II. The holoenzyme, which has no kinase activity, is a tetramer composed of two regulatory and two catalytic subunits. The catalytic subunit is identical in both types, but the regulatory subunits are different. When 2 cAMP molecules bind to each regulatory subunit, the catalytic subunits dissociate and have maximum catalytic activity (see reference 21 for a review). Our findings indicate that gangliosides in the low micromolar concentration range inhibit the kinase activity of the free catalytic subunit. Our results from *in vitro* studies using histone IIA, demonstrate that GM1 inhibits cAK in a manner which is competitive with respect to substrate. Consistent with this, GM1 inhibits autophosphorylation of cAK even more effectively than it inhibits cAK phosphorylation of substrate proteins. Our findings indicate that GM1 at low micromolar concentrations produces a direct inhibition of cAK. The biological significance of this effect in intact cells is uncertain, because of the lack of data on concentrations of soluble gangliosides in specific subcellular compartments. However, 2–5 % of total ganglioside is present in the cytosol of brain (36, 37) and cultured cells (38). Unlike most other mammalian tissues, nervous tissues contain significant amounts of cAMP-dependent protein kinase associated with the particulate fraction (39, 40). Whether or not membrane associated ganglioside can interact with and regulate the activity of membrane-bound cAK is uncertain, but this possibility must be considered in both normal and neoplastic neural cells which contain significant amounts of ganglioside.

The level of intracellular cAMP is the major determinant of cAK activity in the intact cell. The concentration of cAMP is the net result of the rates of synthesis and degradation of cAMP. Adenylate cyclase catalyses the biosynthetic step converting ATP to cAMP, and the rate of this reaction is influenced by several factors. Several ligand-receptor interactions activate G-proteins which stimulate or inhibit adenylate cyclase (41). PKC activates adenylate cyclase in rat adipocyte membranes (42). Gangliosides have been reported to activate adenylate cyclase in rat brain membranes (43) and to inhibit this enzyme in human thyroid membranes (44), but the effect of gangliosides on adenylate cyclase has not been studied in any tumors.

The hydrolysis of cAMP to form 5'AMP is catalyzed by 3',5'-cyclic nucleotide phosphodiesterase (PDE). It was demonstrated previously that a mixture of gangliosides isolated from bovine brain caused a two-fold activation over basal activity of both calcium-dependent and calcium-independent PDE from rat brain (45). This occured at a ganglioside concentration of 63 μM for the former and 6.3 μM for the latter. Calmodulin in the presence of Ca^{2+} activated the calcium-dependent enzyme to levels twice that obtained by gangliosides either in the presence or absence of Ca^{2+}. In our system (19), saturating amounts of calmodulin activate calcium-calmodulin dependent

PDE 40-fold. GM1 (1×10^{-6}M) is essentially equally effective as calmodulin in activation of PDE even in the absence of calcium. GM1 stimulation of PDE activity could result in major decreases in the intracellular concentrations of cAMP, with subsequent reductions in cAK activity.

Our findings indicate that ganglioside may regulate cAK activity through two different mechanisms: One direct, and the other indirect. At submicromolar concentrations ganglioside could indirectly decrease cAK activity by activating cyclic nucleotide PDE and hydrolyzing cAMP. At micromolar concentrations gangliosides might produce a direct inhibition of cAK resulting in a blockade of cAMP dependent processes.

Taken together, the information available indicates that the effects of both endogenously synthesized and exogenously administered gangliosides on protein phosphorylation and subsequent biological events in the intact cell is extremely complex. As with the effects of administered cAMP, the cellular responses to gangliosides will undoubtedly depend upon cell types, growth conditions, levels of intracellular cAMP and the phase of the cell cycle during which they are acting (10). Some biological phenomena will be affected at lower concentrations of gangliosides through the stimulation of cyclic nucleotide phosphodiesterase. Other events may be altered by higher ganglioside concentrations which directly inhibit cAK. An example of this may be the stellation effect of cultured astrocytes which is induced by compounds which elevate levels of intracellular cAMP (2). Exogenously administered gangliosides inhibit this process without altering cAMP levels. It seems likely that ganglioside could directly inhibit cAK in these cells in the same way as we have demonstrated with GM1 inhibition of cAK phosphorylation of nerve membrane proteins and histone IIA as substrates.

In summary, we have found that ganglioside in submicromolar concentration stimulates cyclic nucleotide phosphodiesterase activity, and in low micromolar concentrations directly inhibits cAK. Both effects would alter signal transduction via any pathway which utilizes cAMP as a second messenger. Furthermore, gangliosides might alter growth factor stimulation of cell growth by inhibiting cAK phosphorylation of growth factor receptor. It is possible that some of the effects of gangliosides on proliferation and differentiation of normal and neoplastic cells may be mediated through these mechanisms.

Acknowledgements

The authors would like to thank Eleanor Borem for typing this manuscript and Julie Dolin for photography. This work was supported by the Department of Pathology and the College of Medicine, OSU, and grants from N.I.H.:NS-10165 (AJY), DK-33727-04 (JDJ) and DE-00188 (JDW). GM1 was a gift of Fidia Research Labs, Italy; GA1 was kindly supplied by Dr. Subhash Basu.

References

1. Svennerholm, L. Ganglioside designation. Adv. Exptl. Med. Biol. 125, 11, 1980.
2. Facci, L., Skaper, S. D., Levin, D. L., and Varon, S. Dissociation of the stellate morphology from intracellular cyclic AMP levels in cultured rat brain astrogial cells: effects of ganglioside GM1 and lysophosphatidylserine. J. Neurochem. 48, 566–573, 1987.
3. Gorio, A., Haber, B. *Neurobiology of Gangliosides.* Alan R. Liss Inc. New York, 1985.
4. Ledeen, R.W., Tettamanti, G., Yu, R. K., Hogan, E. L., and Yates, A. J. *New Trends in Ganglioside Research: Neurochemical and Neuroregenerative Aspects.* Liviana Press/Springer Verlag, in press.
5. Byrne, M. C., Ledeen, R.W., Roisen, F. J., Yorke, G., and Sclafani, J. R. Ganglioside-induced neuritogenesis: verification that gangliosides are the active agents, and comparison of molecular species. J. Neurochem. 41, 1214–1222, 1983.
6. Leskawa, K. C. and Hogan, E. L. Quantitation of the in vitro neuroblastoma response to exogenous, purified gangliosides. J. Neurosci. Res. 13, 539–550, 1985.
7. Sparrow, J. R. and Grafstein, B. Sciatic nerve regeneration in ganglioside-treated rats. Exp. Neurol. 77, 230–235, 1982.
8. Spero, D. A., Roisen, F. J. Gangliosides induce microfilament-dependent changes in membrane surface activity of neuro-2a neuroblastoma cells. Int. J. Devl. Neurosci. 3, 631–642, 1985.
9. Goldenring, J. R., Otis, L. C., Yu, R. K., and DeLorenzo, R. J. Calcium/ganglioside-dependent protein kinase activity in rat brain membrane. J. Neurochem. 44, 1229–1234, 1985.
10. Boynton, A. L. and Whitfield, J. F. The role of cyclic AMP in cell proliferation: A critical assessment of the evidence. In: *Advances in Cyclic Nucleotide Research Vol. 15,* Greengard, P. and Robison, G. A. (eds), Raven Press, New York, pp 193–294, 1983.
11. Keenan, T.W., Schmid, E., Franke, W.W., and Wiegandt, H. Exogenous glycosphingolipids suppress growth rate of transformed and untransformed 3T3 mouse cells. Exp. Cell Res. 92, 259–270, 1975.
12. Bremer, E. G. and Hakomori, S.-I. GM3 ganglioside induces hamster fibroblast growth inhibition in chemically-defined medium: Ganglioside may regulate growth factor receptor function. Biochem. Biophys. Res. Com. 106, 711–718, 1982.
13. Icard-Liepkalns, C., Liepkalns, V. A., Yates, A. J., Rodriguez, Z. R., and Stephens, R. E. Effect of exogenous gangliosides on human neural cell division. J. Cell Physiol. 113, 186–191, 1982.
14. Chou, K. H., Nolan, C. E., and Jungalwala, F. B. Composition and metabolism of gangliosides in rat peripheral nervous system during development. J. Neurochem. 39, 1547–1558, 1982.
15. Lowry, O. H., Rosebrough, N. J., Farr, A. L., Randall, R. J. Protein measurement with the Folin phenol reagent. J. Biol. Chem. 193, 265–275, 1951.
16. Laemmli, U. K. Cleavage of structural proteins during the assembly of the head of bacteriophage T4. Nature 227, 680–685, 1970.
17. Reimann, E. M. and Beham, R. A. Catalytic subunit of cAMP-dependent protein kinase. Methods in Enzymol. 99, 51–55, 1983.
18. Sharma, R. K., Taylor, W. A., and Wang, J. H. Use of calmodulin affinity chromatography for purification of specific calmodulin-dependent enzymes. Methods in Enzymology 102, 210–219, 1983.
19. Johnson, J. D., Walters, J. D., and Mills, J. S. A continuous fluorescence assay for cyclic nucleotide phosphodiesterase hydrolysis of cyclic GMP. Anal. Biochem. 162, 291–295, 1987.

20. Walker, A. C. and Schmidt, C. L. Studies on histidase. Arch. Biochem. 5, 445–467, 1944.
21. Edelman, A. M., Blumenthal, D. K., and Krebs, E. G. Protein serine/threonine kinases. Ann. Rev. Biochem. 56, 567–614, 1987.
22. Nestler, E. J. and Greengard, P. *Protein Phosphorylation in the Nervous System.* John Wiley and Sons, New York, 1984.
23. Yarden, Y. and Ullrich, A. Growth Factor Receptor Tyrosine Kinases. Ann. Rev. Biochem. 57, 443–478, 1988.
24. Hunter, T. The proteins of oncogenes. Scientific American 25, 70–79, 1984.
25. James, R. and Bradshaw, R. A. Polypeptide growth factors. Ann. Rev. Biochem. 53, 259–292, 1984.
26. Nishizuka, Y. Studies and perspectives of protein kinase C. Science 233, 305–312, 1986.
27. Farooqui, A. A., Farooqui, T., Yates, A. J., and Horrocks, L. A. Regulation of protein kinase C activity by various lipids. Neurochem. Res. 13, 499–511, 1988.
28. Chan, K.-F. J. Ganglioside-modulated protein phosphorylation in myelin. J. Biol. Chem. 262, 2415–2422, 1987a.
29. Chan, K.-F. J. Ganglioside-modulated protein phosphorylation. J. Biol. Chem. 262, 5248–5255, 1987b.
30. Chan, K.-F. J. Ganglioside-modulated protein phosphorylation. J. Biol. Chem. 263, 568–574, 1988.
30a. Roisen, F. J., Murphy, R. A., and Braden, W. G. Neurite development *in vitro.* I. The effects of adenosine 3′,5′-cyclic monophosphate (cyclic AMP). J. Neurobiol. 3, 347–368, 1972.
31. Prashad, N., Lotan, D., and Lotan, R. Differential effects of dibutyryl cyclic adenosine monophosphate and retinoic acid on the growth, differentiation and cyclic adenosine monophosphate-binding protein of murine neuroblastoma cells. Cancer Research 47, 2417–2424, 1987.
32. Gunning, P. W., Letourneau, P. C., Landreth, G. E., and Shooter, E. M. The action of nerve growth factor and dibutyryl adenosine cyclic 3′,5′-monophosphate on rat pheochromocytoma reveals distinct stages in the mechanisms underlying neurite outgrowth. J. Neurosci. 10, 1085–1095, 1981.
33. Gershenbaum, M. R. and Roisen, F. J. The effects of dibutyryl cyclic adenosine monophosphate on the degeneration and regeneration of crush-lesioned rat sciatic nerves. Neuroscience 5, 1565–1580, 1980.
34. Kilmer, S. L. and Carlsen, R. C. Forskolin activation of adenylate cyclase *in vivo* stimulates nerve regeneration. Nature 307, 455–457, 1984.
35. Yates, A. J., Wood, C. L., Halterman, R. K., Stock, S. M., Walters, J. D., and Johnson, J. D. Effects of gangliosides, calmodulin, protein kinase C and copper on phosphorylation of protein in membranes of normal and transected sciatic nerve, in press.
36. Sonnino, S., Ghidoni, R., Marchesini, S., and Tettamanti, G. Cytosolic gangliosides: occurrence in calf brain as ganglioside-protein complexes. J. Neurochem. 33, 117–121, 1979.
37. Sonnino, S., Ghidoni, R., Masserini, M., Aporti, F., and Tettamanti, G. Changes in rabbit brain cytosolic and membrane-bound gangliosides during prenatal life. J. Neurochem. 36, 227–232, 1981.
38. Miller-Podraza, H. and Fishman, P. H. Soluble gangliosides in cultured neurotumor cells. J. Neurochem. 41, 860–867, 1983.
39. Hofman, F., Bechtel, P. J., and Krebs, E. G. Concentrations of cyclic AMP-dependent protein kinase subunits in various tissues. J. Biol. Chem. 252, 1441–1447, 1977.
40. Rubin, C. S., Rngel-Aldao, R., Sarkar, D., Erlichman, J., and Fleischer, N. Characterization and comparison of membrane-associated and cytosolic cAMP-dependent protein kinases. J. Biol. Chem. 254, 3797–3805, 1979.
41. Dunlap, K., Holz, G. G., and Rane, S. G. G proteins as regulators of ion channel function. Trends in Neuroscience 10, 241–244, 1987.

42. Naghshineh, S., Noguchi, M., Huang, K.-P., and Londos, C. Activation of odipocyte adenylate cyclase by protein kinase C. J. Biol. Chem. 261, 14535–14538, 1986.

43. Partington, C. R. and Daly, J.W. Effect of gangliosides on adenylate cyclase activity in rat cerebral cortical membranes. Molecular Pharmacology 15, 484–491, 1979.

44. Dacremont, G., DeBaets, M., Kaufman, J. M., Elewaut, A., and Vermeulen, A. Inhibition of adenylate cyclase activity of human thyroid membranes by gangliosides. Biochim. Biophys. Acta 770, 142–147, 1984.

45. Davis, C.W. and Daley, J.W. Activation of rat cerebral cortical 3′,5′-cyclic nucleotide phosphodiesterase activity by gangliosides. Mol. Pharmacol. 17, 206–211, 1980.

46. Kim, J.Y.H., Goldenring, J. R., DeLorenzo, R. J., and Yu, R. K. Gangliosides inhibit phospholipid-sensitive Ca^{2+}-dependent kinase phosphorylation of rat myelin basic proteins. J. Neurosci. Res. 15, 159–166, 1986.

47. Kreutter, D., Kim, J.Y. H., Goldenring, J. R., Rasmussen, H., Ukomadu, C., DeLorenzo, R. J., and Yu, R. K. Regulation of protein kinase C activity by gangliosides. J. Biol. Chem. 262, 1633–1637, 1987.

48. Bremer, E. G., Hakomori, S.-I., Bowen-Pope, D. F., Raines, E., and Ross, R. Ganglioside-mediated modulation of cell growth, growth factor binding, and receptor phosphorylation. J. Biol. Chem. 259, 6818–6825, 1984.

49. Bremer, E. G., Schlessinger, J., and Hakomori, S.-I. Ganglioside-mediated modulation of cell growth. Specific effects of GM3 on tyrosine phosphorylation of the epidermal growth factor receptor. J. Biol. Chem. 261, 2434–2440, 1986.

50. Yates, A. J., Walters, J. D., Wood, C. L., Johnson, J. D. Ganglioside modulation of cAMP dependent protein kinase and cyclic nucleotide phosphodiesterase. Submitted.

6. General Concept of Tumor-associated Carbohydrate Antigens: Their Chemical, Physical, and Enzymatic Basis

Sen-itiroh Hakomori

Tumor-associated antigen: How specific should it be?

There is a striking discrepancy between immunological specificity and chemical detectability of antigens. It is well known that "specific antibodies" called Wasserman antibodies, detected in patients with syphilis, were widely utilized for diagnosis of syphilis by Wasserman reaction or its modification. The antigen was originally isolated from syphiloma of fetal liver and was considered to be specific for *Trepanoma pallidum*. The antigen, however, was found subsequently to be a normal cellular component identified as diphosphatidylglycerol (cardiolipin) (1). The lipid antigen is cryptic in normal cells and tissues; our current knowledge indicates that cardiolipin is only present in the mitochrondrial membrane, but absent from the cell surface. However, the antigen could be surface-exposed in syphilis lesions, causing an immune response to this lipid antigen. This famous classical finding has been almost forgotten in current tumor immunology. In the past decade, a number of studies with monoclonal antibodies (MAbs) applied in analysis of tumor-associated antigens have clearly indicated that many of them are directed to carbohydrates, particularly glycosphingolipids. Antigens defined by such antibodies, showing "specific" or "preferential" reactivity with tumor cells, have been found to be (a) relatively novel structures present in minor quantities in normal tissues but greatly accumulated in tumors, or (b) well-known common structures present in both normal and tumor tissues, but showing a reactivity at the tumor cell surface quantitatively and qualitatively distinct from that of the same antigen at the normal cell surface. Strictly speaking, there are no "tumor-specific" structures on a chemical basis. A summary of the general concept of tumor-associated antigens is presented in Table 1.

Table 1. Immunochemical basis of tumor-specificity.

A. There is no "tumor-specific" struc}cture characterized on a chemical basis.

B. However, MAbs have been established after immunization of mice with tumor cells, or tumor cell membranes, and antibody-secreting hybridomas have been selected on the basis of preferential reactivity with tumor cells (or tissue) over normal cells.

C. "Tumor-associated" structures defined by these MAbs are:

   1) Relatively novel structures expressed highly at the tumor cell surface. The same structures are absent in progenitor cells, but can be found in other normal tissues (e. g., GD_3 in melanoma; di- or trimeric Le^x; sialyl-dimeric Le^x; sialyl Le^a in gastrointestinal cancer).

   2) Highly restricted structures immunologically detectable only in tumor cells (e. g., incompatible A, Tn in various cancers).

   3) Common structures abundant in normal cells or tissue, but with a very high concentration in tumors; antibodies can recognize this high density (e. g. GM_3 in melanoma).

Chemical and structural basis of tumor-associated carbohydrate antigens

Tumor-associated carbohydrate antigens can be created by three basic processes as shown in Table 2, i.e., incomplete synthesis, neosynthesis, and organizational changes. The general directions of aberrant glycosylation found in each type of carbohydrate chain are indicated in Table 3. Enhanced synthesis of precursor structure coupled with blocked synthesis of complex structure in ganglio- and globo-series glycolipids has been clearly observed, resulting in accumulation of precursors for ganglio- and globo-structures. In contrast, "neosynthesis" often occurs in lacto-series type 1 and type 2 chains, as well as in blood group A, Lewis and P determinants, resulting in the synthesis of "incompatible blood group antigens". A most striking accumulation of precursors due to blocked synthesis is found in mucin-type O-linked carbohydrate chains, resulting in accumulation of T, Tn, and sialyl-Tn (see Table 3).

Tumor-associated carbohydrate antigens can be classified into three groups as shown in Figure 1, i.e., epitopes expressed on both glycolipids and glycoproteins, those expressed exclusively on glycolipids, and those expressed exclusively on glycoproteins. The first group essentially belongs to the lacto-series structure and is found most abundantly in the most common human cancers such as lung, gastrointestinal, breast, colorectal, liver and pancreatic cancer. The structure has a common backbone consisting of Galβ1$\rightarrow$3GlcNAcβ1$\rightarrow$3Gal (type 1) or Galβ1$\rightarrow$4GlcNAcβ1$\rightarrow$3Gal (type 2) (see for review 2, 3). The novel structures of this group, and their defining MAbs established in this laboratory, are listed in Table 4. All these structures are characterized by unbranched linear type 2 chains with internal fucosylation as the backbone (Table 4, structures 1, 2, and 5), albeit terminal fucosylation (structure 3) or sialylation (structure 4) may also be found. Of particular interest in this structural series was the

---

Table 2. Basic changes in glycolipids associated with oncogenic transformation.

1. *Incomplete synthesis with or without accumulation of precursor glycolipids.*

    ○ Gb_3 in Burkitt's lymphoma

    ○ GD_2 and GD_3 in melanoma, neuroblastoma, and T-cell leukemia

    ○ Gg_3 in Hodgkin's lymphoma, and mouse lymphoma and sarcoma

2. *Enhanced synthesis of neoglycolipids*

    ○ Dimeric or trimeric Le^x, trifucosyl Le^y, sialyl Le^x, and sialyl Le^a in various adenocarcinomas (gastrointestinal, pulmobronchial, genitourinary)

3. *Organizational changes of glycolipids in membranes*

    ○ occurs in all types of tumors

    ○ high exposure due to loss of crypticity, which is influenced by:

      – adjacent glycoconjugates which interact with glycolipids
      – density of glycolipids
      – ceramide composition:
        short-chain fatty acid < long-chain f. a. < alpha-OH f. a.

Table 3. Directions of aberrant glycosylation.

Changes in ganglio-series

Accumulation of GM_3, GD_2, GM_2, GD_3, etc. in melanoma, neuroblastoma, etc.
LacCer $\rightarrow$ GM_3 $\rightarrow$ GD_3 $\rightarrow$ GD_2 $-\!\!/\!\!\rightarrow$ GD_{1b} $\longrightarrow$ GT_{1b}
Fucosyl GM_1 synthesis: GM_1 $\rightarrow$ Fuc-GM_1

Changes in globo-series

Accumulation of Gb3 in Burkitt lymphoma, esophageal cancer
LacCer $\rightarrow$ Gb3 $-\!\!/\!\!\rightarrow$ Gb4
Neosynthesis of extended globo-series, e. g., globo-H

Changes in lacto-type 1 chain

Enhanced synthesis of: 2$\rightarrow$3sialyl Le^a, 2$\rightarrow$3, 2$\rightarrow$6 sialyl Le^a, Le^a, Le^b, 2$\rightarrow$3 sialyl Lc_4;
coexpression of Le^a, Le^b

Changes in lacto-type 2 chain

Enhanced chain elongation without branching (i)
nLc_4, nLc_6, nLc_8, etc.
Le^x, Le^y, dimeric Le^x, trimeric Le^x, sialyl Le^y, sialyl dimeric Le^x, etc.

Synthesis of incompatible:

A antigen in O or B tumor
Le^a, Le^b
P_1, P, p^k in p tumor

Mucin glycoprotein

T, Tn, sialyl Tn

Oncofetal fibronectin, defined by MAb FDC-6

-Val-Thr-His-Pro-Gly-Tyr- no activity
-Val-Thr-His-Pro-Gly-Tyr- strong activity
              |
              O
              |
          GalNAc
polypeptide conformation is converted to antigenically active by GalNAc addition.

expression of real A antigen (type 1 chain A, i.e., ALe^b and ALe^d) in tumors of blood group 0 or B individuals (4). The structures (not shown in the table) are defined by combinations of MAbs that are able to distinguish various A antigens carried by different carbohydrate chains (5–7). The second group of epitopes, expressed exclusively on glycolipids, has been found mainly on ganglio- or globoseries structures (2, 3). These antigens (shown in Table 5) are abundantly expressed in specific types of human cancer such as melanoma, Burkitt's lymphoma, neuroblastoma, and small cell lung carcinoma, but not in common human cancers. The third group of epitopes,

Table 4. Lacto-series structures: Antigens expressed in both glycoproteins and glycolipids.

Structure	Name	MAbs
Type 2 chain		

1. Galβ1→4GlcNAcβ1→3Galβ1→4Glcβ1→1Cer
          3
          ↑
        Fucα1
	difucosyl y₂ (dimeric Le^x)	FH4 (16, 17)

2. Galβ1→4GlcNAcβ1→3Galβ1→4GlcNAcβ1→3Galβ1→4Glcβ1→1Cer
          3   3
          ↑   ↑
        Fucα1   Fucα1
	trimeric Le^x	FH5 (16, 17)

3. Galβ1→4GlcNAcβ1→3Galβ1→4Glcβ1→1Cer
        2   3
        ↑   ↑
      Fucα1 Fucα1
	trifucosyl Le^y	AH6, KH1 (11, 18, 19)

4. Galβ1→4GlcNAcβ1→3Galβ1→4Glcβ1→1Cer
        3   3
        ↑   ↑
    NeuAcα2 Fucα1
	sialosyl difucosyl Le^x	FH6 (20)

5. Galβ1→4GlcNAcβ1→3Galβ1→4GlcNAcβ1→3Galβ1→4Glcβ1→1Cer
          3
          ↑
        Fucα1
		ACFH-18 (21)

Table 5. Globo- or ganglio-series structures: Antigens expressed exclusively in glycolipids.

	Structure	Source/Name	MAbs
Globo-series			
1.	Galα1→4Galβ1→4Glcβ1→1Cer	Burkitt's lymphoma	anti-BLA (22)
2.	Fucα1→2Galβ1→3GlcNAcβ1→4Galα1→3Galα1→4Glcβ1→1Cer	breast cancer (globo-H antigen)	MBr1 (23)
3.	Fucα1→2Galβ1→3GlcNAcβ1→3Galα1→4Galβ1→4Glcβ1→1Cer $\overset{3}{\underset{\uparrow}{}}$ GalNAcα1	colorectal cancer (globo-A antigen)	HH5 (24)
4.	GalNAcα1→3GlcNAcβ1→3Galα1→4Galβ1→4Glcβ1→1Cer	gastric/lung cancer Forssman antigen	(25)
Ganglio-series			
5.	NeuAcα2→3Galβ1→4GlcCer	human/mouse melanoma GM$_3$ ganglioside or lactone DH2 (26)	M2590 (14, 15) DH2 (26)
6.	NeuAcα2→8NeuAcα2→3Galβ1→4GlcCer	human melanoma GD$_3$ ganglioside	4.2 (27)
7.	NeuAcα2→8NeuAcα2→3Galβ1→4GlcCer $\overset{4}{\underset{\uparrow}{}}$ GalNAcβ1	neuroblastoma, melanoma GD$_2$ ganglioside	
8.	Fucα1→2Galβ1→3GlcNAcβ1→4Galβ1→4GlcCer $\overset{3}{\underset{\uparrow}{}}$ NeuAcα2	small cell lung carcinoma fucosyl GM$_1$	

Table 6. Tn and sialyl Tn structures: Antigens expressed exclusively in glycoproteins.

Structure	Source/Name	MAbs
GalNAcα1→O-Ser/Thr (polypeptide)	Tn	NCC-Lu35 and -81 (28) Cu-1 (29)
GalNAcα1→O-Ser/Thr (polypeptide) 6 ↑ NeuAcα2	sialyl Tn	TKH1 and -2 (30)

expressed exclusively in glycoproteins, has been recently identified as Tn and sialosyl Tn, the precursors of O-linked carbohydrate chains. These structures and their defining antibodies are shown in Table 6.

In addition to these three groups, a new type of tumor-associated epitope (Figure 1, item 4) has been found recently in "oncofetal fibronectin" (8). The epitope is a peptide maintained in an active state by glycosylation (9).

1. **Epitopes expressed on both glycolipids and glycoproteins**

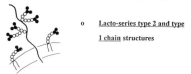

    o   Lacto-series type 2 and type 1 chain structures

2. **Epitopes expressed exclusively on glycolipids**

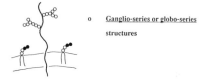

    o   Ganglio-series or globo-series structures

3. **Epitopes expressed exclusively on glycoproteins**

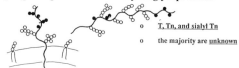

    o   T, Tn, and sialyl Tn
    o   the majority are unknown

4. **Peptide epitope is maintained in active state by glycosylation (i.e., glycosylation as activator of polypeptide epitope)**

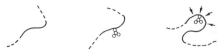

Figure 1. Tumor-associated carbohydrate antigens, and epitopes influenced by glycosylation.

Enzymatic basis of aberrant glycosylation

The enzymatic basis of most of these carbohydrate changes, with a few exceptions, has not been investigated. However, three basic changes in glycolipids associated with oncogenic transformation have been studied extensively, as shown in Table 2. They are: i) incomplete synthesis with or without accumulation of precursor glycolipid; ii) enhanced synthesis of neoglycolipid essentially absent in progenitor cells; iii) organizational changes in the cell membrane, observed in essentially all tumors. A typical example, GM_3 ganglioside highly expressed in human and mouse melanoma, will be discussed subsequently.

An important enzymatic basis for the accumulation of lacto-series type 2 chain glycolipid (Table 4) in colon cancer is the enhancement of $\beta1\rightarrow3GalNAc$ transferase, rather than any other glycosyltransferase (10). Thus, unbranched core structure, to which sialosyl or fucosyl substitution could occur, accumulates greatly. There is no indication in colon cancer of enhanced sialosyl- or fucosyltransferase.

Organizational and physical basis of "tumor specificity"

All glycolipid antigens may share a common physical structure organized in the lipid bilayer. Recent analysis of the conformational structure of glycosphingolipid antigens

1. **Rigid structures formed by GalNAc, GlcNAc, Fuc branch, disialyl residue**

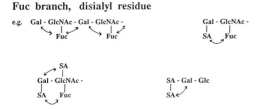

2. **Hydrophobic area surrounded by hydrophilic area**

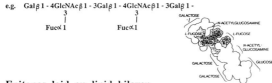

3. **Epitopes laid on lipid bilayer**

   Hydrophobic area on the surface of lipid bilayer

4. **High density ⟶ conformational change**

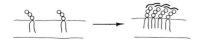

Figure 2. Physical basis of "tumor-specificity".

clearly indicates that the axis of the ceramide is perpendicular to the axis of the carbohydrate chain (11, 12). Furthermore, hydrophobic structures such as the N-acetyl group of GalNAc or GlcNAc are oriented towards the upper surface of the carbohydrate chain, while hydrophilic groups are more abundant on the lower surface. Thus, epitopes carried by glycosphingolipids could constitute the hydrophobic area on the surface of carbohydrate chains laid on the lipid bilayer (Figure 2, item 3). This property is not limited to tumor-associated glycolipid antigens, but is common to all types of glycolipid antigens. However, highly immunogenic tumor-associated antigens are the rigid structures formed by GalNAc or GlcNAc with fucosyl or sialosyl substitution (Figure 2, item 1). These structures show high rigidity due to steric hindrance (conformations based on hard sphere ex-anomeric [HSEA] calculation), and form large hydrophobic areas surrounded by hydrophilic areas (Figure 2, item 2).

Anomalous conformations specific to tumors may also be formed by common structures such as GM_3 or Le^x when they are organized in high density at the surface membrane. Typical examples are shown in antibody M2590, which was established after immunization of C57/BL16 mice with syngeneic B16 melanoma. The antibody reacts only with mouse, human, and hamster melanomas, but not with other types of cells (13). It was shown to be directed to GM_3 (14), although GM_3 is found in essentially all types of normal cells as well as melanomas. The cell surface reactivity of various cell lines with M2590 correlates closely with the quantity of GM_3 and its surface density. An abrupt loss of over 90 % of the cell surface reactivity of M2590 with melanoma results from a 10 % loss of surface GM_3 by sialidase treatment. Antibody reactivity does not change with further hydrolysis of GM_3 by sialidase. Solid-phase antibody binding assay and liposome lysis assay indicate the existence of a threshold GM_3 density that allows the antibody to react maximally with GM_3.

These results all indicate that the conformation of GM_3 at the melanoma cell surface is aberrant and recognized specifically by antibody M2590 due to high GM_3 density (15). Because M2590 shows much higher affinity with GM_3 lactone than with free GM_3, and because GM_3 lactone was detected in melanoma cells, it is assumed that GM_3 lactone is the real immunogen, or that GM_3 at high density mimics the conformation of GM_3 lactone (15).

References

1. Davis, B. D., Dulbecco, R., Eisen, H., Ginsberg, H. S., Wood, W. B. The spirochetes. In: *Microbiology,* pp. 880–896, Harper & Row, New York 1967.
2. Hakomori, S. Tumor associated carbohydrate antigens. Ann. Rev. Immunol. 2, 103–126, 1984.
3. Hakomori, S. Aberrant glycosylation in cancer cell membranes as focussed on glycolipids: Overview and perspective. Cancer Res. 45, 2405–2414, 1985.
4. Clausen, H., Hakomori, S., Graem, N., Dabelsteen, E. Incompatible A antigen expressed in tumors of blood group 0 and B individuals: Immunochemical, immunohistologic, and enzymatic characterization. J. Immunol. 136, 326–330, 1986.

5. Clausen, H., Levery, S. B., McKibbin, J. M., Hakomori, S. Blood group A determinants with mono- and difucosyl type 1 chain in human erythrocyte membranes. Biochemistry 24, 3578–3586, 1985.

6. Clausen, H., McKibbin, J. M., Hakomori, S. Monoclonal antibodies defining blood group A variants with difucosyl type 1 chain (ALe^b) and difucosyl type 2 chain (ALe^y). Biochemistry 24, 6190–6194, 1985.

7. Abe, K., Levery, S. B., Hakomori, S. The antibody specific to type 1 chain blood group A determinant. J. Immunol. 132, 1951–1954, 1984.

8. Matsuura, H., Hakomori, S. The oncofetal domain of fibronectin defined by monoclonal antibody FDC-6: Its presence in fibronectins from fetal and tumor tissues and its absence in those from normal adult tissues and plasma. Proc. Natl. Acad. Sci. USA 82, 6517–6521, 1985.

9. Matsuura, H., Takio, K., Titani, K., Greene, T., Levery, S. B., Salyan, M. E. K., Hakomori, S. The oncofetal structure of human fibronectin defined by monoclonal antibody FDC-6: Unique structural requirement for the antigenic specificity provided by a glycosylhexapeptide. J. Biol. Chem. 263, 3314–3322, 1988.

10. Holmes, E. H., Hakomori, S., Ostrander, G. K. Synthesis of type 1 and 2 lacto series glycolipid antigens in human colonic adenocarcinoma and derived cell lines is due to activation of a normally unexpressed $\beta 1 \rightarrow 3$N-acetylglucosaminyltransferase. J. Biol. Chem. 262, 15649–15658, 1987.

11. Kaizu, T., Levery, S. B., Nudelman, E., Stemkamp, R. E., Hakomori, S. Novel fucolipids of human adenocarcinoma: VI. Monoclonal antibody specific for trifucosyl Le^y (III^{3}FucV^{3}Fuc-VI^{2}FucnLc$_6$), and a possible three-dimensional epitope structure. J. Biol. Chem. 261, 11254–11258, 1986.

12. Hakomori, S. Glycosphingolipids. Sci. Am. 254, 44–53, 1986.

13. Taniguchi, M., Wakabayashi, S. Shared antigenic determinant expressed on various mammalian melanoma cells. Jap. J. Cancer Res. 75, 418–426, 1984.

14. Hirabayashi, Y., Hanaoka, A., Matsumoto, M., Matsubara, T., Tagawa, M., Wakabayashi, S., Taniguchi, M. Syngeneic monoclonal antibody against melanoma antigen with interspecies cross-reactivity recognizes GM$_3$, a prominent ganglioside of B16 melanoma. J. Biol. Chem. 260, 13328–13333, 1985.

15. Nores, G. A., Dohi, T., Taniguchi, M., Hakomori, S. Density-dependent recognition of cell surface GM$_3$ by a certain anti-melanoma antibody, and GM$_3$ lactone as a possible immunogen: Requirements for tumor-associated antigen and immunogen. J. Immunol. 139, 3171–3176, 1987.

16. Hakomori, S., Nudelman, E., Levery, S. B., Kannagi, R. Novel fucolipids accumulating in human adenocarcinoma: I. Glycolipids with di- or trifucosylated type 2 chain. J. Biol. Chem. 259, 4672–4680, 1984.

17. Fukushi, Y., Hakomori, S., Nudelman, E., Cochran, N. Novel fucolipids accumulating in human adenocarcinoma: II. Selective isolation of hybridoma antibodies that differentially recognize mono-, di-, and trifucosylated type 2 chain. J. Biol. Chem. 259, 4681–4685, 1984.

18. Abe, K., McKibbin, J. M., Hakomori, S. The monoclonal antibody directed to difucosylated type 2 chain (Fuc$\alpha 1 \rightarrow 2$Gal$\beta 1 \rightarrow 4$[Fuc$\alpha 1 \rightarrow 3$]-GlcNAc$\beta 1 \rightarrow$R; Y determinant). J. Biol. Chem. 258, 11793–11797, 1983.

19. Nudelman, E., Levery, S. B., Kaizu, T., Hakomori, S. Novel fucolipids of human adenocarcinoma: Characterization of the major Le^Y antigen of human adenocarcinoma as trifucosylnonaosyl Le^Y glycolipid (III^{3}FucV^{3}FucVI^{2}FucnLc$_6$). J. Biol. Chem. 261, 11247–11253, 1986.

20. Fukushi, Y., Nudelman, E., Levery, S. B., Rauvala, H., Hakomori, S. Novel fucolipids accumulating in human cancer: III. A hybridoma antibody (FH6) defining a human cancer-associated difucoganglioside (VI^{3}NeuAcV^{3}III^{3}Fuc$_2$nLc$_6$). J. Biol. Chem. 259, 10511–10517, 1984.

21. Nudelman, E. D., Levery, S. B., Stroud, M. R., Salyan, M. E. K., Abe, K., Hakomori, S. A novel tumor-associated, developmentally-regulated glycolipid antigen defined by monoclonal antibody ACFH-18. J. Biol. Chem., in press.
22. Nudelman, E., Kannagi, R., Hakomori, S., Parsons, M., Lipinski, M., Wiels, J., Fellous, M., Tursz, T. A glycolipid antigen associated with Burkitt lymphoma defined by a monoclonal antibody. Science 220, 509–511, 1983.
23. Bremer, E. G., Levery, S. B., Sonnino, S., Ghidoni, R., Canevari, S., Kannagi, R., Hakomori, S. Characterization of a glycosphingolipid antigen defined by the monoclonal antibody MBrl expressed in normal and neoplastic epithelial cells of human mammary gland. J. Biol. Chem. 259, 14773–14777, 1984.
24. Dabelsteen, E., Graem, N., Clausen, H., Hakomori, S. Structural variations of blood group A antigens in human normal colon and carcinomas. Cancer Res. 48, 181–187, 1988.
25. Hakomori, S., Wang, S. M., Young, W.W. Jr. Isoantigenic expression of Forssman glycolipid in human gastric and colonic mucosa: Its possible identity with "A-like antigen" in human cancer. Proc. Natl. Acad. Sci. USA 74, 3023–3027, 1977.
26. Dohi, T., Nores, G. A., Hakomori, S. An IgG$_3$ monoclonal antibody established after immunization with GM$_3$ lactone: Immunochemical specificity and inhibition of melanoma cell growth in vitro and in vivo. Cancer Res., in press.
27. Nudelman, E., Hakomori, S., Kannagi, R., Levery, S. B., Yeh, M.-Y., Hellstrom, K. E., Hellstrom, I. Characterization of a human melanoma-associated ganglioside antigen defined by a monoclonal antibody, 4.2. J. Biol. Chem. 257, 12752–12756, 1982.
28. Hirohashi, S., Clausen, H., Yamada, T., Shimosato, Y., Hakomori, S. Blood group A cross-reacting epitope defined by monoclonal antibodies NCC-Lu-35 and -81 expressed in cancer of blood group 0 or B individuals: Its identification as Tn antigen. Proc. Natl. Acad. Sci. USA 82, 7039–7043, 1985.
29. Takahashi, H. K., Metoki, R., Hakomori, S. Immunoglobulin G3 monoclonal antibody directed to Tn antigen (tumor-asociated α-N-acetylgalactosaminyl epitope) that does not cross-react with blood group A antigen. Cancer Res. 48, 4361–4367, 1988.
30. Kjeldsen, T., Clausen, H., Hirohashi, S., Ogawa, T., Iijima, H., Hakomori, S. Preparation and characterization of monoclonal antibodies directed to the tumor-associated O-linked sialosyl-2-6 α-N-acetylgalactosaminyl (sialosyl-Tn) epitope. Cancer Res. 48, 2214–2220, 1988.

7. Cellular Expression of Glycolipids after Oncogene Transfection; Oncogene-type Specific Changes of Gangliosides in Rat 3Y1 Cells

Y. Sanai, and Y. Nagai

Introduction*

Drastic und characteristic alterations of the cell glycolipid profile during onco-genesis, in vitro as well as in vivo, have been well documented (1). The mode of these alterations is believed to be determined in part by the type of progenitor cells from which the tumor cells were derived, being classified as either incomplete synthesis or neosynthesis. Neoplastic transformation-associated alterations of the ganglioside pro-file are under the control of transforming genes of DNA or RNA tumor viruses (2–12). In a previous study (6) we reported that neosynthesis of the ganglioside GD3 was induced by transfection of rat 3Y1 cells with the human adenovirus type 12 early gene, E1A. This suggested that expression of GD3 in rat transformed cells was under the control of the function of adenovirus E1A gene products and raised the question of whether or not the same type of change in the ganglioside profile can be induced by transfection of 3Y1 cells with other transforming genes coding for products with func-tions different from those of the adenovirus E1A gene products. In the present paper, we present evidence that characteristic changes of the ganglioside profile can be induced by transfection of rat 3Y1 cells with cloned DNA encoded oncogenes derived from Rous sarcoma virus (*src*), feline sarcoma virus (*fes*) and cellular homologue to Harvey murine sarcoma virus (activated c-H-*ras*), respectively.

Materials and Methods

Cells and DNA transfections. 3Y1 cells, a fibroblast cell line derived from Fisher rat embryo (13), were cultured in Dulbecco's modifed minimal essential medium contain-ing 6% fetal calf serum. Rous sarcoma virus (RSV) DNA was a gift from J. M. Bishop (University of California, San Francisco) (14). Gardner-Arnstein feline sarcoma virus (GA-FeSV) DNA was obtained from C. J. Sherr (St. Jude's Children Research Hospi-tal, Memphis) (15) and human c-H-*ras* DNA carring a point mutation at the 61st codon was provided by Y.Yuasa (Gunma University School of Medicine, Maebashi, Japan) (16). DNA transfection into 3Y1 cells was carried out by a method involving polybrene (17). Before DNA transfection, RSV DNA was purified from pBR322-SRA-2-RSV DNA by digestion with SalI and then religated. GA-FeSV and human c-H-*ras* plasmid DNAs were directly used for DNA transfection, since the structure of these genes are not permuted. 50 to 100 ng of DNA was used per 6 cm-diameter culture dish, in which 1.5×10^5 3Y1 cells were seeded. Transformed foci were obtained 3 weeks after DNA transfection. The transfectants were propagated under the same conditions as for 3Y1 cells and then used for ganglioside analysis.

Isolation and analysis of gangliosides from cells. Cells were harvested in the late logarithmic growth phase using 0.05% EDTA in phosphate buffered saline (PBS),

---

*Abbreviations used: the ganglioside nomenclature used followed Svennerholm's system (32). GM3, NeuAcα2-3Galβ1-4Glcβ1-1ceramide; GM2, GalNAcβ1-4(NeuAcα2-3)Galβ1-4Glcβ1-1 ceramide; GM1,Galβ1-3GalNAcβ1-4(NeuAcα2-3)Galβ1-4Glcβ1-1ceramide; GD1a, NeuAcα2-3Galβ1-3GalNcβ1-4(NeuAcα2-3)Galβ1-4Glcβ1-1ceramide; GD 1b, Galβ1-3GalNAcβ1-4(NeuAcα2-8NeuAcα2-3)Galβ1-4Glcβ1-1ceramide; GT1b, NeuAcα2-3Galβ1-3GalNAcβ1-4(NeuAcα2-8NeuAcα2-3)Galβ1-4Glcβ1-1cera-mide; sialosylparagloboside, NeuAcα2-3Galβ1-4GlcNAcβ1-3Galβ1-4Glcβ1-1ceramide. src-3Y1, transfec-tants with RSV DNA; fes-3Y1, transfectants with RA-FeSV DNA; ras-3Y1, transfectants with c-H-*ras*DNA.

washed twice with PBS, and pelleted by centrifugation. The cell pellet (about 5×10^8) was extracted successively with an appropriate volume of chloroform-methanol-water (1:1:0.1, by volume) and then with two chloroform-methanol mixtures (2:1, 1:1, by volume) at 40°C each for 1 hr. The combined extracts were evaporated to dryness. The residue was disolved with chloroform-methanol-water (30:60:8, by volume, solvent A) and then applied to a DEAE-Sephadex A-25 column (acetate form). The DEAE column was successively rinsed with 10 column volumes of solvent A and then with 5 column volumes of methanol to ensure complete removal of all neutral lipids. The acidic lipids were then eluted with 10 column volumes of 0.2 M sodium acetate in methanol. The eluant was concentrated by rotary evaporator and the residue was basetreated with 0.1 M sodium hydroxide in methanol for 1 hr at 40°C. The reaction mixture was evaporated to dryness and the residue was disolved in water and then neutralized with 0,5 M acetic acid. The solution was diluted with water to adjust the salt concentration to 0.1 M. The ganglioside fraction was purified with a C_{18} Sep-Pak cartridge according to Kundu and Suzuki (18). Ganglioside compositions were analyzed by thin-layer chromatography (TLC)-densitometry according to Ando et al. (19). Individual gangliosides were identified by comparing their mobilities with those of the reference standards derived from human brain.

Results and Discussion

Several reports dealing with the relationship between cellular expression of glycolipids and oncogene transfection have appeared since 1983 (Table 1). These papers have demonstrated the usefulness of this relatively new technique in evaluating the genetic background of glycolipid expression (2–3). Little is known about the functional difference of oncogene products and glycolipid expression. The objective of this study was to determine whether or not the expression of specific transforming genes can induce characteristic alteration of the ganglioside profile in the transformed cells. Thus, we examined ganglioside expression in several transformed cells that had been clonally derived from the same ancestral normal rat 3Y1 cells, after transfection with either v-*src*, v-*fes* or activated c-H-*ras* DNA. This strategy was necessary because it is

Table 1. Glycolipid alterations accompanying gene transfection.

Cells	Oncogene	Glycolipids affected	Reference
JB6	mos	GT ↑, GD1a ↑	(8)
NIH3T3	ras	asialoGM2 ↑	(5)
NIH3T3	ras	GM3 ↓	(12)
BALB/c3T3	myc + ras	polysialogangliosides(PSG) ↑	(5)
3Y1	adenovirus E1A + E1B	GM3 ↓, GD3 ↑	(6)
3Y1	src	sialosylparagloboside ↑, PSG ↑	(10)
3Y1	ras	sialosylparagloboside ↑, PSG ↑	(10)
3Y1	fes	sialosylparagloboside ↑, PSG ↑	(10, 11)
3Y1	myc	GM3 ↓, GD3 ↑	(9)
3Y1	fps	sialosylparagloboside ↑, PSG ↑	(10)

↑, increase; ↓, decrease.

well known that different cell types frequently express different patterns of gangliosides; expression of glycosphingolipids is species- and tissue- specific (20).

As shown in Figure 1, 3Y1, src-3Y1, fes-3Y1 and ras-3Y1, cells each exhibited a characteristic TLC pattern of gangliosides. In 3Y1 cells, with were used as host for the
DNA transfection, only a doublet of GM3 was detected. In contrast, GM3 proportion-
ally decreased in accord with the appearance of a new ganglioside species with longer
carbohydrate portions, which was unequivocally observed in all of the transforming
genetransfected cells examined.

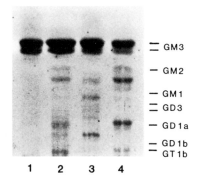

= GM3

– GM2

– GM1
= GD3

– GD1a

– GD1b
= GT1b

1   2   3   4

Figure 1. Thin-layer chromatogram of gangliosides from oncogene-transfected transformed
cells: (1) 3Y1, (2) src-3Y1 (3) fes-3Y1, and (4)
ras-3Y1. Each of the lanes containing 10 μg of
sialic acid equivalents. Solvent system,
chloroform-methanol-water   (55 : 45 : 10)
containing 0.02 % (w/v) of CaCl $_2$H$_2$O.
Plate, Merck precoated silica gel 60. All bands
were purple after spraying with resorcinol
reagent (31).

In one clone of src-3Y1 cells (D611), at least five new resorcinolpositive bands were
detected in addition to GM3 (Figure 2). Three of them had the same motilities as
GM2, GD1a, and GT1b. As to the other two unidentified species, designated as X1
and X3, X1 migrated between GM2 and GM1, and X3 between GD1a and GD1b. In
another clone of src-3Y1 cells (612), GM2, X1, and GD1b were detected but GD1a and
X3 were not detected as major bands under our experimental conditions. In a clone of
fes-3Y1 cells (T3-1), X1, X3 and another unidentified species, X2, which migrated to a
position nearly coinciding with that of GM1a, were detected. Other *fes*-transfected
clones (T1 and T2) also expressed these three species of gangliosides, but also an adi-
tional unknown trisialosylganglioside fraction. In ras-3Y1 clone (H-ras, 27–41 and
27–42), gangliosides that comigrated with GM3, GM2, X1, and GD1a were unequivocally expressed. Recently we identified the structure of X1, X2, and X3 as sialosylparagloboside, GM1b and GD1α (9–11). The results described here demonstrate that
all retrovirus-related oncogenes examined induced more glycosylated gangliosides in
3Y1 cells during neoplastic transformation. This suggests that stimulation of the neosynthesis of gangliosides, most probably by activation of glycosyltransferases, can be
triggered by the action of transforming gene products.

Recent progress in molecular oncology has shown that transforming genes (or
oncogenes) can be categorized according to the functions of their gene-products
(Table 2). It has been shown that the 60kDa product of v-*src* can catalyze the phosphorylation of proteins on tyrosine residues (21, 22). The transforming protein of GA-
FeSV was synthesized as a fused protein (p95) and also exhibited tyrosine kinase activity itself (23). The c-H-*ras* gene encodes a 21kDa peripheral membrane protein (24)
which has GTP binding (25, 26) and GTPase activities (27, 28). Therefore, it seems
possible that the divergent and characteristic changes of ganglioside expression of cells

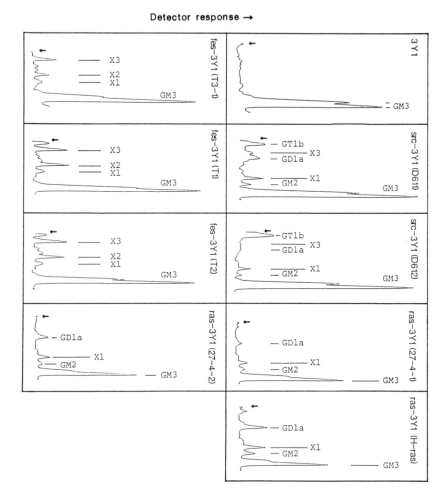

Figure 2. TLC-densitometric analysis of gangliosides from individual clones of oncogene-transfected rat cells.

after oncogene-transfection are due to differences in the actions of individual oncogene products. Although the activity of UDP-GalNAc : GM3 N-acetylgalactosaminyl transferase (GM2 synthetase) was enhanced by factors that stimulate cAMP-dependent protein kinase and that of CMP-NeuAc : lactosylceramide sialyltransferase (GM3 synthetase) is reduced by dephosphorylation and enhanced by ATP and cAMP-dependent protein kinase (28, 29), it remains to be determined whether or not the chances in ganglioside synthesis induced by oncogenes presented here are mediated via the phosphorylation mechanism.

It has been thought that the mode of transformation-associated changes of gangliosides in cells transformed by DNA or RNA tumor viruses or emical carcinogens is determined by the type of cells. Blocked synthesis of GM3 caused by polyoma virus, SV40 as well as RSV, was found in BHK transformed cells, whereas mouse fibroblast

Table 2. The products of viral oncogenes.

Oncogene	Proposed localization(s) of product	Proposed function(s)
Adenovirus		
E1A	Nucleus; cytoplasm	Regulates transcription
E1B(21KDa)	Nuclear envelop; endoplasmic reticulum; plasma membrane	unknown
E1B(55KDa)	Nucleoplasm; perinuclear cytoplasm; Cell-cell contacts	Binds and stabilizes p53
v-src	Plasma membrane; juxtanuclear membranes	Protein-tyrosine kinase
v-fes/fps	Plasma membrane	Protein-tyrosine kinase
v-ras	Plasma membrane	Regulates adenylate cyclase
v-myc	Nucleus	Regulates transcription

3T3 showed blocked synthesis of higher gangliosides caused by polyoma, SV40, and murine sarcoma virus (1). In rat 3Y1 cells, on the contrary, the neosynthetic type of alterations in ganglioside profile was induced by transfection with the adenovirus transforming gene (6), myc (9) and also with RNA tumor virus oncogenes (10, 11). It is likely that the underlying molecular mechanism which leads to the differential expression during neoplastic transformation of gangliosides in cells responding with blocked ganglioside synthesis such as mouse 3T3 cells and in cells responding with ganglioside neosynthesis such as rat 3Y1 cells in the present experiment is closely associated with the molecular background for the generation of animal species-, tissue- and cell-specificity of the phenotypic expression of gangliosides and other glycolipids. Approaches involving oncogene transfection will provide important information about this issue.

Summary

The ganglioside compositions of rat 3Y1-derived transformed cells transfected with three types of cloned retrovirus oncogene DNAs derived from Rous sarcoma virus, *src*, feline sarcoma virus, *fes*, and an activated cellular oncogene homologue to Harvey sarcoma virus, c-H-*ras*, were investigated. The ganglioside composition of 3Y1 cells was quite simple, consisting exclusively of GM3, NeuAcα2-3Galβ1-4Glcβ1-1Cer. The oncogene-transfected and transformed cells, however, exhibited more glycosylated gangliosides in addition to GM3. Their molecular profiles characteristically dependant upon the transfected oncogene species. These results strongly suggest that the mode of neoplastic transformation-associated changes of gangliosides is determined in part by the type of oncogene products.

This work was supported in part by a Grant-in-Aid from the Ministry of Education, Science and Culture, Japan, and also by a Grant-in-Aid for Cancer Research from the Ministry of Education, Science and Culture, Japan.

References

1. Hakomori, S. Glycosphingolipids in cellular interaction, differentiation, and oncogenesis. Annu. Rev. Biochem. 50, 733, 1981.
2. Nagai Y., H. Nakaishi, and Y. Sanai, Gene transfer as a novel approach to the gene-controlled mechanism of the cellular expression of glycosphingolipids. Chem. Phys. Lipids 42, 91, 1986.
3. Nagai, Y., Y. Sanai, and H. Nakaishi. Fundamentals of genetic control of gangliosides: The enigma of carbohydrate chain diversity in glycosphingolipids, in NATO ASI series 1. "Gangliosides and Modulation Neurological Functions", Ced. H. Rahmann) p275, Springer Verlag, 1987.
4. Hakomori, S., J. Nyke, and P. K. Vogt. Glycolipids of chick embryo fibroblasts infected with temperature-sensitive mutants of avian sarcoma viruses. Virology 76, 485, 1977.
5. Tsuchiya, S., and S. Hakomori. Cell surface glycolipids of transformed NIH3T3 cells transfected with DNA's of human bladder and lung carcinomas. EMBO J. 2, 2323. 1983.
6. Nakakuma, H., Y. Sanai, K. Shiroki, and Y. Nagai. Generegulated expression of glycolipids: appearance of GD3 ganglioside in rat cells on transfection with transforming gene E1 of human adenovirus type 12 DNA and its transcriptional subunits. J. Biochem. 96, 1471, 1984.
7. Takimoto, M., T. Hirakawa, T. Oikawa, M. Naiki, I. Miyoshi, and H. Kobayashi. Synergistic effects of the myc and ras oncogenes on ganglioside synthesis by BALB/c 3T3 fibroblasts. J. Biochem. 100, 813, 1986.
8. Srinivas, L., and N. H. Colburn. Reduced trisialoganglioside synthesis in chemically but not mostransformed mouse epidermal cells. Cancer Res. 44, 1510, 1984.
9. Nakaishi, H., Y. Sanai, K. Shiroki, and Y. Nagai. Analysis of cellular expression of ganglioside by gene transfection I. GD3 expression in myc-transfected and transformed 3Y1 corelates with anchorage-independent growth activity. Biochem. Biophys. Res. Commun. 150, 760, 1988.
10. Nakaishi, H., Y. Sanai, M. Shibuya, and Y. Nagai. Analysis of cellular expression of ganglioside by gene transfection II. rat 3Y1 cells transformed with several DNA's containing oncogene (fes, fps, ras, and src) invariably express sialosylparagloboside. Biochem. Biophys. Res. Commun. 150, 760.
11. Nakaishi, H., Y. Sanai, M. Shibuya, M. Iwamori, and Y. Nagai. Neosynthesis of neolacto- and novel ganglio-series gangliosides in a rat fibroblastic cell line brought about by transfection with the v-fes oncogene-containing Gardner-Arnstein strain feline sarcoma virus-DNA. Cancer Res. 48, 1753, 1988.
12. Matyas, G. R., S. A. Aaronson, R. O. Brady, and P. H. Fishman. Alteration of glycolipids in ras-transfected NIH 3T3 cells. Proc. Natl. Acad. Sci. USA 84, 6065, 1987.
13. Kimura, G., A. Itagaki, and J. Summers. Rat cell line 3Y1 and its virogenic polyoma- and SV40-transformed derivatives. Int.J. Cancer 15, 694, 1975.
14. De Lorbe,W. H., P. A. Luciw, H. M. Goodman, H. E. Varmus, and J. M. Bishop. Molecular cloning and characterization of avian sarcoma virus circular DNA molecules. J. Virology 36, 50, 1980.
15. Fedele, L. A., J. Even, C. F. Garon, Donner, and C. J. Sherr. Recombinant bacteriophages containing the integrated transforming provirus of Gardner-Arnstein feline sarcoma virus. Proc. Natl. Acad. Sci. USA 78, 4036, 1981.
16. Yuasa, Y., S. K. Srivastava, C.Y. Dunn, J. S. Rhim, E. P. Reddy, and S. A. Aaronson. Acquisition of transforming properties by alternative point mutations within c-bas/has human protooncogene. Nature 303, 775, 1983.

17. Kawai, S., and M. Nishizawa. New procedure for DNA transfection with polycation and dimethylsulfoxide. Mol. Cell. Biol. 4, 1172,1984.

18. Kundu, S. K., and A. Suzuki. Simple micro-method for the isolation of gangliosides by reversed-phase chromotography. J. Chromatogr. 224, 2491981.

19. Ando, S., N.-C. Chang, and R. K. Yu. High-performance thin-layer chromatography and densitometric determination of brain ganglioside compositions of several species. Anal. Biochem. 89, 437, 1978.

20. Hakomori, S., and J. N. Kanfer. Sphingolipid Biochemistry, Plenum Press, New York, 1983.

21. Purchio, A. F., E. Erikson, J. S. Brugge, and R. L. Erikson. Identification of a polypeptide encoded by the avian sarcoma virus src gene. Proc. Natl. Acad. Sci. USA 75, 1576, 1978.

22. Collet, M. S. and R. L. Erikson. Protein kinase activity associated with the avian sarcoma virus src gene product. Proc. Acad- Sci. USA 75, 2021, 1978.

23. Hampe, A., I. Laprevotte, F. Galibert, L. A. Fedele, and C. J. Sherr. Nucleotide sequences of feline retroviral oncogenes (v-fes) provide evidence for a family of tyrosinespecific protein kinase genes. Cell 30, 775, 1982.

24. Willingham, M. C., I. Pastan, T.Y. Shih, and E. M. Scolnik. Localization of the src gene product of the Harvey strain of MSV to plasma membrane of transformed cells by electron microscopic immunocytochemistry. Cell 19, 1005, 1980.

25. Scolnik, E. M., A. G. Papageorge, and T.Y. Shih. Guanine nucleotide-binding activity as an assay for src protein of ratderived murine sarcoma viruses. Proc. Natl. Acad. Sci. USA 76, 5355, 1979.

26. Shih, T.Y., A. G. Papageorge, P. E. Stokes, M. O. Weeks, and E. M. Scolnik. Guanine nucleotide-binding and autophosphorylating activities associated with the p21^{src} protein of Harvey murine sarcoma virus. Nature 287, 686, 1980.

27. McGrath., J. P., D. J. Capon, D.V. Goeddell, and A. D. Levinson. Comparative biochemical properties of normal and activated human ras p21 protein. Nature 310, 644, 1984.

28. Gibbs, J. B., I. S. Sigal, M. Poe, and E. M. Scolnik. Intrinsic GTPase activity distinguishes normal and oncogenic ras p21 molecules. Proc. Natl. Acad. Sci. USA 81, 5704 1984.

29. Dawson, G., R. McLawhon, and R. J. Miller. Inhibition of sialoglycosphingolipid (Ganglioside) biosynthesis in mouse clonal lines N4TG1 and NG108–15 byβ-endorphin, enkephalins, and opiates. J. Biol. Chem. 255, 129, 1980.

30. Burczak, J. D., R. M. Soltysiak, and C. C. Sweeley. Regulation of membrane bound enzymes of glycosphingolipid biosynthesis. J. Lipid. Res. 25, 1541, 1984.

31. Svennerholm, L. Quantitative estimation of sialic acids II. A colorimetric resorcinol-hydrochloric acid method. Biochim. Biophys. Acta 24, 604, 1957.

32. Svennerholm, L. Chromatographic separation of human brain gangliosides. J. Neurochem. 10, 613, 1963.

8. Diversity of Ganglioside Expression in Human Melanoma

M. H. Ravindranath, T. Tsuchida, and R. F. Irie

Introduction

Melanoma is a tumor of the melanocytes, the melanin producing cells, distributed in the skin as well as in other organs such as the uveal tract, meninges, ectodermal mucosal and internal visera. These cells are derived from the neural crest early in embryonic development. The prominant features of the melanocytes, in addition to their unique ability to synthesize melanin, is their motility in early life. These cells can be cultured under laboratory conditions.

Melanocytes express gangliosides, the qualitative pattern of which is somewhat characteristic of other extra-neutral tissues. The quantity of the gangliosides is higher than that of other extra-neutral tissues. GM3 is the most predominant ganglioside; the oligosaccharide sequence linked to the ceramide is Siaα2-3Galβ1–4Glcβ1-1Cer (1). Other gangliosides of the melanocytes, which include GD3, GM2, GD1a, and GT1b, constitute less than 10 % of the total (1). The presence of GD1a and GTb in melanocytes are indicative of its neural crest origin.

The onset of the neoplastic transformation of melanocytes triggers the enzyme machinery associated with glycosylation, particularly that related to addition of sialic acid (Sia) and N-acetyl galactosamine (GalNAc). Adding sialic acid to the preexisting sialic acid of GM3 results in the formation of GD3 (1). This transfer of sialic acid is facilitated by CMP-NeuAc: α2–8 sialyl-transferase (2). GD3 accumulation is an important event associated with the growth and proliferation of melanoma.

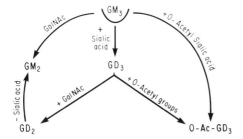

Figure 1.

At some stage of GD3 accumulation, two important events leading its modification may occur (Figure 1). UDP-GalNAc transferase is activated to transfer GalNAc to GD3, resulting in the formation of GD2 (3). As a sequel, GM2 levels also increase in melanoma. Another event is the formation of O-acetyl GD3 (4–6), through the addition of O-acetyl group to the terminal sialic acid of GD3 or the addition of O-acetyl sialic acid to GM3. Both these mechnisms may operate in O-acetylated sialomucins (7). Thus it may be noted that malignant melanoma expresses a small but sequential group of gangliosides.

Analysis of Melanoma Biopsy

Most observationes concerning the ganglioside profiles of melanorma are restricted to cultured melanoma cells, which may or may not reflect the true picture of the ganglioside changes associated with neoplasms. Information on the ganglioside profiles of biopsied melanoma have been scarce and fragmentary; they conform to the general pattern of gangliosides described above (8, 9). In order to detect diversity, if any, in the ganglioside profile of melanoma tumor tissue *in situ*, we have analysed more than 50 biopsied melanoma specimens obtained from our clinic (10). Table 1 summarizes our results regarding incidence and quantiative pattern of the gangliosides. The gangliosides GM3, GD3, and GM2 are found in 100 % of the biopsies, whereas GD2 and alkali-labile gangliosides are found in 71 and 83 % of the biopsies respectively. Other gangliosides that are reminiscent of the neural crest origin of melanoma are either absent or occur in traces, indicating that the enzyme machinary concerned with their production is either shut down or "silent". The range of gangliosides in biopsies indicates that GM3 and GD3 are the major melanoma gangliosides characteristic of melanoma tumor tissue. GM2 and GD2 rarely exceeded 15 % each of the total gangliosides. Alkali-labile gangliosides, which have escaped attention because of the conventional methodology followed for purification of gangliosides, maintained a low profile. These gangliosides may signify the presence of gangliosides with inner lactones or gangliosides containing O-acetyl sialic acids. Using a O-acetyl sialic acid specific lectin and chromatographic mobility before and after base treatment of an isolated alkali-labile ganglioside in a biopsied specimen, we identified the alkali-labile ganglioside as O-acetyl GD3 (6).

Figure 2 and 3 throughly document the diversity in GM3 and GD3 ratio in human melanoma biopsies. A comparision of ganglioside ratios in the biopsies reveals that

Table 1. Incidence and relative proportion of gangliosides found in human melanoma. (Modified from Tsuchida, Saxton, Morton and Irie, 1987: Ref; 10).

Gangliosides	Incidence (%)		Percentage of total gangliosides* (Range and mean in parenthesis)	
	Biopsies (n = 52)	Cell lines (n = 28)	Biopsies	Cell lines
GM3	100	100	14.0–90.3 (43.2)	10.6–83.9 (38.6)
GM2	100	100	0.5–14.1 (3.2)	1.7–47.4 (13.6)
GD3	100	100	5.7–73.3 (47.7)	3.6–62.9 (34.6)
GD2	71	79	0.0–9.7 (2.0)	0.0–32.4 (7.8)
Alkalilabile	83	54	0.0–12.6 (3.7)	0.0–5.7 (1.6)
Others**	15–42	7–68	(3.9)	(5.1)
total	–	–	33.0–302.0 (100.0)	34.0–183.0 (104.0)

* Percentage of gangliosides refer to relative intensity of resorcinol positivity as measured by densitometry.
** Other gangliosides include, GD1a, GD1b, GT1, GQ and an unidentified ganglioside fraction. n refers to sample size.

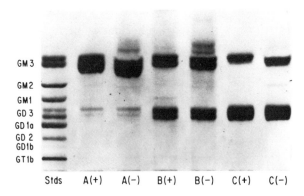

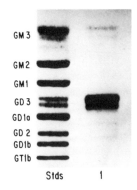

Figure 2.

Figure 3.

the GM3 : GD3 ratio may shift from 19 : 1 to 19 : 1. One of the biopsies maintained a ganglioside profile strikingly similar to the ganglioside pattern of normal melanocytes (Figure 2). One of the biopsies exhibited a unique ratio of 1 : 19 (Figure 3). GM2 and GD2 showed interindividual variability. In some biopsies, both GM2 and GD2 (Figure 4) were found to be high. The same is true for O-acetyl GD3; while normally it does not exceed 10 % of the total gangliosides it may reach as high as 20 % (Figure 5 and 6). These observations indicate that the enzyme machinery involved with the conversion of GM3 to GD3 and the formation of GM2 and GD2 and of O-acetyl GD3 were activated in melanoma tumor tissues.

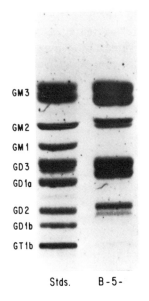

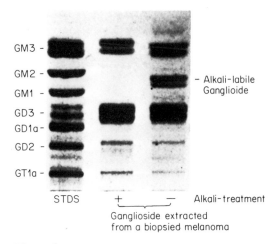

Figure 5.

Figure 4.

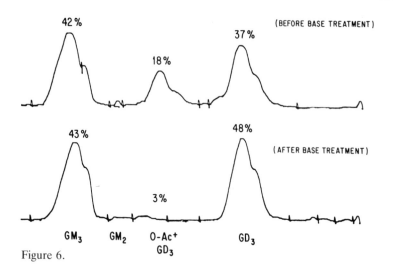

42 %

37 %

(BEFORE BASE TREATMENT)

18 %

43 %

48 %

(AFTER BASE TREATMENT)

3 %

GM₃   GM₂   O-Ac⁺   GD₃
                GD₃

Figure 6.

Analysis of Cultured Melanoma Cell Lines

In our laboratory, we maintain cultures of melanoma cells derived from the surgical specimens of the patients visiting our clinic. This facilitated comparisions of the ganglioside profiles of pairs of biopsies nd cells grown *in vitro* (10, 11). Table 1 summarizes our results. The most striking difference observed between biopsies and their corresponding cell lines was an increase in the levels of GM2 and GD2 and a decrease in alkali-labile gangliosides in melanoma grown *in vitro*. It is obvious that the tumor-associated, GalNAc-containing sialyllactosyl ceramides are sensitive to the surrounding environment. To assess the possibility of reverting these *in vitro*-induced changes,

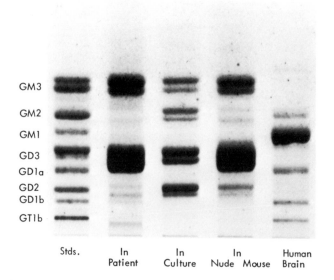

GM3

GM2

GM1

GD3
GD1a

GD2
GD1b

GT1b

Stds.   In   In   In   Human
         Patient   Culture   Nude Mouse   Brain   Figure 7.

we implanted the cultured melanoma cells into immunedeficient nude mice (11). Interestingly, the ganglioside profiles of the tumors grown in nude mice showed a reversion to the biopsied condition (Figure 7). These studies elucidated four important issues regarding the gangliosides' diversity in melanoma: the expression of gangliosides on melanoma tissues is susceptible to environmental alterations; the differences between cells grown *in vitro* and *in vivo* are not to the selection of some particular cell population; the characteristics of ganglioside expression can be conserved after many passages *in vivo* and/or *in vitro*; and the inter-individual diversity in the ganglioside expression of melanoma may be governed primarily by the genomic machinery of the melanocytes that have undergone neoplastic transformation. The observations of Fredman and coworkers (12) on the ganglioside profile of gliomas obtained *in vitro*, from biopsies, and from cultured cells grown in nude mice support our findings.

Cellular Function and Diversity of Gangliosides in Melanoma

The uniformity in the pattern of melanoma-associated gangliosides in spite of their diversity in different biopsies and cultured cell lines as well as the sequential transformation of GM3 into various other melanoma-associated-gangliosides, indicates that the expression of the gangliosides in melanoma is primarily governed by the sequential "switching on" of the enzymes involved in the transfer of sugar residues. Still unclear is the homeostatic role, the tumor-associated-gangliosides may play in the sequential change of the ganglioside profile of melanoma.

When the cell surface ganglioside pattern is changed during neoplastic transformation, one may expect these changes to be reflected in the functional characteristics of the cell. The normal melanocyte, motile during early life, ceases to be motile until it is transformed into a malignant cell. The motility of the neoplastic cell is responsible for the radial and vertical migration and metastasis of melanoma. Metastasis further involves an interaction with the basement membrane components leading to infiltration through the limiting membrane (basement membrane). The ganglioside pattern of primary melanoma, both at radial and vertical migratory phases, and of metastatic melanoma reveal that there is a progressive increase in GD3 and GD2 from the radial to the vertical phase and from the vertical phase to the metastatic phase; this suggests that motility commences with the formation of the disialoganglioside, GD3 (13). The role of the disialogangliosides of melanoma in the spreading and infiltration of tumor cells has been proposed; the monoclonal antibodies directed against the carbohydrate moieties of GD3 and GD2 on melanoma cells inhibited attachment of the cells to various basement membrane components (substrate adhesion proteins) such as collagen, fribronectin, vitronectin, and laminin (14, 15).

There is a noteworthy difference in the proliferative capiabilities of melanoma cells grown in tumor *in situ* and those grown under culture condition. It is noteworthy that the levels of GalNAc containing gangliosides (GM2 and GD2) in cells grown under *in vitro* conditions are higher than in those grown *in situ* and *in vivo* (11). A similar observation was made on gliomas (12).

We have observed that the melanoma cells rich in GM2 or GM2 plus Gd2 are highly tumorigenic when implanted into nude mice system, in contrast to GM2-poor melanoma cells (16). Table 2 compares the tumorigenicity of GM2-rich and GM2-poor melanoma cell lines in nude mice. Several reasons are attributed for the tumorigenicity of GM2-rich cells (16). One of the noteworthy reasons is that the expression of GM2 may signify a dedifferentiated state of the malignant cells. The ability of the neoplastically transformed cells to recapitulate the functional capabilities characteristic of early embryonic melanocytes, such as proliferation, motility and migration support such a contention. In this connection, it would be of interest to know the ganglioside pattern of early embryonic melanocytes. Association of GM2 with embryonic tissues is well exemplified in the ganglioside pattern of fetal human brain tissues, which differ from the adult brain in expressing high level of GM2 (17).

Table 2. Relationship between tumorigenicity in nude mice and GM2 content in melanoma cell lines (Modified from Tsuchida, Saxton, Irie, 1987: Ref: 16).

Melanoma cell lines	No of mice with tumor/ No of mice tested	GM2 (nMol/g)*	Total lipid-bound sialic acid (µg/g)*
GM2-rich:			
M-24	6/6	219.0	143
M-101	6/6	53.7	177
M-14	6/6	88.3	183
M-10	6/6	46.8	73
M-111	4/6	87.7	80
GM2-poor:			
M-109	1/6	12.3	164
M-21	0/6	5.8	103
M-112	0/6	14.9	103
M-25	0/6	8.4	78
M-15	0/6	5.5	98

*values refer to gram of wet tissue
All analyses were carried out from tumor removed from nude mice after day 36 of subcutaneous inoculation of 1 X 10-6 cells.

Clinical Aspects of Diversity of Gangliosides in Melanoma

In further examining the association of the diversity of gangliosides on melanoma with the natural history of melanoma development and progression, we found that the ganglioside pattern of biopsied melanoma do not show any correlation with sex, age, tumor size, and tumor stages II and III of the patients. We also compared the ganglioside profiles of biopsied melanoma obtained at different times and sites within the same patients. Both the GM3 : GD3 and GM2 : GD2 ratios remained basically the same in biopsies obtained at different times and from different sites of metastasis within the same individuals. However, when the histological types of the primary melanoma originally developed by the patients were assessed, there was a significant difference in the total lipid-bound-sialic acid content and alkali-labile gangliosides between superficially spreading melanoma and nodular melanoma. The total gangliosides content was also higher in melanotic melanoma than in amelanotic melanoma (18).

The clinical usefulness of the diversity of membrane-bound-gangliosides on melanoma is appreciated in cellular und humoral immunotherapie. We have shown that GM2, functions as a target cell receptor for natural killer cells (19, 20). The identification of the cytotoxic cell clone(s) capable of recognizing GM2 on target cells would valuable in adaptive immunotherapy.

The importance of diversity of the gangliosides in humoral immunotherapy is realized in melanoma vaccine trials undertaken in our division (21). The melanoma cell vaccine consists of irradiated cells of three different melanoma cell lines that express melanoma associated gangliosides on their cell surfaces. We found antibodies against GD2 and GM2 in the sera of melanoma patients immunized with the vaccine, indicating that these gangliosides present on melanoma cells are capable of being recognized as antigens by patients (22). The immunogenicity of tumor-associated gangliosides in melanoma patients is also confirmed using purified gangliosides as antigens (23).

The anti-ganglioside aaantibodies are involved in complement-dependant cytotoxicity (CDC) and/or in antibody-dependant cellular cytotoxicity (ADCC) of tumor cells (24–26). These studies have prompted phase I clinical trials with melanoma patients having malignant melanoma, using the murine monoclonal anti-GD3 and anti-GD2 antibodies (27–32). In these studies patients developed anti-murine IgG antibodies, which may limit the repeated administration of murine monoclonal antibodies (28, 29). We have developed human monoclonal antibodies against melanoma associated GD2 and GM2 (17, 33). We have observed a strong cytotoxic effect of human monoclonal antibody L72, which binds specifically with ganglioside GD2 in the presence of complement (34). Intralesional injection of the antibodies on patients with cutaneous melanoma caused significant regression in all tumors, except in two patients whose tumors had low antigenicity. These initial series of clinical trials using anti-ganglioside antibodies highlight the therapeutical usefulness of the diversity of melanoma associated gangliosides.

We have also studied the relationship between the sensitivity of tumor cells to anti-cancer treatments and the expression of gangliosides on the tumor cells (35). The effect of anti-tumor treatment was assessed through the colony-forming ability of cells *in vitro*. The results reveal that a decrease in GM3 content of the melanoma cells increases sensitivity to exposure to radiation and vincristine treatment. In contrast, there was a positive correlation between GD2 content of the tumor cells and sensitivity to these phase-specific treatment. These observations suggests that GM3 and GD2 may be useful as marker to determine individuals insusceptible or susceptible to phase-specific anti-cancer treatment in melanoma (35). We could not oberserve any significant correlation between ganglioside expression and the effect of other anti-cancer drugs such as Cisplatin, Bleomycin and DTIC on the colony-forming ability of melanoma cell lines.

Shedding of gangliosides has been demonstrated *in vivo* and *in vitro* (33, 36) and the ganglioside levels in the plasma correlates with the tumor burden in melanoma (36). A four-fold increase in GD3, observed in the plasma of melanoma patients before surgery, declined significantly after tumor excision (36). Shed gangliosides may be incorporated directly onto the surface of normal cells; this is demonstrated by a ganglioside analysis of erythrocytes obtained from melanoma patients (36). In neuroplastoma patients, the level of circulating tumor-associated gangliosides is also found to correlate with tumor burden (37). Recently, Portoukalian has found that the lower bands of GM3 and GD3 (containing mostly C16 to C20 fatty acids) are shed readily from the melanoma tumor tissues and was incorporated onto lymphocytes (38). A strong inhibition of lectin-induced and mixed-lymphocyte reaction-induced proliferations of patients' lymphocytes was noticed (38, 39). It is also known that shed gangliosides such as GD3 may bind to interferons (40, 41) and circulating antibodies (42). Preferential interactions of specific melanoma gangliosides with lymphocytes on IL-2 stimulation were found to promote immunosuppression (39). While GM2 and GD2 enhanced the lymphocyte response to IL-2, GM3, and GD3 significantly inhibited it. Since different gangliosides can up-regulate and down-regulate lymphocyte responses to IL-2, it has been suggested that the ganglioside phenotype of melanoma cells may play a major role in determining whether an individual tumor causes immune stimulation and suppression (39).

Conclusion

The diversity of melanoma-associated-gangliosides is unique in that it is a result of sequential transformation of GM3. The diversity could be predetermined at the onset of neoplastic transformation of melanocytes, or may reflect tumor progression. However, our studies on ganglioside profiles of more than fifty biopsied melanoma specimens revealed that the ratio of GM3 to total gangliosides ranged from 95 %, as in normal melanocytes to less than 10 % within the metastatic melanoma. In addition, the ganglioside pattern remained the same in specimens obtained at different time and from different sites within the same individual patients, indicating that the observed diversity is governed by individual genotypic differences. The differences in the ganglioside profile of neoplastically transformed melanocyte correlates with the changes in the functional characteristics of the malignant cell, namely, proliferation, migration, adhesion to basement membrane components, infiltration and metastasis.

Shedding of these gangliosides in the light of their affinity to lymphokines on one hand, and their ability to suppress or enhance immune responses on the other, suggests their role in immunoregulation against melanoma. The immunogenic gangliosides of melanoma either in purified state or in association with other membrane components as in melanoma cell vaccine are valuable therapeutic agents in immunotherapy. The ability of the anti-ganglioside antibodies to partake in complement mediated cytotoxicity and antibody-dependent cytotoxicity enhances therapeutic application of these antibodies.

Acknowledgements

This work is supported by Public Health Service Grants CA-12582, CA-36064, and CA-42396 from National Cancer Institute; and by a grant from Cancer Research Institute (M.H.R.).

References

1. Carubia, J. M., Yu, R. K., Macala, L. J., Kirkwood, J. M., Varga, J. M. Gangliosides of normal and neoplastic human melanocytes. Biochem. Biophys. Res. Commun. 120, 500–504, 1984.
2. Rosenberg, J. M., Cheresh, D. A. Increased activity of cytidine-5'-monophospho-N-acetyl-neuraminic acid: GM3 sailyltransferase leads to the enhanced expression of GD3 on human melanoma cells derived from a metastatic lesion. Proc. Am. Soc. Biol. Chem. 45, 1822–1827, 1986.
3. Thurin, J., Thurin, M., Elder, D. E., Steplewski, Z., Clark, W. H., Kaprowski, H. GD2 ganglioside biosynthesis is a distinct biochemical event in human melanoma tumor progression. FFBS Letters 208, 17–22, 1986.
4. Cheresh, D. A., Varki, A. P., Varki, N. M., Stallcup, W. P. Levine, J., Reisfeld, R. A. A monoclonal antibody recognizes an O-acetyl sialic acid in a human melanoma-associated ganglioside. J. Biol. Chem. 259, 7453–7459, 1984.
5. Thurin, J., Herlyn, M., Hindegaul, O., Stromberg, N., Karlsson, K-A., Elder, D., Steplewski, Z., Koprowski, H., Proton NMR and fast-bombardment mass spectrometry analysis of the melanoma-associated ganglioside 9-O-acetyl GD3.
   J. Biol. Chem. 260, 14556-14653, 1985.
6. Ravindranath, M. H., Paulson, J. C., Irie, R. F. Human melanoma associated antigen O-acetyl ganglioside GD3 is recognized by *Cancer antennarius* lectin. J. Biol. Chem. 263, 2079–2086, 1988.
7. Higa, H., Paulson, J. C. Sialylation of glycoprotein oligosaccharides with N-Acetyl-, N-Glycolyl-, and N-O-Diacetylneuraminic acids. J. Biol. Chem. 260, 8838–8849, 1985.
8. Portoukalian, J., Zwingelstein, G., Dore, J-F., Borgoin, J-J. Studies of a ganglioside fraction extracted from human malignant melanoma. Biochemie 58, 1285–1287 (1976).
9. Pukel, C. S., Lloyd, K. O., Travassos, L. R., Dippold, W. G., Oettgen, H. F., Old, L. J. GD3, a prominent ganglioside of human melanoma: Detection and characterization of mouse monoclonal antibody. J. Exp. Med. 155, 1133–1147, 1982.
10. Tsuchida, T. Saxton, R. E., Morton, D. L., Irie, R. F. Gangliosides of human melanoma. J. Natl. Cancer Inst. 78, 45–54, 1987.
11. Tsuchida, T., Ravindranath, M. H., Saxton, R. E., Irie, R. F. Gangliosides of human melanoma: Altered expression *in vivo* and *in vitro*. Cancer Res. 47, 1278–1281, 1987.
12. Fredman, P., von Holst, H., Collines, V. P., Ammar, A., Dellheden, B., Wahren, B., Granholm, L., Svennerholm, L. Potential ganglioside antigens associated with human gliomas. Neurol. Res. 8, 123–126, 1986.
13. Herlyn, M., Thurin, J., Balaban, G., Bennicelli, J. L., Herlyn, D., Elder, D. E., Bondi, E., Guerry, D., Nowell, P., Clark, W. H., Koprowski, H. Charcteristics of cultured human melanocytes isolated from different stages of tumor progression. Cancer Res. 45, 5670–5676, 1985.

14. Cheresh, D. A., Pierschbacher, M. D., Herzig, M. A., Mujoo, K. Disialogangliosides GD2 and GD3 are involved in extracellular matrix proteins. J. Cell Biol. 102, 688–696, 1986.
15. Cheresh, D. A., Klier, F. G. Disialoganglioside distributes preferentially into substrate associated microprocesses on human melanoma cells during their attachment to fibronectin. J. Cell Biol. 102, 1877–1897, 1986.
16. Tsuchida, T., Saxton, R. E., Irie, R. F. Gangliosides of human melanoma GM2 and tumorigenicity. J. Natl. Cancer Inst. 78, 55–60, 1987.
17. Tai, T., Paulson, J. C., Cahan, C. D., Irie, R. F. Ganglioside GM2 as a human tumor antigen (OFA-I-1). Proc. Natl. Acad. Sci. 102, 688–696, 1986.
18. Tsuchida, T., Saxton, R. E.; Morton, D. L., Irie, R. F. Gangliosides of human melanoma II. Cancer (in press).
19. Ando, I., Hoon, D. S. B.. Suzuki, Y., Saxton, R. E., Golub, S. H., Irie, R. F. Ganglioside GM2 on the K562 cell line is recognized as a target structure by human natural kill cells. Int. J. Cancer 40, 12–17, 1987.
20. Ando, I., Hoon, D. S. B., Pattengale, P. K., Golub, S. H., Irie, R. F. Ganglioside GM2 as a target structure recognized by human natural killer cells. J. Clin. Lab. Anal. 1, 209–213, 1987.
21. Morton, D. L., Nizze, J. A., Gupta, R. K., Famatiga, E., Hoon, D. S. B., Irie, R. F. Active specific immunotherapy of malignant melanoma. In: Current status of cancer control and therapy, eds: Kim J. P., Kim, B. S. Park, J. P. pp. 152–161, 1987.
22. Tai, T., Cahan, L. D., Tsuchida, T., Morton, D. L., Irie, R. F., Immunogenicity of melanoma associated gangliosides in cancer patients. Int. J. Cancer 35, 607–612, 1985.
23. Livingston, P. O., Natoli, E. J., Calves, M. J., Stockert, E., Oettgen, H. F., Old, L. J. Vaccines containing purified GM2 ganglioside elicit GM2 antibodies in melanoma patients. Proc. Natl. Acad. Sci. USA 84, 2911–2915, 1987.
24. Hellstrom, I., Brankovan, V., Hellstrom, K. E., Strong antitumor activities of IgG 3 antibodies to a human melanoma-associated ganglioside. Proc. Natl. Acad. Sci. USA, 82, 1499–1502, 1985.
25. Cheresh, D. A., Honsik, C. J., Staffeleno, L. K., Jung, G., Reisfeld, R. A. Disialoganglioside GD3 on human melanoma serves as a revelant target antigen for monoclonal antibody-mediated tumor cytolysis. Proc. Natl. Acad. Sci. USA, 82, 5155–5159, 1985.
26. Cheresh, D. A., Harper, J. R., Schulz, G., Reisfeld, R. A. Localization of gangliosides GD2 and GD3 in adhesion plaques and on the surface of human melanoma cell. Proc. Natl. Acad. Sci. USA 81, 5767–5771, 1984.
27. Dippold, W., Knuth, A., Meyer zum Büschenfelde, K.-H. Inflammatory response at the tumor silte after systemic application of monoclonal anti-GD3 ganglioside antibody to patients with malignant melanoma. Am. Assoc. Cancer Res. 978, 247, 1984.
28. Houghton, A. N., Mintzer, D., Cordon-Cardo, C., Welt, S., Fliegel, B., Vadhan, S., Carswell, E., Melamed, M. R., Oettgen, H. F., Old, L. J. Mouse monoclonal IgG3 antibody detecting GD3 ganglioside: A phase I trial in patients with malignant melanoma. Proc. Natl. Sci. USA 82, 1242–1246, 1985.
29. Cheung, NV., Lazarus, H., Miraldi, F. D., Abramowsky, C. R., Kallick, S., Saarinen, U. M., Spitzer, T., Strandjord, S. E., Coccia, P. F., Berger, N. A. Ganglioside GD2 specific monoclonal antibody 3F8: A phase I study in patients with neuroblastoma and malignant melanoma. J. Clin. Oncol. 5, 1430–1440, 1987.
30. Bajorin, D., Chapman, P., Kunicka, J., Cordon-Cardo, C., Welt, K., Mertelsmann, R., Melamed, M., Oettgen, H. F., Houghton, A. H. Phase I trial of a combination of R-24 mouse monoclonal antibody and recombinant interleukin-2 in patients with melanoma. Amer. Assoc. Cancer Res. 827, 210, 1987.

31. Lichtin, A. E., Guerry, D., Elder, D. E., Hamilton, R., LaRossa, D., Herlyn, D., Iliopoulos, D., Thurin, J., Steplewski, A. A phase I study of monoclonal antibody therapy in disseminated melanoma. Proc. 8th Interntl. Pigment cell Confer. Tucson, Arizona, 1986.

32. Goodman, G. E., Hellstrom, I., Hummel, D., Brodzinsky, L., Yeh, M.Y., Hellstrom, K. E. Phase I trail of monoclonal antibody MG-21 directed against a melanoma assoiciated GD3 ganglioside antigen. Proc. Am. Soc. Clin. Oncol. 6 A823 1987.

33. Cahan, L. D., Irie, R. F., Singh, R., Cassidenti, A., Paulson, J. C. Identification of a human neuroectodermal tumor antigen (OFA-I-2) as ganglioside GD2. Proc. Natl. Acad. Sci. USA 79, 7629–7633, 1982.

34. Irie, R. F., Morton, D. L. Regression of cutaneous metastatic melanoma by intralesional injection with human monoclonal antibody to ganglioside GD2. Proc. Natl. Acad. Sci. USA 83, 8694–8698, 1986.

35. Kono, K., Tsuchida, T., Kern, D. H., Irie, R. F. Relationship of ganglioside expression on melanoma cells and response to anti-tumor treatment in the human tumor colonyforming assay. Fed. Amer. Soc. Exp. Biol. 46, 1057, 1987.

36. Portoukalian, J., Zwingelstein, G., Abdul-Malek, N., Dore, J. F. Alteration of gangliosides in plasma and red cells of human bearing melanoma tumors. Biochem. Biophys. Res. Commun. 85, 916–920, 1987.

37. Ladisch, S., Wu, Z-L., Feig, S., Ulsh, L., Schwartz, E., Floutsis, G., Wiley, F., Lenarsky, C., Seeger, R. Shedding of GD2 ganglioside by human neuroblastoma. Int. J. Cancer 39, 73–76, 1987.

38. Portoukalian, J. Immunoregulatory activity of gangliosides shed by melanoma tumors. In: Present Status of Gangliosides in Oncology, Biosymposia (abstr.) 1988.

39. Hoon, D. S. B., Irie, R. F., Cochran, A. J. Gangliosides from human melanoma immunomodulate response of T-cells to interleukin-2. Cell Immunol. 111, 1–10, 1988.

40. Ankel, H., Krishnamurthi, C., Besancon, F., Stefano, S., Falcoff, E. Mouse fibroblast (type I) and immune (type II) interferons: Pronounces differences in affinity for gangliosides and in antiviral and antigrowth effects on mouse leukemia L-1210R cells. Proc. Natl. Acad. Sci. USA 77, 2528–2532, 1980.

41. MacDonald, H. S., Elconin, H., Ankel, H. Leukemic cells sensitive or resistant to beta-interferon have identical ganglioside patterns. FEBS letters 141, 267–270, 1982.

42. Hakansson, L., Fredman, P., Svennerholm, L. Gangliosides in serum immune complexes from tumor-bearing patients. J. Biochem. 98, 843–849, 1985.

9. A GM3 Epitope Expressed in Tumor Infiltrating Macrophages is Generated in Phagocytizing Monocytes in vitro

F. Schriever, R. D. Dennis,
B. Pallmann, G. Riethmuller, and
J. P. Johnson

Introduction

Gangliosides are a major component of melanoma cells and antibodies produced against human tumors either by mice or by the patients themselves frequently are directed against these molecules (1, 2). Gangliosides have recently been shown to play an important role in modulating the interaction of melanoma cells with the extracellular matrix (3). Since aberrations in the interaction with the extracellular matrix are characteristic of malignant cells and are speculated to contribute to invasion and metastases (4), it was of interest to search for differences in the gangliosides expressed between melanoma cells and the nevus cells which comprise benign melanocyte tumors. Previous studies have shown that it is possible to identify differences in protein antigen expression between benign and maligant melanocytes by searching for monoclonal antibodies which show differential reactivity with these cells in situ (5, 6). Using this approach, monoclonal antibody (Mab)* MacG1 which reacts with GM3 ganglioside preparations was isolated (7). In contrast to other antibodies directed to GM3, MacG1 which shows differential reactivity with melanoma and nevi in tissue sections, does not stain the melanoma cells themselves but rather granules associated with tumor infiltrating macrophages. In vito studies suggest that the MacG1 epitope is generated during phagocytic degradation of ganglioside rich cellular debris.

Materials and Methods

Antibodies, Cells, and Tissues. Mab MacG1 was produced as described (7) from a C57BL/6 x BALB/C mouse injected with 100 mg lipid A (day 0), and liposomes containing 100 µg melanoma gangliosides (day 1). The spleen was removed on day 4 and the cells fused with mouse myeloma P3X63 Ag8.653 using standard procedures.

Mabs 63D3 (anti-macrophage marker) and GAp 8.3 (anti CD45, T200) were obtained from the American Type Culture Collection (Rockville, MD). Mab Leu 7 (anti HNK-1) was purchased from Becton- Dickinson (Mountain View, CA). Mabs T15.1 (anti CD4), T301 (anti CD3), T910 (anti CD2), T811 (anti CD8), M522 (anti macrophage marker), M42 (anti macrophage marker) were kindly provided by E. P. Rieber in our institute. The myeloma protein UPC10 (IgG2a) was purchased from Sigma Chemical Company (St. Louis, MO) as were all chemicals where not otherwise specified.

Tissues were snap frozen in liquid nitrogen after removal and stored at −70 °C.

Antibody Binding Assays. Tissue sections and cell lines were tested for antibody binding with standard immunohistochemical procedures using peroxidase, alkaline phosphatase or gold labelled second antibodies as described (7, 8). Antibody binding to TLC plates was performed essentially as described by Dippold et al (9) using a peroxidase labelled second antibody.

---

*Abbreviations: Mab, monoclonal antibody; ELISA, enzyme-linked immunosorbent assay; GM3, NeuACα2-3Galβ1-4G1c-Cer; TLC, thin layer chromatography.

Glycolipids. The gangliosides GT1b, GD1a, GD1b, GM1, GM2, and GD3 purified from bovine brain were purchased from Fidia (Abano Terme, Italy). Glucosyl ceramide was purchased from Sigma and additional glycolipids were obtained from Dr. Pallmann KG, Munich.

Gangliosides were extracted from a human malignant melanoma lymph node metastasis using chloroform : methanol : H_2O (10 : 10 : 1) and chloroform : methanol : 0.8M aqueous sodium acetate (60 : 35 : 8) as described (7). Separation of the gangliosides from neutral glycolipids was performed on a DEAE-Sephadex A25 column (10) and final purification was achieved using middle pressure chromatography on Iatrobeads 6 (RS-8060 column). Reactive gangliosides were eluted with a solvent gradient of chloroform : methanol : H_2O (70 : 25 : 4 to 65 : 25 : 4).

Thin layer chromatography was performed as described (7) using a solvent system of chloroform : methanol : 0.2 % $CaCl_2$ (60 : 35 : 8) for gangliosides and chloroform : methanol : H_2O (60 : 25 : 4) for neutral glycolipids. Gangliosides were identified with resorcinol/HCl and neutral glycolipids with orcinol/H_2SO_4.

Phagocytosis Assay. Plastic adherent peritoneal cells from CBA x DBA/2 mice were activated with 1 µg/ml lipopolysaccharide (LPS, Difco Laboratories, Detroit MI) and exposed for up to 3 hours to antibody coated sheep red blood cells (SRBC; anti SRBC antiserum, Ambozeptor, Behringwerke, Marburg, FRG), liposomes (containing 1400 µg dimyristoyl phosphatidyl choline, 580 βg cholesterol, 120 µgdicetyl phosphate; 7) or iron particles (Lymphocyte separator reagent, Technicon, Tarrytown, N.Y.) as described (8). Cells were harvested at different times thereafter and examined for Mab binding.

Results and Discussion

Mab MacG1 distinguishes between malignant melanoma and benign melanocytic nevi in tissue sections. Mab MacG1 (IgG2a) was obtained following immunization with a mixture of gangliosides prepared from a melanoma lymph node metastasis. In addition to reacting with the immunizing glycolipids, MacG1 stained frozen tissue sections containing malignant melanoma and this staining was abrogated by treatment of the section with neuraminidase (data not shown). Analysis of a large panel of melanocytic lesions revealed that MacG1 was unreactive with epidermal melanocytes and benign melanocytic nevi but stained approcimately 50 % of the melanomas examined (Table 1; Figure 1). The staining was heterogeneous, ranging from less than 10 to more than 100 reactive cells per section. Although no correlation was found tumor stage (i.e. the Clark or Breslow levels), reactivity occurred more often in heavily pigmented tumors. The staining was cytoplasmic and often appeared to be associated with granules rather than entire cells. Examination of a variety of normal and malignant tissues revealed that MacG1 reactivity was not restricted to melanomas nor to malignant cells (Table 2). Reactivity was observed with occasional carcinomas and the 4 tested hepatomas were reactive in contrast to normal liver. Among nonmalignant tissues, reactivity was observed with most neural tissues and structures but as well in the red pulp of the spleen. As opposed to the granule-like staining of the spleen and the majority of tumors, the neural structures were uniformly stained.

Table 1. Reactivity of Mab MacG1 with malignant melanoma and benign nevi.

Lesion	Positive/tested
Melanocytic nevi	
Dermal	0/11
Junctional	0/10
Compound	1/20
Congenital nevi	0/ 3
Spitz nevi	0/ 2
Dysplastic nevi	0/ 5
Malignant melanoma	
Primary tumors	9/20
Metastases	15/26

Reactivity determined by immonoperoxidase staining of frozen tissue sections. Positive tissues had at least 10 stained cells.

Mab MacG1 reactivity is associated with a minor subpopulation of tissue macrophages. Although 50% of melanomas examined in situ were reactive with Mab MacG1, no reactivity could be detected with the 7 melanoma cell lines examined. Serial sections of tumors stained with an antibody directed to CD45, the T200 antigen common to all cells of the hematopoietic lineage (11), indicated that MacG1 reactivity was associated with the presence of mononuclear cell infiltrate. Comparison of serial sections stained with antibodies to T cell and macrophage markers revealed that the MacG1 reactive areas were rich in cells with a macrophage phenotype. In one bronchial carcinoma reactivity of MacG1 was localized to granules which, since they could be identified in unstained sections, could be shown to be present in cells bearing

Fig. 1

a   b

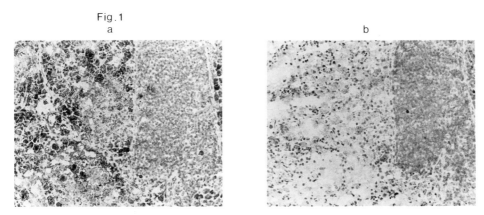

Figure 1. Reactivity of MacG1 with malignant melanoma. a, Mab MacG1; b, isotype control UPC10. Immunoperoxidase staining of a melanoma lymph node metastasis. x125.

Table 2. Reactivity of MacG1 with non-melanocytic cells and tissues.

Malignant	Normal
Reactive tissues	
hepatomas (4/4)*	spleen (2/2)
bronchial carcinome (1/1)	kidney tubules (5/5)
glioblastoma (2/3)	cortex parietalis (2/2)
renal cell carcinoma (1/2)	cerebellum (1/2)
Unreactive tissues	
carcinomas:	colon, stomach, liver, skin, bone marrow,
ovarian, breast, thyroid, basal cell,	thymus, thyroid
gastric neuroblastoma, astrocytoma	

Reactivity determined by immunoperoxidase staining of frozen tissue sections. Positive tissues hat at least 10 stained cells.
* For positive tissues, number positive/number tested.

macrophage markers. These cells were stained with antibodies directed to CD45, CD4, HLA-DR, and the macrophage markers 63D3, M522, and M42. They were unreactive with antibodies directed against CD2, CD3, CD8, and the natural killer cell marker, HNK-1 (7). These observations suggest that the MacG1 reactivity observed in situ is with tumor infiltrating macrophages rather than with the melanoma cells themselves. MacG1 cannot however be a general marker of tissue macrophages since many tumors (e.g. the breast carcinomas) contained large numbers of infiltrating cells with macrophage phenotypes but were nevertheless unreactive with MacG1. In addition MacG1 showed no reactivity with tissue macrophages such as Kupffer cells in the liver or with cultured peripheral blood monocytes or monoblastic cell lines (7). In comparison to the staining observed with antibodies directed to macrophage markers, MacG1 reactive cells account for only a very minor fraction (P1%) of the tumor infiltrating macrophages.

Generation of MacG1 Epitope in Phagocytic Adherent Monocytes in vitro. One possible explanation for the observed MacG1 reactivity in tissue sections is that it is generated during phagocytosis of ganglioside rich cellular debris. If this is true, it should be possible to reproduce this effect in vitro. Since erythrocytes contain high amounts of gangliosides and since epitopes on these molecules are generally not species specific, a heterologous system was used to test this possibility. Murine peritoneal cells were activated with LPS and exposed to antibody coated SRBC. In the presence of LPS alone, no reactivity of the cells with MacG1 was observed. However, in the presence of SRBC, which are themselves negative, MacG1 staining of the monocytes was observed as soon as 1 hour and was detectable as late as 5 days after SRBC exposure (8; Figure 2a). Other antibodies of the IgG2a isotype did not bind to these cells, ruling out Fc receptor mediated binding of MacG1 (8). The expression of MacG1 epitope, which was found on 80–90% of the adherent cells, was dependent on catabolism. In the presence of 0.1 mmd chloroquine, which which interfereses with catabolism by increasing

a

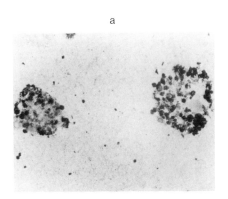

b

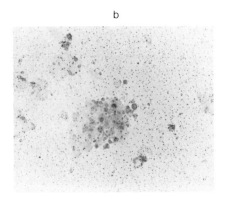

Figure 2. Effect of chloroquine on the generation of the MacG1 epitope in phagocytic monocytes. Immunogold reactivity of MabMacG1 with monocytes incubated with SRBC in the
absence (a) or presence (b) or 0,1 mnd chloroquine.

Table 3. Expression of MacG1 epitope on adherent mononuclear cells.

Incubation conditions	MacG1 binding
–	<1%*
LPS 1 µg/ml	<1%
LPS + iron particles	<1%
LPS + liposomes	<1%
LPS + antibody-SRBC	80–90%
LPS + antibody-SRBC + 0.1 mM chloroquine	<1%

*% positive cells as determined with immunohistochemical staining of cytospin preparations.

lysosomal pH (12), no expression of the MacG1 epitope was observed (Figure 2b). As
can be seen, phagocytosis of the SRBC was not prevented by this treatment. The
expression of MacG1 was also not induced when the cells were allowed to ingest iron
particles or liposomes (Table 3). While this observation argues that the MacG1 epitope
originates from the ingested the SRBC, themselves were not stained by the antibody,
suggesting that the MacG1 epitope is created or exposed by lysosomal enzymes.

The MacG1 epitope is localized to a subfraction of GM3 molecules. Mab MacG1 was
shown to react with the immunizing glycolipid extract in a solid phase ELISA. When
this material was separated by TLC, MacG1 stained a single band which migrated in
the region of the GM3 standard. No evidence could be obtained for reactivitys of
MacG1 with a glycoprotein (7). The melanoma lymph node gangliosides were further
fractionated using ion exchange chromatography on DEAE Sephadex and middle
pressure chromatography on Iatrobeads and the various factions tested in immuno-
TLC for MacG1 reactivity. Reactivity was only observed with the GM3 fraction. Reactivity was also observed with a preparation of GM3CNeuGc) from bovine brain
(Figure 3, lanes 2a, 2b) but not with GM3(NeuGc) (lanes 3a, 3b) GM3 lactone (not
shown) or any other of the ganglioside standards (lanes 4a, 4b). Reactivity of Mab
MacG1 with both melanoma lymph node and standard GM3 was abrogated after neur-

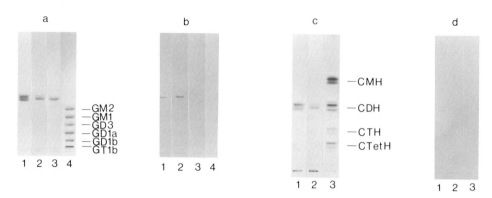

Figure 3. Mab MacG1 reactivity with gangliosides and neutral glycolipids. Effect of neuramini-dase treatment.

TLC plates a and b and c and d were run under identical conditions with the same amounts of glycolipids.

a (resorcinol staining) and b (MacG1 immunoreactivity): lane 1, GM3 melanoma fraction; lane 2, GM3 bovine brain; lane 3, GM3(NeuGc9; lane 4, standard gangliosides;

c (resorcinol staining) and d (MacG1 immunoreactivity): lane 1, GM3 melanoma neuramini-dase treated; lane 2, GM3 bovine brain neuraminidase treated; lane 3, standard neutral glyco-lipids. CMH, ceramide monohexoside; CDH, ceramide dihexoside; CTH, ceramide trihexo-side; CTetH, ceramide tetrahexoside.

aminidase treatment (Figure 3c, d) suggesting that this is indeed the antigen recog-nized by MacG1 in melanoma tissue sections. The GM3 specificity of Mab MacG1 on TLC conflicts with its reactivity pattern on tissue sections. Melanoma cells are not stained by MacG1 although they contain large amounts of GM3 and react with other antibodies directed to GM3 (13, 14). However, as can be seen in Figure 3 (lanes 1a, 1b), the reactive band appears to be only a minor component of the melanoma lymph node GM3 fraction, suggesting that the MacG1 epitope may be localized to a subpopulation of GM3 molecules. This is further supported by the observation that MacG1 negative as well as MacG1 positive GM3 fractions were isolated from the melanoma lymph node gangliosides and both fractions were shown to have the identical sugar sequence (NeuAc-GA1β-Glc) by sequential enzymatic hydrolysis (Schriever et al., manuscript in preparation).

Although further biochemical studies are needed to determine the exact structure of the MacG1 epitope, the data presently available suggest that it is generated in phagocytic monocytes during the enzymatic degradatiion of MacG1 negative ganglio-sides and appears to represent a modified GM3. The preferential association of the MacG1 epitope with melanomas as opposed to nevi in situ is likely to reflect the increased amount of gangliosides and cellular debris in the tumors rather than a struc-tural difference in these molecules.

Summary

Murine monoclonal antibody MacG1 was obtained following immunization with a mixture of gangliosides extracted from a fresh human melanoma metastasis. In frozen tissue sections, Mab MacG1 showed preferential reactivity with malignant tissues, staining 25 of 46 tested melanomas and 4 of 4 hepatomas but showing no reactivity with benign melanocytic nevi and normal hepatocytes. Closer examination of the sections revealed that the tumor cells themselves were not stained but that Mab MacG1 reacted instead with granules associated with cells expressing the phenotypic markers of macrophages. In vitro studies with murine peritoneal adherent cells revealed that the MacG1 epitope is expressed in phagocytic granules following the phagocytosis and degradation of MacG1 negative sheep red blood cells. Stimulation of adherent cells phogocytosis alone did not lead to the expression of the MacG1 epitope suggesting that it is generated during phagocytic degradation. MacG1 reacted with a single band of thin layer chromatography separated melanoma metastases gangliosides and this band was found in the GM3 fraction. When tested with a panel of purified gangliosides and neutral glycosphingolipids, MacG1 bound only to a preparation of bovine GM3. Lack of reactivity with GM3-lactone, GM3(NeuGc) as well as other GM3 preparations suggests that Mab MacG1 may detect a variant GM3.

Acknowledgements

This work was supported in part by a grant from the Deutsche Krebshilfe, Mildred Scheel Stiftung, Bonn, West Germany. We thank Professor H. Wiegandt, Marburg, West Germany, for helpful discussions.

References

1. Herlyn, M., and H. Koprowski. Melanoma antigens: immunological and biological characterization and clinical significance. Ann. Rev. Immunol. 6, 283, 1988.
2. Tai, T., J. C. Paulson, L. D. Cahan, and R. F. Irie. Ganglioside GM2 as a human tumor antigen (OFA-I-1). Proc. Natl. Acad. Sci. USA 80, 5392, 1983.
3. Cheresh, D. A., M. D. Pierschbacher, M. A. Herzig, and K. Mujoo. Disialogangliosides GD2 and GD3 are involved in the attachment of human melanoma and neuroplastoma cells to extracellular matrix proteins. J. Cell Biol. 102, 688, 1986.
4. Liotta, L. A., Tumor invasion and metastases-role of the extracellular matrix. Cancer Res. 46, 1, 1986.
5. Holzmann, B., J. P. Johnson, P. Kaudewitz, and G. Riethmüller. In situ analysis of antigens on malignant and benign cells of the melanocyte lineage. Differential expression of two surface molecules gp75 and p89. J. Exp. Med. 161, 366, 1985.

6. Lehmann, J. M., B. Holzmann, E.W. Breitbart, P. Schmiegelow, G. Riethmüller, and J. P. Johnson. Discrimination between benign and malignant cells of the melanocytic lineage by two novel antigens, a glycoprotein with a molecular weight of 113,000 and a protein with a molecular weight of 76,000. Cancer Res. 47, 841, 1987.

7. Schriever, F., R. D. Dennis, G. Riethmüller, and J. P. Johnson. MacG1, a mouse monoclonal antibody detecting a monosialoganglioside expressed in tumor-infiltrating macrophages. Cancer Res. 48, 2524, 1988.

8. Schriever, F., G. Riethmüller, and J. P. Johnson. Enzymatic degradation in phagocytic monocytes generates the ganglioside epitope defined by antibody MacG1. Hybridoma 7, 249, 1988.

9. Dippold, W. G., R. Klingel, H. Bernhard, H.-P. Dienes, A. Knuth, and K.-H. Meyer zum Büschenfelde. Secretory epithelial cell marker on gastrointestinal tumor and in human secretions by a monoclonal antibody. Cancer Res. 47, 2092, 1987.

10. Ledeen, R.W., R. K. Yu, and L. F. Eng. Gangliosides of human myelin: sialosylgalactosylceramide as a major component. J. Neurochem. 21, 829, 1973.

11. Omary, M. B., I. S. Trowbridge, and H. A. Battifora. Human homologue of murine T200 glycoprotein. J. Exp. Med. 152, 842, 1980.

12. Ohkuma, S., and B. Poole. Fluorescence probe measurement of the intralysosomal pH in living cells and the perturbation of pH by various agents. Proc. Natl. Acad. Sci. USA 75, 3327, 1978.

13. Tsuchida, T., R. E. Saxton, D. L. Morton, and R. F. Irie. Gangliosides of human melanoma. J. Natl. Cancer Inst. 78, 45, 1987.

14. Nores, G., T. Dohi, M. Taniguchi, and S.-I. Hakomori. Density dependent recognition of cell surface GM3 by a certain anti-melanoma antibody, and GM3 lactone as a possible immunogen: requirements for tumor-associated antigen and immunogen. J. Immunol. 139, 3171, 1987.

10. Monoclonal Antibody Detection of Ganglioside Expression in Human Neuroblastoma

N.-K. V. Cheung, N. Usmani,
C. Cordon-Cardo, A. N. Houghton,
J. Biedler, and H. F. Oettgen

Abstract

The expression of gangliosides GD2, GD3, and GM2 were analyzed by indirect immunofluorescent staining of neuroplastoma cell lines and fresh tissue sections. The antibody 3F8 (specific for GD2), R24 (specific for GD3) and 10–11 (specific for GM2) were used as primary antibodies. Thirty-one neuroblastoma tumors (including primary, metastatic, obtained at diagnosis and after chemotherapy treatments) and 7 cell lines were studied. While all the neuroplastic cell lines (N-lines) were positive for GD2, the epithelial subclones (5S and 6S, both from LAN-1) showed decreased GD2 expression. GM2 was present in both N and S subclones. All fresh neuroblastoma tumors from children were GD2 positive, and GM2 negative. There was no significant heterogeneity of GD2 expression within tumors and among tumors. The expression of GD3 was variable. The pattern of expression of gangliosides in neuroblastomas may reflect differences in cellular origin or their degrees of differentiation. They may have therapeutic implications in future clinical trials using antibodies 3F8 and R24.

Introduction

Neuroblastoma, the most common extra-cranial solid tumor of childhood, is difficult to eradicate using currently known methods (1). In order to explore alternative treatment methods using targeted immunotherapy and radiotherapy (2), surface antigens on neuroblastoma cells are actively studied using monoclonal antibodies. Disialoganglioside antigens have been detected in human neuroblastomas using biochemical and immunological methods (3–6). Their restricted distribution in the human body may have therapeutic advantages for targeted therapies (7). However, tumor heterogeneity among tumors and within tumors pose obstacles preventing complete tumor elimination. In addition, the density of antigens on tumor cells may be low such that the total number of binding sites for a specific monoclonal antibody may be inadequate for efficient complement or cell-mediated cytotoxicity. Although biochemical methods have provided estimates of ganglioside expression (10^7 molecules per cell) in human neuroblastoma tissues (4), information on their expression in individual cell in fresh tumors and cell lines was not available. Murine monoclonal antibodies specific for GD2 (6), GD3 (8), and GM2 (9) have recently been described. They are useful reagents for studying the cellular distribution of gangliosides in normal tissues as well as in human tumors. In this report we describe the expression of these disialoganglioside antigens detected by the use of these monoclonal antibodies in human neuroblastoma tissues and cell lines, with respect to tumor antigen heterogeneity both within and among tumors.

Material and Methods

Source of Tissues and Cell lines. Tissues were obtained from autopsies of patients at diagnosis, relapse and second look surgery. Normal tissues were obtained from autopsy patients or from surgical specimens within 1–2 hours of resection. Tissue was placed in OCT compound (Miles, Naperville, IL), snapfrozen in isopentane chilled in liquid-nitrogen and stored at −70 °C. Five um sections were cut on a cryostat, fixed in acetone, stored at 4 °C and washed in Tris buffered salind (TBS) pH 7.4 prior to use. LA-N-1, LA-N-2, and LA-N-5 were obtained from Dr. Robert Seeger, UCLA, Los Angeles, CA. IMR32, SKNSH, and SKNMC were provided by the American Type Culture Collection (ATCC), Bethesda, MA. The subclones of LA-N-1 have been previously published (10).

Immunohistochemistry. Specificities of the various monoclonal antibodies have been previously described: 3F8 for GD2 (6), R24 for GD3 (8), and 10–11 for GM2 (9). In the indirect immunofluorescence method, sections were first reacted with 1 % calf serum in PBS, washed with TBS and then incubated with the monoclonal antibody (3F8: 20 μg/ml, R24: 30 μg/ml, 10–11: 20 μg/ml) for one hour at room temperature. Control monoclonal mouse antibody NS.7 (TIB 114, an IgG3) was obtained from American Type Culture Collection (ATCC), Rockville, MA. After washing with TBS, the slides were incubated with goat anti-mouse IgG labeled with fluorescein isothiocyanate (FITC) (Tago Laboratories, Burlingame, CA) diluted to 1 : 25 in 0.5 % Bovine Serum Albumin (BSA) in PBS. After washing in Tris HCl pH 7.4, the sections were mounted in Permaflour (Lipshaw Corporation, Detroit, MI) and examined under a fluorescent microscope (Table 1).

Table 1. Detection of neuroblastoma ganglioside antigens by immunostaining.

Total number of neuroblastoma patients	Positivity* of		
	G_{D2}	G_{D3}	G_{M2}
31	31	14	0

* Positivity is defined as homogenous staining $\geq 2+$ (scale of 1–3) for staining intensity.

Immunofluorescence. Neuroblastoma cell lines grown in 10 % calf serum (Hyclone, Logan, UT) in 1640 RPMI were harvested with 2mM EDTA and washed in cold Phosphate Buffered Saline (PBS) containing 0.02 % sodium azide. 5×10^5 cells were reacted with 100 μl of the primary monoclonal antibody for 45 minutes on ice. Cells were underlaid with 500 μl calf serum and washed in cold buffer. After two more washes and centrifugation at 200 x g for 10 minutes, the cells were reacted with 100 μl of FITC-goat anti-mouse antibody (Tago, Burlingame, CA) diluted in 1 : 25 in 0.5 % BSA in PBS. After 45 minutes on ice, the cells were underlaid with 500 μl of calf serum and washed in cold PBS before fixation in 1 % formaldehyde in PBS. Stained cells were analysed by flow cytometry using the Facscan from Becton-Dickinson, San Diego, CA (Table 2).

Table 2. Analysis of surface gangliosides in neuroblastoma by flow cytometry.

Antigen	G_{D2}		G_{D3}		G_{M2}	
	%[a]	FI[b]	%	FI	%	FI
NMB7	95	1.00	17	0.09	97	0.53
LAN-1	90	0.48	14	0.10	68	0.24
LA1-15n	98	1.45	5	0.08	87	0.22
LA1-19n	97	0.96	3	0.09	96	0.96
LA1-21n	93	0.63	4	0.07	84	0.25
LA1-22n	95	0.72	67	0.14	93	0.45
LA1-23n	93	1.31	28	0.11	95	0.58
LA1-5s	25	0.42	7	0.18	28	0.24
LA1-6s	3	0.18	5	0.10	52	0.46
SKNSH	3	0.06	3	0.10	60	0.38
SKNMC	5	0.18	12	0.22	37	0.17
LAN-2	95	0.69	7	0.19	90	0.34
LAN-5	87	1.05	57	0.25	65	0.31
IMR-32	95	0.75	7	0.09	81	0.33

[a] Percentage of cells positive.
[b] FI = fluorescence intensity (scale 10^0 to 10^4), relative to 3F8 (anti-G_{D2}) staining of NMB-7 neuroblastoma cells.

Results and Discussion

A total of 31 human neuroblastomas were examined by immunohistology using monoclonal antibodies specific for gangliosides. All 31 of the tumors showed expression of GD2 (3F8) on tumor cell surface as well as cytoplasm. The expression was rather uniform within tumors and among tumors. In contrast, only 14 of the tumors had homogeneous staining using R24 (GD3). In addition, R24 tended to show weaker staining of neuroblastomas than 3F8. These patterns of ganglioside expression seemed to bear no apparent relationship to the stage of disease or whether the tumor was obtained at diagnosis, after chemotherapy or at relapse. No surface expression of GM2 was found using the antibody 10–11 on fresh human neuroblastomas.

Indirect immunofluorescence was also used to study neuroblastoma cell lines. LA-1-15n,21n,22n,23n,5s,6s were all derived from the parental clone LAN-1 as previously described (10). Fluorescence was analyzed by flow cytometry, and expressed on a 4-decaded logarithmic scale. The fluorescence channel beyond which the control antibody TIB114 showed P5 % staining was used as the cutoff for positive staining. Mean fluorescence was calculated in log fluorescence units for the population of cells beyond the cutoff, and then expressed as a ratio of the fluorescence intensity of 3F8 binding to NMB-7 cells. Except for SKNSH and SKNMC (a neuroepithelioma), GD2 expression was more uniform and more intense among these cell lines when compared to GD3. There was quite a variability of relative fluorescence intensity with respect to GD2 among the subclones (0.18–1.45). Both epithelial subclones 5s and 6s, which have been reported to have decreased tumorigenic potentials in vitro as well as in athymic nude mice (10), have smaller percentages of positive cells and lower fluoroscence intensities among the positive cell populations. Unlike in human neuroblastoma tissues, GM2 was detected in cell lines. However, the mean fluorescence intensity was lower than that for GD2. Although the FITC-goat anti-mouse antibody reacts with both mouse IgM and IgG3 antibodies, the difference in affinities toward individual antibody class is not known and has rendered the comparison of antigen densities (GD2 versus GM2) based on mean fluorescence intensities impossible.

References

1. Kushner, B. H., N. K.V. Cheung. Treatment of neuroblastoma. In: V.T. DeVita, S. Hellman, S. A. Rosenberg, eds. Cancer Updates, Vol 2., Philadelphia Lippincott, 1988.
2. Cheung, N. K., D. Munn, B. H. Kushner, N. Usmani, and S. D. J. Yeh. Targeted radio-therapy and immunotherapy of human neuroblastoma with GD2 specific monoclona anti-bodies. In: Eckelman, W. C., et al. (eds), In Vivo Diagnosis and Therapy of human tumor with monoclonal antibodies. Pergamon Press, London, 1988 (in press).
3. Schultz, G., D. A. Cheresh, N. M. Varki, A. Yu, L. K. Staffileno, R. A. Reisfeld. Detection of ganglioside GD2 in tumor tissues and sera of neuroblastoma patients. Can. Res. 44, 5914, 1984.
4. Wu, Z. L., E. Schwartz, R. Seeger, S. Ladisch. Expression of GD2 ganglioside by untreated primary human neuroblastomas. Can. Res. 46, 440, 1986.
5. Schengrund, C. L., M. A. Repman, S. Shochat. Ganglioside composition of human neuro-blastoma: correlation with prognosis, a pediatric oncology group study. Cancer 56, 2640, 1985.
6. Cheung, N. K.V., U. M. Saarinen, J. Neely, B. Landmeier, D. Donavan, P. F. Coccia. Monoclonal antibodies to a glycolipid antigen on human neuroplastoma cells. Cancer Res. 45, 2642, 1985.
7. Cheung, N. K.V., F. D. Miraldi. Iodine 131 labelled GD2 monoclonal antibody in the diagno-sis and therapy of human neuroblastoma. In: Advances in Neuroblastoma Research 2. Evans, A. E., et al.,(ed) Alan R. Liss, Inc., New York, p. 595, 1988.
8. Pukel, C. S., K. O. Lloyd, L. R. Travassos, W. G. Dippold, H. F. Oettgen, L. J. Old. GD3, a prominent ganglioside of human melanoma. Detection and characterization by mouse monoclonal antibody. J. Exp. Med. 155, 1133, 1982.
9. Natoli, E. J., P. O. Livingston, C. S. Pukel, K. O. Lloyd, H. Wiegandt, J. Szalay, H. F. Oett-gen, L. J. Old. A murine monoclonal antibody detecting N-acetyl and N-glycolyl-GM2: charcterization of cell surface reactivity. Can. Res. 46, 4116, 1986.
10. Biedler, J. L., B. A. Spengler, T. Chang, R. A. Ross. Transdifferentiation of human neuro-blastoma cells results in coordinate loss of neuronal and malignant properties. In: Advances in neuroblastoma research 2, Evans, A. E., et al. (Ed), Alan R. Liss, Inc. New York, N.Y:, p. 265, 1988.

11. Gangliosides of Human Gliomas in vivo and in vitro.

P. Fredman

Introduction

Human malignant gliomas have a poor prognosis and 50 % of the patients are dead within one year after diagnosis. Modern therapy has not improved the survival and there is a need for new approaches in both diagnosis and therapy of these tumors. Gangliosides are cell surface molecules proposed to play a role in cellular differentiation, growth control and invasiveness, and tumor-associated gangliosides have been characterized in both tumor tissues and established tumor cell lines (1, 2).

Earlier studies (3–8) on gangliosides in human glioma tissue have shown increased proportions, as compared with normal adult brain tissue, of the gangliosides GM3, GM2 and in particular GD3. In one study (8) the amount of GD3 was found to be correlated to the malignancy of the tumor. In our studies (9, 10) we could, beside these quantitative alterations as compared to adjacent normal brain, detect gangliosides that appeared to be glioma-associated. However, isolation and characterization of these potential glioma-associated gangliosides from biopsy or autopsy material was rendered difficult as these tumors grow infiltratively (11), and tumor cells are mixed with normal brain cells.

One possible way to circumvent this problem is to work with human glioma cell lines, which provide a continous source of tumor cells that are not contaminated with normal brain cells. The established cell lines might also be used as an experimental model for studies on the regulation and functional roles of gangliosides. However, there are some features of the established glioma cell lines that have to be considered.

Human gliomas are heterogeneous and show both genotypic and phenotypic differences not only between tumors but also within one tumor (12, 13). The establishment of a glioma cell line involves a selection of one or few of the clones from the original tumor, and only the most malignant clones will grow (12, 14). Moreover it is known that both genotypic and phenotypic characteristics might be altered during culture (12, 15). These factors might also involve the expression of glioma associated gangliosides and the gangliosides isolated from the cell lines might not represent antigens of the original tumor.

Gangliosides of Human Glioma Cell Lines

Eleven human glioma cell lines were analysed with regard to their ganglioside composition by thin-layer chromatography, sialidase hydrolysis and detection of ganglioside antigens with specific monoclonal antibodies. The results showed large differences between the cell lines (Figure 1). Most ganglioside bands appeared in all cell lines but in various proportions. However, some gangliosides appeared to be specific for individual cell lines.

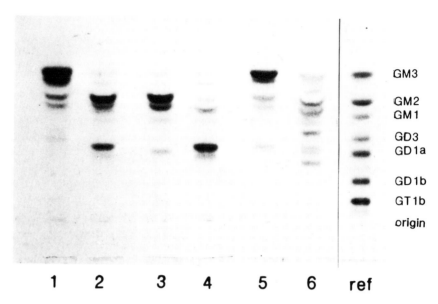

Figure 1. Thin-layer chromatographic seperation of gangliosides from various human glioma cell lines grown in culture. The gangliosides were extracted and separated according to the procedure described by Svennerholm et al. (21). The chromatographic solvent was chloroform/methanol/0.25 % KCL in water (50 : 50 : 10, by vol) and the ganglioside bands were visualized with the resorcinol reagent.

Isolation and Characterization of Potential Glioma-associated Gangliosides from the Human Glioma Cell Line D-54MG

Preliminary analyses by thin-layer chromatography had revealed that human glioma biopsies contained gangliosides that were not detected in normal adult human brain (9). At least some of these were also detected in an established glioma cell line (9). The D-54MG cell line had shown a relatively simple ganglioside pattern with one major component. This ganglioside band comigrated with one of the potential glioma-associated gangliosides detected in glioma tissue specimens. It appeared therefore likely that this cell line could be used for the isolation and characterization of one potential glioma-associated ganglioside.

In some cases human glioma cell lines could also be grown as solid tumors in nude mice (14, 16). This provides a sufficiently large and consistent source of tissue for ganglioside extraction, free of dilution by normal brain gangliosides. The D-54MG cell line grown as solid tumors in nude mice was therefore used as source for extraction and characterization of glioma-associated gangliosides (17).

The major gangliosides, constituting approximately 60 % of the total sialic acid, was 3'-isoLM1 (Figure 2). It should be noted that 90 % of the sialic acid was of the N-glycolyl form, which does not occur in human tissue. This reflects the influence of

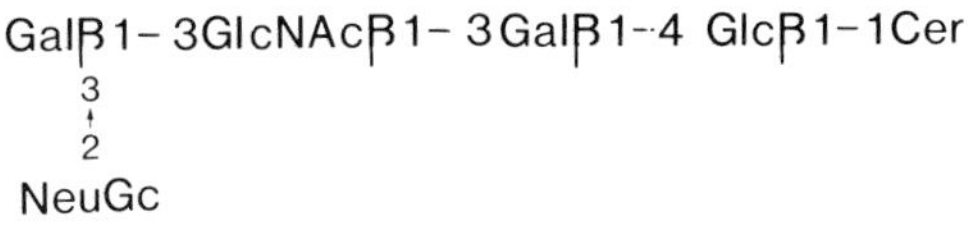

Galβ1– 3GlcNAcβ1– 3Galβ1–4 Glcβ1–1Cer
    3
    ↑
    2
NeuGc

Figure 2. Structure of the major ganglio-side, 3'-isoLM1, in the D-54MG cell line grown as solid tumors in nude mice.

the host on ganglioside metabolism and might limit the usefulness of nude mouse tumors for isolation of human glioma-associated ganglioside antigens. However, in our hands many monoclonal antibodies to gangliosides have shown the same reactivity with N-glycolyl and N-acetylneuraminic acid containing structures.

Determination of the Potential Glioma-associated Ganglioside 3'-isoLM1 in Human Glioma Tissue Specimens

The occurrence of 3'-isoLM1 in individual human glioma tissue specimens could only be shown by immunological techniques. We had previously produced a mono-clonal antibody to Fuc-3'-isoLM1, which crossreacted with 3'-isoLM1 (18). This anti-body was used for determination of the 3'-isoLM1 in biopsy material.

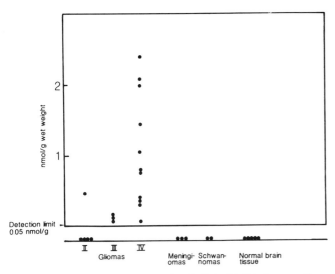

Figure 3. Occurrence of the ganglioside 3'-isoLM1 in human glioma biopsies. The determination was performed by radioimmunodetection of the antigen after separation of the ganglioside frac-tions on tlc-plates (10) using the C-50 antibody (18). The developing solvent was chloroform/methanol/2.5M ammonia (50:40:10, by vol). Ganglioside extract corresponding to 25 mg of tumor tissue and 100 mg of normal adult brain tissue was applied to the plate.

All biopsies were taken at operation and part of the material used for histopatho-logical analyses. The antigen was determined by radioimmunodetection after separation of the gangliosides on thin-layer plates (10). The results are illustrated in Figure 3 and 14/14 biopsies of grades III or IV (10) were positive, which means more than 0.05 nmol of 3'-isoLM 1/g tissue. The number of grade II tissue specimens was small but only one out of four was positive. Normal adult brain tissue did not show any detectable amounts of the antigen. Schwannomas and meningiomas were also negative.

The amount of antigen in the tissue specimens did not allow isolation and characterization of ganglioside from one individual, but when several specimens were pooled 3'-isoLM1 could be isolated and its structure verified by fast atom bombardment-mass spectrometry (10).

The ganglioside 3-isoLM1 or sialyllactotetraosylceramide has also been found in brain tissue from children who had died from infantile neuronal ceroid lipofuscinosis (INCL), also named polyunsaturated fatty acid lipidosis (PFAL) (19), a disease which is characterized by an intense reactive astrocytosis and astrogliosis (20). It is therefore suggested that 3'-isoLM1 is associated with proliferating astroglial cells and might be a marker for human malignant gliomas.

Summary

Human glioma cell lines could be used for isolation and characterization of glioma-associated gangliosides provided they still express those gangliosides. Ganglioside 3'-isoLM1 initially characterized in the D-54MG human glioma cell line was demonstrated by immune thin-layer chromatography in 14/14 glioma biopsies of grades III and IV. It is suggested to be a marker for human malignant gliomas.

References

1. Feizi, T.: Demonstration by monoclonal antibodies that carbohydrate structures of glyco-proteins and glycolipids are oncodevelopmental antigens. Nature 314, 53, 1985.
2. Hakomari, S. I.: Tumor-assoziated glycolipid antigens, their metabolism and organization. Chem. Phys. Lipid 42, 209, 1986.
3. Slagel, D. E., Dittmer, J. C., Wilson, C. B.: Lipid Composition of human glial tumor and adjacent brain. J. Neurochem. 14, 89, 1967.
4. Kosti'c, D., Bucheit, F.: Gangliosides in human brain tumors. Life Sci. 9, 589, 1970.
5. Yates, A. J., Thompson, D. K., Boesel, C. P., Albrightson, C., Hart, R.W.: Lipid composition of human neural tumors. J. Lipid Res. 20, 428, 1979.
6. Traylor, T. D., Hogan, E. L.: Gangliosides of human cerebral astrocytomas. J. Neurochem. 34, 216, 1980.
7. Eto, T., Shinoda, S.: Gangliosides and neutral glycosphingolipids in human brain tumors: specificity and their significance. Adv. Exp. Med. Biol. 152, 279, 1982.

8. Berra, B., Gaini, S. M., Riboni, L.: Correlation between ganglioside distribution and histological grading of human astrocytomas. Int. J. Cancer 36, 363, 1985.

9. Fredman, P., von Holst, H., Collins, V. P., Ammar, A., Dellheden, B., Wahren, B., Granholm, L., Svennerholm, L.: Potential ganglioside antigens associated with human gliomas. Neurol. Res. 8, 123, 1986.

10. Fredman, P., von Holst, H., Collins, V. P., Granholm, L., Svennerholm, L.: Sialyllactotetraosylceramide, a ganglioside marker for human malignant gliomas. J. Neurochem. 50, 912, 1988.

11. Russel, D. S., Rubistein, L. J. In: Pathology of the tumours of the nervous system, 4th edition 171.

12. Bigner, D. D., Bigner, S. H., Pontén, J., Westermark, B., Mahaley, M. S., Ruoslathi, E., Herschman, H., Eng, L. F., Wikstrand, C. J.: Heterogeneity of genotypic and phenotypic characteristics of fifteen permanent cell lines derived from human gliomas. J. Neuropath. Exp. Neurol. 40, 201, 1981.

13. Collins, V. P.: Cultured human glial and glioma cells. Exp. Rev. Exp. Pathology 24, 135, 1983.

14. Bigner, S. H., Bullard, D. E., Pegram, C. E., Wikstrand, C. J., Bigner, D. D.: Realtionship of in vitro morphology and growth characteristics of established human glioma-derived cell lines to their tumorgenicity in athymic mice. J. Neuropath. Exp. Neurol. 40, 309. 1981.

15. Markwell, M., Fredman, P., Svennerholm, L.: Receptor ganglioside content of three hosts for Sendai virus MDBK, HeLa and MDCK cells. Biochim. Biophys. Acta 775, 7, 1984.

16. Bullard, D. E., Bigner, D. D.: The heterotransplantation of human craniopharyngiomas in atymic nude mice. Neurosurgery. 4, 308, 1979.

17. Månsson, J.-E., Fredman, P., Bigner, D. D., Molin, K., Rosengren, B., Friedman, H. S., Svennerholm, L.: Characterization of new gangliosides of the lactotetraose series in murine xenografts of a human glioma cell line. FEBS Lett. 201, 109, 1986.

18. Nilsson, O., Månsson. J.-E., Lindholm, L., Holmgren, J., Svennerholm, L.: Sialyllactotetraosylceramide, a novel ganglioside antigen detected in human carcinomas by a monoclonal antibody. FEBS Lett. 182, 398, 1985.

19. Svennerholm, L., Fredman, P., Ljungbjer, B., Månsson, J.-E., Rynmark, B.-M., Boström, K., Hagberg, L., Norén, L., Santavouri, P.: Large alterations in ganglioside and neutral glycosphingolipid patterns in brains from cases with infantile neuronal ceroid lipofuscinosis/polyunsaturated fatty acid lipidosis (INCL/PFAL). J. Neurochem. 49, 1771, 1987.

20. Hagberg, L., Haltia, M., Sourander, P., Svennerholm, L., Eeg-Olofsson, O.: Polyunsaturated fatty acid lipidosis. Infantile form of so-called neuronal ceroidlipofuscinosis. I. Clinical and morphological aspects. Acta Paediatr. Scand. 63, 753, 1974.

21. Svennerholm, L., Fredman, P.: A procedure for the quantitative isolation of brain gangliosides. Biochim. Biophys. Acta 617, 97, 1980.

12. Exo-1, a Neutral Glycolipid of Human Epithelial Cells Expressed at Certain Stages of Spinous Cell Differentiation of Human Keratinocytes

R. Klingel, K.-H. Meyer zum Büschenfelde, and W. Dippold

Introduction

The instability of the transformed phenotype results from many epigenetic changes, deregulated differentiation programs and abnormal microenvironmental interactions (1, 2). Glycolipids are essential cellular structures involved in immunomodulatory events (3, 4), in the regulation of cell growth and proliferation (5–7), and in the regulation of the attachment of cells to a matrix (8, 9). They undergo significant changes in expression during embryonic and fetal development, differentiation and malignant transformation of cells (for review: 5, 10).

Exo-1, a polar neutral glycolipid was defined by the monoclonal antibody Pa G-14, which was raised against the human pancreatic cancer cell line Capan-1 (11). Especially with respect to its tissue distribution Exo-1 is a novel antigen of epithelial cells different from other glycolipid antigens like CA-50, MBr-1, SSEA-1 and novel fucolipids of human adenocarcinomas (12–16). As revealed by immunoelectron microscopy of duodenal microvilli which showed apical surface staining Exo-1 is a cell surface antigen especially of exocrine secretory epithelial cells and their derivative neoplastic cells (11).

To obtain further information about the biological significance of the Exo-1 antigen in epithelial cells we studied the changes in the expression of Exo-1 during human epidermal keratinocyte differentiation and development of benign and malignant neoplasia by immunohistochemistry.

Materials and Methods

Preparation of tissues: All tissue samples were snap-frozen and stored in liquid nitrogen until sectioned according to standard procedures.

Monoclonal antibodies and immunocytochemical staining: Mouse monoclonal antibody Pa G-14 (IgM) was raised against the human pancreatic cancer cell line Capan-1 (11). A pool of 5 : 1 concentrated hybridoma culture supernatant (Ig concentration 200 µg/ml) was used throughout the whole study.

Fresh frozen, non-fixed tissue sections (4–6 µm) were 1–2 h airdried and stained with Pa G-14 by an indirect immunoperoxidase method essentially as described previously (17). The immunochemical reaction was developed with the red stain 3-amino-9-ethylcarbazole. A monoclonal antibody to the mouse lymphocyte antigen Lyt. 1.1 (IgM) served as a negative control. The anti–HLA-A, B, C MoAb W6/32 was used as positive control for the immunochemical procedure (18).

Results and Discussion

In order to assess the biological significance of the Exo-1 antigen in human epithelial cells we studied the Exo-1 expression in human keratinocytes by immunohistochemical analysis of 106 non-fixed tissue specimens of human skin. Included were human skin at different stages of fetal development, normal adult human skin and different benign and malignant neoplastic skin lesions.

The results for normal adult and fetal human skin and benign neoplastic lesions are summarized in Table 1. In normal regularly stratified adult human epidermis Exo-1 was not detectable in basal or spinous cell layers (Figure 1A). In 25 tissue specimens tested staining was only seen in the areas of the inner root sheath and the matrix of the hair follicle, but not in the sebaceous gland. Luminal and apical cytoplasmic reactions were present in the eccrine sweat gland in accordance with the results for other secretory epithelial cells like salivary gland, breast and pancreas (11).

In the fetal epidermis membrane-bound and cytoplasmic staining was seen in intermediate cell layers at the 14th week of gestation (Figure 1B). At the 24th week of gestation the reaction was also present but restricted to the top layers of the intermediate cells. Enlargement of the spinous cell layer in adult skin is accompanied with the appearance of Exo-1 as revealed by staining of 24 specimens from ancanthosis, psoriasis and verruca vulgaris. Acanthotic epidermis for example enclosing or surrounding nevus cell nevi showed Exo-1 staining in spinous cell layers mainly accentuating the cell

Table 1. Exo-1 expression in normal adult and fetal human skin, hyperproliferative epidermis and benign epidermal neoplasia.

Tissue	Number tested	Exo-1 reactivity
normal adult skin	25	
basal cell layer		—
spinous cell layer		—
fetal skin	3	
(14th/24th week gestational age)		
basal cells		—
intermediate cells		+
Acanthosis	15	
basal cell layer		—
spinous cell layer		+
Psoriasis	5	
basal cell layer		(+)
spinous cell layer		+
Verruca vulgaris	4	
basal cell layer		—
spinous cell layer		+
Basal cell papilloma	4	—
Nevus cell nevus	15	—

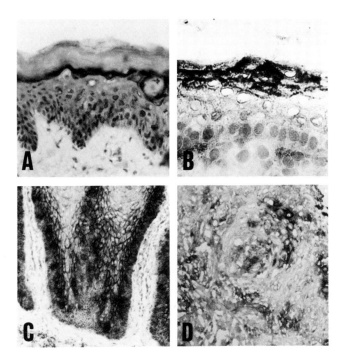

Figure 1. Exo-1 expression (A) in normal adult human skin staining negative: (B) in the intermediate cells of fetal skin at the 14th week of gestational age; (C) in spinous cell layers of a verruca vulgaris, and (D) in tumor cells of a moderately differentiated squamous cell carcinoma.

membrane. The same pattern was seen in verruca vulgaris (Figure 1C) and in psoriasis. In the psoriatic lesion additionally to the positive spinous cells the reaction started weakly in basal cells. As in the normal basal cells of regularly stratified epidermis Exo-1 was not detectable in the cells of 4 basal cell papillomas and 15 nevus cell nevi.

In regard to malignant epidermal neoplasia 4 specimens of Morbus Bowen, 6 squamous cell carcinomas, 10 basal cell epitheliomas, and 15 malignant melanomas were tested (Table 2). Precancerous skin lesions of the Morbus Bowen appeared histologically above an intact basement membrane but the regular stratification was broken off. Distributed in an unarranged manner about 50 % of the tumor cells were Exo-1 positive. The staining as well developed on the cell membrane as cytoplasmic. Keratinization or fusiform growth behaviour are morphological criteria to describe the differentiation of spinous cell carcinomas. The 6 moderately to low differentiated squamous cell carcinomas tested were heterogeneously composed of keratinizing and more anaplastic parts. Loss of differentiation was accompanied with a shift from cell membrane to cytoplasmic Exo-1 staining and the absolute number of positive cells decreased from 30–50 % to 10–30 % (Figure 1D). Where keratinization occurred typical membrane bound Exo-1 reactions were seen. Tumor cells of the basal cell epithelioma (10 specimen) and the malignant melanoma (15 specimen) were completely negative.

Table 2. Exo-1 expression in precancerous and malignant epidermal lesions.

Tissue	Number tested	Exo-1 reactivity (staining characteristics)
Precancerous Lesions/ Morbus Bowen	4	+ (app. 50% of cells; cytoplasmic staining; cell membrane staining partly confined to lower cell layers)
Squamous cell carcinomas	6	+ (10–50% of cells; spinous like cells typical staining accentuating the cell membrane)
Basal cell epithelioma	10	–
Malignant melanoma	15	–

The changes of Exo-1 expression during fetal development, differentiation and neoplastic transformation of human keratinocytes can be explained as part of a differentiation program that can be deregulated when neoplasia originates. Fetal keratinocytes of the intermediate cell type express the Exo-1 determinant cytoplasmic and membrane bound. In adult skin abnormal proliferative activity in spinous cells leads to a mainly membrane bound reemergence of the antigen. In general the concentration of neutral lipids and ceramides increases towards the surface layers of normal epidermis (19). Exo-1, however, was not detectable in the horny layer or in the sebaceous gland, so it should not be one of the skin lipids involved in the epidermal barrier function (20). Reexpression of this fetal antigen is not necessarily connected with malignant transformation as it is documented for the carcinoembryonic antigen or the alpha-1-fetoprotein, although the shift to more cytoplasmic expression in low differentiated squamous cell carcinomas contributes to an oncofetal character. This pattern has a certain similarity with the expression of the carbohydrate chain of the blood group antigen Le y, but which in its general tissue distribution differs from Exo-1 (21, 22, 23, 24). The weak Exo-1 staining in the basal cell layer of psoriatic skin lesions could point to a premature beginning of spinous cell differentiation. This disease entity is characterized by a short duration of the germinative cell cycle, a doubling of the proliferative cell population and an increase of the growth fraction (25). The development of malignancy may also lead to an abnormally localized expression of Exo-1 in the lower layers of an epidermal neoplasia, as it was deteced in some parts of the Morbus Bowen specimens, where the typical Exo-1 membrane bound reaction was confined to lower cell layers despite any morphological correlation. Exo-1 expression seems to be under control or at least under direct influence of transforming genes, as revealed by results with a spontaneously immortalized, non-tumorigenic human keratinocyte cell line (26). Grown under organotypical culture conditions the cells built up cell layers similar to normal adult human epidermis and did not express the Exo-1 determinant. Cells rendered tumorigenic by the Ha-ras oncogene or the SV 40 virus (P. Boukamp, unpublished data), stained positive for Exo-1 like squamous cell carcinoma tissues (data not shown).

Therefore Exo-1, a polar neutral glycolipid represents a novel antigenic determinant of human epithelial cells, which undergoes characteristic changes in expression during fetal development, at certain stages of spinous cell differentiation in adult human skin and in benign and malignant neoplasia. The functional role of its regulation in normal cells and wheather deregulated expression may contribute to neoplastic transformation will be the subject of further investigation.

Summary

Exo-1, a polar neutral glycolipid was defined by the monoclonal antibody Pa G-14. It is expressed on the apical cell surface of secretory epithelial cells, especially in the gastrointestinal tract. Further information about the biological significance of the Exo-1 antigen in epithelial cells was achieved by studying its expression in human keratinocytes undergoing cell differentiation and development of benign and malignant neoplasia. During fetal skin development Exo-1 is detectable in the intermediate cells. It is not present in normal adult, regularly stratified epidermis. Exo-1 reemergence occurred when development of benign or malignant neoplasia was based upon spinous like differentiated cells. Hyperproliferative spinous cells typically express Exo-1 membrane bound, whereas tumor cells showed a more cytoplasmic antigen expression or were negative. Therefore Exo-1 appears to be expressed in certain stages of spinous cell differentiation of normal and neoplastic human keratinocytes.

Acknowledgements

This work was supported by a grant from the BMFT DI/KN 01GA054.

References

1. Marks, P. A., Sheffery, M., Rifkind, R. A. Induction of transformed cells to terminal differentiation and the modulation of gene expression. Cancer Research 47, 659–666, 1987.
2. Sutherland, R. M. Cell and invironment interactions in tumor microregions: The multicell spheroid model. Science 249, 177–184, 1988.
3. Marcus, M. D. A review of the immunogenic and immunomodulatory properties of glycosphingolipids. Molecular Immunology 21, 1083–1091, 1984.
4. Dyatlovitskaya, E.V., L. D. Bergelson. Glycosphingolipids and antitumor immunity. Biochemica Biophysica Acta 907, 125–143, 1987.
5. Hakomori, S.-I. Aberrant glycosylation in cancer cell membranes as focussed on glycolipids: Overview and perspectives. Cancer Research 45, 2405–2414, 1985.
6. Spiegel, S., P. H. Fishman. Gangliosides as bimodal regulators of cell growth. Proc. Natl. Acad. Sci. USA 84, 141–145, 1987.

7. Kreutter, D., J.Y.H. Kim, H.R. Goldenring, H. Rasmussen, C. Ukomadu, R.J. deLorenzo, R.K. Yu. Regulation of protein kinase C activity by gangliosides. J. Biol. Chem. 262, 1633–1637, 1987.

8. Dippold, W.G., A. Knuth, K.-H. Meyer zum Büschenfelde. Inhibition of human melanoma cell growth in vitro by monoclonal anti-GC3-ganglioside antibody. Cancer Research 44, 806–810, 1984.

9. Cheresh, D.A., M.D. Pierschbacher, M.A. Herzig, K. Mujoo. Disialogangliosides GD2 and GD3 are involved in the attachment of human melanoma and neuroblastoma cells to extracellular matrix proteins. J. Cell Biol. 102, 689–696, 1986.

10. Feizi, T. Demonstration by monoclonal antibodies that carbohydrate structures of glycoproteins and glycolipids are onco-developmental antigens. Nature 314, 53–57, 1985.

11. Dippold, W.G., R. Klingel, H. Bernhard, H.-P. Dienes, A. Knuth, K.-H. Meyer zum Büschenfelde. Secretory epithelial cell marker on gastrointestinal tumors and in human secretions defined by monoclonal antibody. Cancer Research 47, 2092–2097, 1987.

12. Fukushi, Y., S.I. Hakomori, E. Nudelman, N. Cochran. Novel fucolipids accumulating in human adenocarcinoma. II. Selective isolation of hybridoma antibodies that differentially recognize mono-, di-, and trifucosylated type 2 chain. The Journal of Biological Chemistry 259, 4681–4685, 1984.

13. Fukushi, Y., E. Nudelman, S.B. Levery, S.-I. Hakomori. Novel fucolipids accumulating in human adenocarcinoma. III. A hybridoma antibody (FH6) defining a human cancer-associated difucoganglioside. The Journal of Biological Chemistry 259, 10511–10517, 1984.

14. Fox, N., I. Damjanov, B.B. Knowles, D. Solter. Immunohistochemical localization of the mouse stage-specific embryonic antigen 1 in human tissues and tumors. Cancer Research 43, 669–678, 1983.

15. Bremer, E.G., S.B. Levery, S. Sonnino, R. Ghidoni, S. Canevari, R. Kannagi, S.-I. Hakomori. Characterization of a glycosphingolipid antigen defined by the monoclonal antibody MBr1 expressed in normal and neoplastic epithelial cells of human mammary gland. The Journal of Biological Chemistry 259, 14773–14777, 1984.

16. Mansson, J.-E., P. Fredman, O. Nilsson, L. Lindholm, J. Holmgren, L. Svennerholm. Chemical structure of carcinoma ganglioside antigens defined by monoclonal antibody C-50 and some allied gangliosides of human pancreatic adenocarcinoma. Biochimica et Biophysica Acta 834, 110–117, 1985.

17. Dippold, W.G., H.-P. Dienes, A. Knuth, K.-H. Meyer zum Büschenfelde. Immunohistochemical localization of ganglioside GD3 in human malignant melanoma, epithelial tumors, and normal tissues. Cancer Research 45, 3699–3706, 1985.

18. Barnstable, C.J., W.F. Bodmer, G. Brown, G. Galfre, C. Milstein, A.F. Williams, A. Ziegler. Production of monoclonal antibodies to group A erythrocytes, HLA and other human cell surface antigens - new tools for genetic analysis. Cell 14, 9–20, 1978.

19. Elias, P.M. Epidermal lipids, barrier function, and desquamation. J. Invest. Dermatol. 80, 044s–049s, 1983.

20. Downing, D.T., M.E. Stewart, P.W. Wertz, S.W. Colton, W. Abraham, J.S. Strauss. Skin lipids: An update. J. Invest. Dermatol. 88, 2s–6s, 1987.

21. Dabelsteen, E., K. Holbrook, H. Clausen, S.-I. Hakomori. Cell surface carbohydrate changes during embryonic and fetal skin development. J. Invest. Dermatol. 87, 81–85, 1986.

22. Fukushi, Y., S.-I. Hakomori, T. Shepard. Localization and alteration of mono-, di-, and trifucosyl L - 3 type 2 chain structures during human embryogenesis and in human cancer. J. Exp. Med. 159, 506–520, 1984.

23. Cordon-Cardo, C., K.O. Lloyd, J. Sakamoto, M.E. McGroarty, L.J. Old, M.R. Melamed. Immunohistologic expression of blood-group antigens in normal human gastrointestinal tract and colonic carcinoma. Int. J. Cancer 37, 667–676, 1986.

24. Kim, Y. S., M. Yuan, S. H. Itzkowitz, Q. Sun, T. Kaizu, A. Palekar, B. F. Trump, S.-I. Hakomori. Expression of LE^Y and extended LE^Y blood group-related antigens in human malignant, premalignant, and nonmalignant colonic tissues. Cancer Research 46, 5985–5992, 1986.
25. Weinstein, G. D., J. L. McCullough, P. A. Ross. Cell kinetic basis for pathophysiology of psoriasis. J. Invest. Dermatol. 85, 579–583, 1985.
26. Boukamp, P., R.T. Petrussevska, D. Breitkreutz, J. Hornung, A. Markham, N. E. Fusenig. Normal keratinization in a spontaneously immortalized aneuploid human keratinocyte cell line. Journal of Cell Biology 106, 761–771, 1988.

13. Hepatoma-associated Gangliosides – Gangliosides with N-Acetyl-neuraminosyl(α2–6)-galactose Structure

T. Taki, K. Ishii, and A. Myoga

Summary

Gangliosides of hepatomas have been analyzed by a monoclonal antibody directed to N-acetylneuraminosyl ($\alpha2$–6)lactoneotetraosylceramide (sialyl[$\alpha2$–6]paragloboside), which was prepared by injecting the monosialoganglioside fraction of human meconium into BALB/c mice. The monoclonal antibody, named MSG-15, was found to bind sialyl ($\alpha2$–6)paragloboside by TCL-immunostaining method, but it failed to react with other ganglioside including GM3, GM2, GM1a, GM1b, GD1a, GD1b, GT1b, N-acetylneuraminosyl [$\alpha2$–3]lactoneoetraosyl ceramide (sialyl[$\alpha2$–3]paragloboside) and "Ii" type gangliosides.* Gangliosides from human hepatomas were analyzed by immunostaining on HPTLC-plate using the monoclonal antibody, MSG-15. All primary hepatoma samples used in the present study (nine samples) were found to contain sialyl ($\alpha2$–6)paragloboside, which accounted for 13–31 % of the monosialoganglioside fractions in the hepatomas. Furthermore, MSG-15 recognized several gangliosides in addition to sialyl($\alpha2$–6)paragloboside. These gangliosides also apparently contain a terminal NeuAC$\alpha2$–6Galβ structure. Bands showing similar mobilities with these gangliosides stained with MSG-15 were also detected in the monosialogangliosides of meconium. From these results, the NeuAc$\alpha2$–6Galβ structure of gangliosides appeared in the hepatoma is assumed to be an oncofetal antigen.

Glycoconjugates on cell surfaces change their chemical composition and metabolism in association with oncogenic transformation (2–4) and cell differentiation (5, 6). Some gangliosides in tumor tissues or cells have been proposed as tumor-associated antigens (7, 9). Glycosphingolipids of meconium have been demonstrated to contain many kinds of oligosaccharide structures including Le^X and Le^Y which are tumor-associated (10–12). Based on these informations, we tried to prepare monoclonal antibodies directed to tumor-associated antigens by immunizing the ganglioside fraction from meconium.

In the present paper, we describe the preparation of monoclonal antibody against sialyl($\alpha2$–6)paragloboside and its application to the detection of the ganglioside in hepatoma samples. We could find various glycolipids containing NeuAc$\alpha2$–6Galβ structure at their nonreducing terminals by a TLC-immunostaining technique in hepatomas and meconium gangliosides.

---

*Abbreviations used are: sialyl($\alpha2$–6)paragloboside, NeuAc$\alpha2$–6Galβ1–4GlcNAcβ1–3Galβ1–4Glcβ1–1Cer; Sialyl($\alpha2$–3)paragloboside, NeuAC$\alpha2$–3Galβ1–4GlcNAcβ1–3Galβ1–4Glcβ1–1Cer; i-ganglioside, NeuAc$\alpha2$–3Galβ1–4GlcNAcβ1–3Galβ1–4GlcNAcβ1–3Galβ1–4Glcβ1–1Cer; I-ganglioside. NeuAc$\alpha2$–3Galβ1–4GlcNAcβ1–3(NeuAc$\alpha2$–3Galβ1–4GlcNacβ1–6)Galβ1–4GlcNAcβ1–3Galβ1–4Glcβ1–1Cer; (other abbrevations for ganglio-series gangliosides are according to Svennerholm[1]); HPTLC, high performance thin layer chromatography.

Materials and Methods

Preparation of Monoclonal Antibody Directed to Monosialoganglioside Fraction from Meconium. Immunization was performed by the method of Young et al. (13). About hundred μg of monosialoganglioside of meconium was suspended in 40 μg of acid treated *S. minnesota* in 0.5 ml of phosphate buffered saline (pH 7.4). The monosialogangliosides suspension was injected subcutaneously in BALB/c mice four times at weekly intervals. Three days after the last injection, the spleen was removed for fusion. Preparation of hybridomas and enzyme linked immunosorbent assay (ELISA) method for antibody detection were performed as described previously (14).

Isolation of Gangliosides from Human Hepatomas and Meconium. Nine samples of primary hepatomas were used in the present study. The wet weight of each sample was about 1–5 g. Hepatoma tissue was homogenized with 20 volumes of a mixture of chloroform/methanol (2 : 1, v/v). The homogenate was filtered. The filtrate was evaporated under reduced pressure in a rotary evaporator. The residue was dissolved in 20 ml of a mixture of chloroform/methanol/water (30 : 60 : 8, v/v/v) and applied to DEAE Sephadex A-25 column (1 : 2 x 10 cm). Neutral lipids, phopholipids and neutral glycolipids were eluted with a mixture of chloroform/methanol/water (30 : 60 :8, v/v/v). Monosialogangliosides were eluted with a mixture of chloroform/methanol/0.05 M sodium acetate, (30 : 60 :8, v/v/v).

Meconium (720g) was homogenized with 7.2 l of the solvent mixture of chloroform/methanol (2 : 1, v/v). The lipid extract was evaporated to dryness under reduced pressure, suspended in distilled water, dialyzed against distilled water and lyophilized. Ten gram of the crude extract was dissolved in 100 ml of the mixture of chloroform/methanol/water (30 : 60 :8, v/v/v). Insoluble materials was removed by centrifugation and washed with the solvent mixture several times. The supernatants were combined and applied to a DEAE Sephadex A-25 column (3.2 x 45 cm). Neutral glycolipids was eluted with the solvent mixture of chloroform/methanol/water (30 : 60 : 8, v/v/v) and monosialoganglioside fraction was eluted with the solvent mixture of chloroform/methanol/0.05 M sodium acetate (30 : 60 : 8, v/v/v). By this procedure, 2.53g of neutral glycolipid fraction and 0.87g of monosialoganglioside fraction were obtained.

High Performance Liquid Chromatography (HPLC). About 10 mg of monosialoganglioside fraction was applied to HPLC (Shimadzu LC-4A) equiped with a Iatrobeads column (6RS 8010, 3 x 180 mm, donated from Iaton Co. Ltd. Tokyo, Japan) which was equilibrated with a mixture of isopropanol/hexane/water (55 : 40 : 5, v/v/v). Ganglioside was dissolved with the solvent mixture of chloroform/methanol (2 : 1, v/v) and subjected to the HPLC. Gangliosides were eluted with a gradient elution manner of mixture of isopropanol/hexane/water (55 : 40 : 5 – 55 : 25 : 20, v/v/v). Flow rate was 1 ml/min, and each fraction contained 1 ml. An aliquot was taken from each fraction and analyzed by thin layer chromatography (TLC).

Immunostaining on HPTLC-plate. Immunostaining of glycolipid on HPTLC-plate was performed as reported by Saito et al. (15) with the following modification; substrate, 3,3'-diaminobenzidine for peroxidase was substituted with 4-chloro-1-naphthol reagent. The substrate solution was prepared as follow: 1 ml of methanol solution of 4-chloro-1-naphthol (3 mg/ml) was mixed with 5 ml of 100 mM NaCl/0.1 M tris-HCl buffer (pH 7.2) and 10 μl of hydrogen peroxide was added. As the first antibody, MSG-15 (IgM type) was used.

Results and Discussion

Monosialogangliosides of Meconium. Seven hybridomas secreting monoclonal antibodies which bound to the monosialoganglioside fraction of meconium were obtained. One of the seven monoclonal antibodies, MSG-15 was selected based on the reactivity and specificity to a monosialoganglioside. In order to determine the structure of the epitope recognized by the MSG-15 antibody, the monosialoganglioside fraction was separated by HPLC. Elution profile was monitored by TLC (Figure 1). Three gangliosides (MG-1, MG-2, and MG-3) were separated as shown in Figure 1. Fractions eluted after fraction number 100 contained several gangliosides. The MG-1 ganglioside was identified as GM3 by TLC. MG-2 showed similar mobility with sialyl(α2–3)paragloboside and MG-3 was suggested to be sialyl(α2–6)paragloboside from its mobility on TLC and also according to the report by Nilsson et al. (12) (Figure 2).

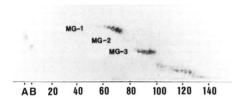

Figure 1. HPLC elution profile of monosialogangliosides of human meconium. The fraction eluted from HPLC were analyzed by TLC. The solvent system was chloroform/methanol/o.2 % CaCl2 (60 : 40 : 9, v/v/v). Gangliosides were visualized by spraying with resorcinol/HCl reagent. Lane A und B show the standard GM3 and the sialyl(α2–3)paragloboside, respectively.

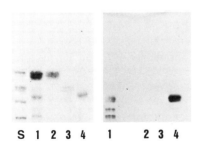

Figure 2. Purified gangliosides and immunostaining with the MSG15 antibody on HPTLC plate. A, TLC of monosialogangliosides and purified monosialogangliosides. B, immunostaining on HPTLC with the MSG15 antibody. Lane S, the standard gangliosides, GM3, sialyl(α2–3)para-globoside, i-ganglioside and I-ganglioside from the top to bottom; lane 1, monosialogangliosides of human meconium; lane 2, MG1; lane 3, MG2; lane 4, MG3.

Structure of MG-3 Ganglioside. Purified gangliosides, MG-1, MG-2, and MG-3 were subjected to immunostaining on HPTLC plate using the MSG-15 antibody. Since MSG-15 was found to bind MG-3 ganglioside as shown in Figure 2, the structure of MG-3 ganglioside was analyzed by glycosidase treatments, NMR spectrum and methylation analysis.

By the treatment of *Cl. perfringens* sialidase, the MG-3 ganglioside was converted to a lipid showing similar mobility with paragloboside on TLC. The asialo-compound of MG3 was converted to lactotriaosylceramide by the treatment of β-galactosidase and then converted to lactosylceramide by β-hexosaminidase treatment.

NMR spectrum of the MG3 ganglioside is shown in Figure 3. Assignments of signals of anomeric protons appeared between 4 and 5 ppm are indicated in the figure. Quartet peaks at 2.69, 2.67, 2.66, and 2.64 ppm were assigned as equatrial 3-H of N-acetyl-

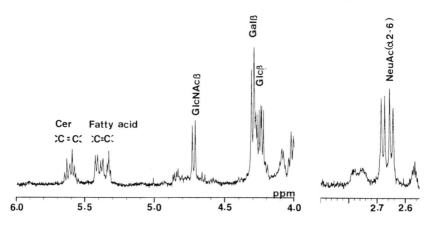

Figure 3. NMR spectrum of MG3. MG3 was dissolved in 0.5 ml of Me_2SO-d_6 containing 10 % D_2O. NMR was obtained by a JEOL Fx-400 spectrometer at 90°C.

neuraminic acid which is attached to 6-C position of hexose or hexosamine. From the area of anomeric proton and equatrial 3-H of NeuAc, the molar ratios of βGal : βGlc-NAc : βGlc : αNeuAc was determined to 2 : 1 : 1 : 1.

Methylation analysis of the MG3 ganglioside by gas chromatography-mass spectrometry indicated the presence of 3-substituted galactose, 4-substitute N-acetyl-glucosamine, 4-substituted glucose, and 6-substituted galactose. Methylation study indicated that N-acetylneuraminic acid is linked to 6-C position of terminal galactose of lactotetraosylceramide. From these data, the structure of MG3 was determined to be NeuAcα2–6Galβ1–4GlcNAcβ1–3Galβ1–4Glcβ1–1Cer (sialyl[α2–6]paragloboside).

Gangliosides Recognized with the MSG15 Monoclonal Antibody. As shown in Figure 2 the MSG15 monoclonal antibody was found to bind MG3 ganglioside, that is, sialyl(α2–6)paragloboside. When monosialoganglioside fraction was stained with MSG15, however, together with the MG3 ganglioside, two additional bands were visualized. Recently, we separated these bands and demonstrated by NMR that these slower migrating gangliosides have the same terminal sequence as MG3 (NeuAcα2–6Galβ). The MSG15 antibody failed to react with other gangliosides including GM3, GM2, GM1a, GM1b, GD1a, GD1b, GT1b, sialyl(α2–3)paragloboside and "Ii" type gangliosides. The result indicate that the antibody is specific for the NeuAcα2–6Galβ structure.

A titration curve of MSG15 obtained by using sialyl(α2–6)paragloboside as antigen is shown in Figure 4. One nanogram of sialyl(α2–6)paragloboside could be visualized by the immunostaining technique on HPTLC-plate.

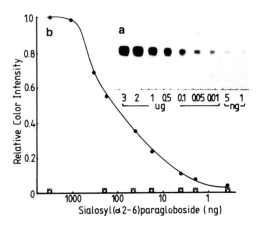

Figure 4. Assay of binding activity of the MSG15 antibody to the sialyl(α2–6)paragloboside. a, various amount of the sialyl(α2–6)paragloboside were applied to TLC and binding activity of the MSG15 antibody to the ganglioside was tested by the immunostaining. b, tritration curve obtained by the immunostaining method. Color intensity was measued by a TLC chromato-scanner (Shimadzu CS-910). ●, sialyl(α2–6)paragloboside; ○, sialyl(α2–3)paragloboside; □, GM$_3$.

The Sialyl(α2–6)paragloboside in Monosialoganglioside Fraction of Primary Hepatomas. Monosialoganglioside fractions from nine primary hepatoma samples were developed on HPTLC plate and subjected to immunostaining with the MSG15 antibody. All hepatoma samples used in the present study found to contain bands stained with the antibody and these bands showed same mobilities as that of the sialyl-(α2–6)paragloboside (Figure 5). Furthermore, five samples (No. 3, 6, 7, 8, and 9) contained some other gangliosides stained with the monoclonal antibody. These bands seemed to be gangliosides containing NeuAcα2–6Galβ structure at their terminals. These gangliosides showed similar mobilities with slower moving meconium gangliosides stained with MSG15 (data not shown here). The sialyl(α2–6)paragloboside content in each monosialoganglioside fraction of hepatomas was determined by densitometric analysis. The concentrations of the sialyl(α2–6)paragloboside were 13–31% of total monosialogangliosides but that of normal liver was only 3%. If the gangliosides stained by the MSG15 antibody were combined, gangliosides with NeuAcα2–6Galβ structure accounted for about 50% in one case (sample No. 9). The major monosialoganglioside in normal liver was GM3 accounting for 87% and the rest was mainly sialyl(α2–3)paragloboside. These results indicate that the activity of sialyltransferase catalyzing the formation of NeuAcα2–6Galβ structure at non-reducing terminal of glycolipid is enhanced in hepatoma tissue, and the NeuAcα2–6Galβ structure is an oncofetal antigen.

Hakomori and his co-workers reported the preparation of a monoclonal antibody directed to NeuAcα2–6Galβ (16). The antibody, named IB9, seemed to have similar specificity to the monoclonal antibody, MSG15. They showed the accumulation of NeuAcα2–6Galβ containing gangliosides in a human liver adenocarcinoma. Nilsson et al. (17) prepared a monoclonal antibody, LM4, directed to sialyl(α2–6)para-globoside, and demonstrated that gangliosides with NeuAcα2–6Galβ substitution were enriched in carcinomas. In the present study, we also found accumulation of the sialyl(α2–6)paragloboside and several other gangliosides containing the terminal NeuAcα2–6Galβ structure in hepatomas and in meconium. The gycolipids containing the NeuAcα2–6Galβ are rarely found in gangliosides. Two types of gangliosides, sialyl(α2–6)paragloboside and sialyl(α2–6)lactoneohexaosylceramide, have been isolated from human red cells (18). But the quantity of these gangliosides was very low (less than 2 % of total gangliosides of human erythrocytes) (18). From this point of view, the gangliosides with NeuAcα2–6Galβ structure seem to be hepatoma asso-ciated gangliosides.

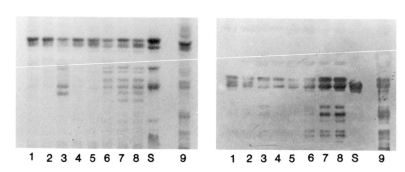

Figure 5. Immunostaining of monosialoganglioside fractions obtained from nine hepatoma samples. a, TLC of monosialogangliosides of hepatoma samples. Gangliosides were visualized by spraying with resorcinol/HCl reagent. b, immunostaining of the hepatoma monosialo-gangliosides with the monoclonal antibody MSG15.

The solvent system was chloroform/methanol/0.2 % CaCl$_2$ (55 : 45 : 10, v/v/v).

Lane 1 to 9 are hepatoma samples; lane S, the standard gangliosides, GM3, sialyl(α2–3)-paragloboside and sialyl(α2–6)paragloboside from the top to bottom.

Acknowledgements

This work was supported by a Grant in Aid from The Ministry of Education, Science and Culture of Japan.

References

1. Svennerholm, L. J. Lipid Res. 5, 145–155, 1964.
2. Yogeeswaran, G. Adv. Cancer Res. 38, 289–350, 1983.
3. Hakomori, S. Ann. Rev. Immunol. 2, 103–126, 1984.
4. Hakomori, S. Cancer Res. 45, 2405–2414, 1985.
5. Hakomori, S. Ann. Rev. Biochem 50, 733–764, 1981.
6. Taki, T., Kawamoto, M., Seto, H., Noro, N., Masuda, T., Kannagi, R., and Matsumoto, M. J. Biochem. 94, 633–644, 1983.
7. Magnani, J. L., Nilsson, B., Brockhouse, M., Zopor, D., Steplewski, Z., Koprowski, H., and Ginsberg, V. J. Biol. Chem. 157, 14365–14369, 1982.
8. Nudelman, E., Hakomori, S., Kannagi, R., Levery, S., Yeh, M. Y., Hellstrom, K. E., and Hellstrom, I. J. Biol. Chem. 257, 12752–12756, 1982.
9. Fukushima, K., Hirota, M., Terasaki, P. I., Wakisaka, A., Togashi, H., China, D., Suyama, N., Fukushi, Y., Nudelman, E., and Hakomori, S. Cancer Res. 44, 5279–5285, 1984.
10. Karlsson, K. A., and Larson, G. J. Biol. Chem 254, 9311–9316, 1979.
11. Karlsson, K. A., and Larson, G. J. Biol. Chem. 256, 3512–3524, 1981.
12. Nilsson, O., Mansson, J. E., Tibblin, E., and Svennerholm, L. FEBS Lett. 133, 197–200, 1981.
13. Young, Jr.W.W., MacDonal, E. M. S., Nowinski, R. C., and Hakomori, S. J. Exp. Med. 150, 1008–1019, 1979.
14. Myoga, A., Taki, T., Arai, K., Sekiguchi, K., Ikeda, I., Kurata, K., and Matsumoto, M. Cancer Res. 48, 1512–1516, 1988.
15. Saito, M., Kasai, N., and Yu, R. K. Anal. Biochem. 148, 54–58, 1985.
16. Hakomori, S., Nudelman, E., Levery, S. B., and Patterson, C. M. Biochem. Biophys. Res. Commun. 113, 791–798, 1983.
17. Nilsson, O., Lindholm, L. Holmgren, J., and Svennerholm, L. Biochim. Biophys. Acta 835, 577–583, 1985.
18. Hakomori, S., Patterson, C. M., Nudelman, E., and Sekiguchi, K., J. Biol. Chem. 258, 11819–11822, 1983.

14. Analysis of Tumor-associated Gangliosides in Acute Leukemic Lymphoblasts Utilizing Anti-GD3 and Anti-GM3 Monoclonal Antibodies

W. D. Merritt, M.-B. Sztein, and G. H. Reaman

Introduction

Lymphoid leukemias of childhood have been subclassified as T-cell and non-T-cell based on the presence or absence to surface antigenic markers. For instance, monoclonal antibodies (mAb) which detect the major cluster group CD7 bind to normal T-cells and thymocytes and are diagnostic for T-cell acute lymphoblastic leukemia (T-ALL)(1). Non-T-ALL appears to be derived from cells of the pre-B stage of lymphoid differentiation based on the presence of pre-B surface markers (2). At present, the significance of the presence of many of these surface antigens is not well understood. Glycolipid antigens, which are homogeneous molecules and can be readily isolated and characterized, offer alternative antigenic sites against which monoclonal antibodies can be directed in this disease.

Analysis of the glycolipid composition of lymphoid malignancies in our previous studies demonstrated the ganglioside GD3 is a major ganglioside of lymphoblasts obtained from children with T-cell ALL, whereas this ganglioside is not found in non-T-ALL blasts (3). Non-T-ALL blasts contained GM3 and varying amounts of sialyl-lactoneotetraosylceramide (sialylparagloboside, SPG) as the major gangliosides. We also showed that a mAb reactive against GD3, R24, detected GD3 in lipid extracts of T-ALL blasts, utilizing the HPTLC immunooverlay technique (4). This report summarizes our studies to date on the immunocytochemical analysis of T-ALL and non-T-ALL with anti-GD3 (R24) antibody. Additionally, we have tested by immunoflourescence the binding to leukemic blasts of the monoclonal antibody M2590, which has specificity for the gangliosides GM3 and SPG (5), and report on the ratio of these two antibodies as a measure of the ganglioside expression in T-ALL and non-T-ALL.

Reactivity of Anti-GD3 Monoclonal Antibodies to T-ALL

Initial studies of the binding of R24 to T-ALL and non-T-ALL blasts by indirect immunofluorescence and FACS analysis showed that GD3 was detected in the T-ALL sample, but not in the non-T-ALL cells (4). We have now extended this study to assess binding of R24 in a large number of T-ALL and non-T-ALL patient samples to determine the ubiquity of R24 binding to T-ALL lymphoblasts, and to determine whether GD3 is indeed absent in non-T-ALL (6). The data from all T-ALL samples studied to date is summarized in Table 1 along with analyses of other surface markers of T-ALL. Out of 50 patients diagnosed with T-ALL, based on reactivity with an anti-CD7 antibody, 37 stained positive for GD3. Comparisons of anti-GD3 reactivity and those of other markers revealed that R24 did not stain the same population of cells stained by any other marker, but rather delineated a novel subpopulation of T-ALL. The closest correlation was observed with staining with anti-CD2, an antibody that reacts with the sheep red blood cell receptor, in that 6 out of 7 CD2$^-$ samples were GD3$^-$, and all GD3$^+$ samples were CD2$^+$. However, the GD3$^-$ population is larger than the CD2$^-$ popula-

Table 1. Surface marker analysis of T-cell-ALL.

Anti-GD$_3$	Anti-CD7	Anti-CD2	Anti-CD3
37/50*	50/50	43/50	12/50
(74%)	(100%)	(86%)	(24%)

* Ratio of positive populations to the total number of patients analyzed for anti-GD$_3$ (R24) and other surface markers.

tion. In contrast to the results with T-ALL, none of the 33 non-T-ALL samples tested reacted with anti-GD3 in an indirect positive immunofluorescence assay (6). This confirmed the results obtained by the HPTLC immunooverlay technique (4) and indicated the absence of GD3 in the subclass of lymphoid leukemia.

Immunofluorescence in each positive sample of T-ALL varied widely with regard to the number of stained lymphoblasts; a range from 11% to 93% was observed (6). In an attempt to determine whether this heterogeneity in staining with R24 was a reflection of varying content of GD3 or a reflection of low anti-GD3 reactivity due to cryptogenicity of the GD3 in the cell surface membrane, we have tested R24 binding in T-ALL and non-T-ALL blasts after treatment with trypsin. Results with 9 T-ALL patients that were widely variant in staining showed that staining was not enhanced after trypsin pretreatment (6). T-ALL cells that did not stain positive with R24 were unaffected by trypsin, and staining of non-T-ALL blasts also was negative after trypsin. These studies suggest that the wide range in R24 binding in T-ALL is due to constitutive differences in the ganglioside content of the blasts rather than due to differences in the cell surface availability of the ganglioside for antibody binding.

In vitro cytotoxicity studies with anti-GD3 mAb in other laboratories show that anti-GD3 mediates both complement and antibody-dependent cytolysis of melanoma target cells (7–10). Treatment of melanoma patients at Sloan-Kettering Institute with the R24 antibody has resulted in partial remissions in phase I trials (11, 12). We therefore have studied the ability of R24 to lyse leukemic lymphoblasts in both complement-mediated lysis (CML) and antibody-dependent (ADCC) assays. Utilizing human serum as the source of complement, lymphoblasts of the T-cell lineage which were positive for R24 binding in immunofluorescence assays, also were lysed by R24 in the CML assay (Reaman et al., manuscript in preparation). The percent of positive cells by immunofluorescence generally correlated with % cytolysis in the CML assay. A second anti-GD3 antibody, C281, which was obtained from Dr. David Cherish, Scripps Institute, bound to T-cell leukemia blasts with nearly the same reactivity as R24. This antibody also was cytolytic in the CML assay. Both antibodies failed to lyse GD3 blasts or blasts from patients with non-T-ALL. R24 was similarly effective in mediating cytolysis of GD3$^+$ T-ALL blasts in the ADCC assay, utilizing human peripheral blood lymphocytes as the effector cell population. ADCC ranged from 18 to 54% cytolysis and no cytolysis occurred in a GD3$^-$T-ALL population. The results show that anti-GD3 mAb are not only cytotoxic for melanoma cells but are also cytotoxic for a large subclass of T-ALL which express GD3 at the cell surface.

M2590 Immunofluorescence Analysis of T-ALL and Non-T-ALL

Due to the heterogeneity in staining of T-ALL with R24 and lack of staining of non-T-ALL, a second anti-ganglioside antibody was sought ich when used in conjunction with anti-GD3 might provide a representative measure of ganglioside expression in lymphoid leukemias. Therefore, the M2590 antibody, which was found to react with GM3 and SPG in lipid extracts of non-T-ALL and GM3 in T-ALL (4), was tested for its ability to stain these blasts by immunocytochemical techniques. A comparison of FACS analysis results of M2590 binding and R24 binding to blasts from a patient with T-ALL and a patient with non-T-ALL is shown in Figure 1. T-ALL blasts were 58.8 % positive for R24 and staining was highly heterogeneous, while no staining of non-T cells was observed (5.5 % positive cells). However, M2590 anti GM3/SPG antibody stained a high percentage of non-T cells (45.4 % positive cells), although staining was dim. A low percentage of T-ALL blasts was positive for M2590 (15.1 %), and staining was also very dim.

The inverse nature of staining of blasts from T-ALL and non-T-ALL with R24 and M2590 antibodies suggested that a ratio of the percent of cells stained positive with these antibodies (R24/M2590) would yield a quantitative measure of GD3 expression in T-ALL relative to non-T-ALL, and may also distinguish a subpopulation of T-ALL which is GD3$^-$. The ratio R24/M2590 in the T-ALL population described above was 3.9, while this ratio in the non-T-ALL sample was 0.12. This ratio in a T-ALL blast pulation that was 10 % positive for R24 binding was 0.07, with R24 staining 2.7 %, and M2590 39.4 %. Since the ratio R24/M2590 in this T-ALL population was similar to that of the non-T-ALL population, it appears that the ratio of these two antibodies defines a subpopulation of T-ALL with low or absent anti-GD3 antibody expression. Although these results are preliminary, we propose that a ratio of R24/M2590 >1.0 in T-ALL defines a GD3$^+$ subpopulation, while a ratio <1.0 defines a non-T-ALL population or a subpopulation of T-ALL which is GD3$^-$.

The effect of trypsin on M2590 staining has also been recently examined in order to assess whether the dim staining of M2590 on T-ALL and non-T-ALL could be due to cryptogenicity of the ganglioside. In three patients studied to date, the low binding of M2590 to T-ALL was not affected by trypsin treatment. On the other hand, binding of M2590 to two non-T-ALL patient blasts was enhanced from 14 to 47 % positive cells and from 19 to 74 % positive cells, suggesting that the gangliosides GM3 and/or SPG in non-T-ALL cells are indeed cryptic in their cell membrane location.

Discussion

A summary of the pathways of lymphoid cell differentiation is presented in Figure 2. While non-T-ALL appears to be the neoplastic counterpart of pre-B lymphocytes, T-ALL results from the malignant transformation of thymocytes at various stages of

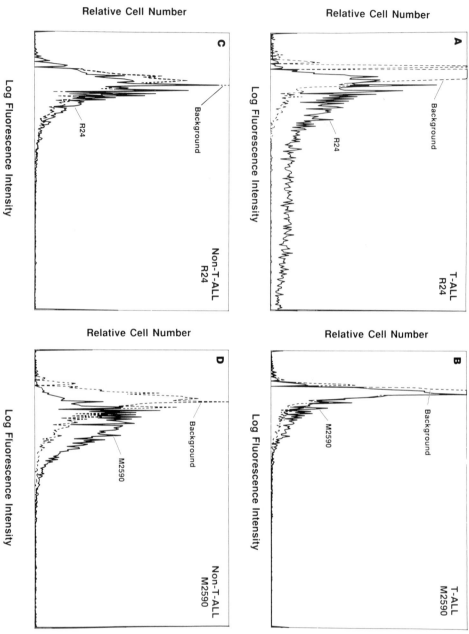

Figure 1. FACS analysis of R24 and M2590 mAb staining of T-ALL and non-T-ALL. Blasts from a T-ALL and a non-T-ALL patient were incubated with R24 or M2590 mAb followed by either FITC-labelled anti-mouse IgG or IgM, respectively. The cells were then washed, fixed with paraformaldehyde, and analyzed by flow cytometry using a FACS IV instrument (Bectin-Dickinson). The percent of positive cells was determined against a background of cells stained with MOPC-21 (an IgG purified protein of unknown specificity derived from a mouse myeloma) or normal mouse 1gM for leukemic cells stained with R24 or M2590, respectively.

Pathways of Hematopoietic Differentiation and Subclasses of Lymphoid Leukemia

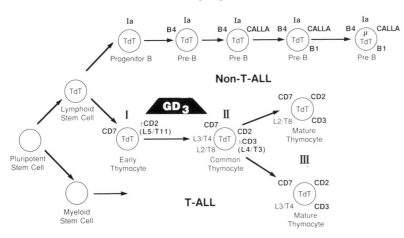

Figure 2. Pathways of hematopoietic differentiation and subclasses of lymphoid leukemia. The surface antigens tested in non-T-ALL (pre-B) and T-ALL are indicated in bold. CD7, CD2, and CD3 appear in progressively mature stages of T-ALL. GD3 apparently appears in a relatively early stage of T-ALL as depicted, in that this ganglioside is found in 74 % of T-ALL cases studied to date (adapted from Foon, 20).

differentiation (I–III). The results of our studies on the ganglioside composition of T-ALL and non-T-ALL cell membranes clearly show that GD3 appears only in leukemic lymphoblasts arising in the T-cell group of lymphoid malignancies of childhood. However, Gd3 expression was not ubiquitous in T-ALL, in that 26 % of 50 patient samples were negative for GD3. Among the common T-cell surface antibodies tested, only the expression of the erythrocyte receptor antigen (CD2) correlated with GD3 expression. Reactivity of anti-GD3 was restricted to the $CD7/CD2^+$ phenotype; however, the $GD3^-$ subclass is larger than the CD2 subclass in that $6 \, CD7^+/CD2^+$ blast populations were negative for GD3. GD3 expression therefore defines a unique subclass of T-ALL.

We have currently begun to assess the expression of GD3 in leukemic lymphoblasts as it relates to expression of two other gangliosides found in these cells, GM3 and SPG. One anti-ganglioside antibody, M2590, was particularly valuable in that it reacted to both these gangliosides in lipid extracts in non-T-ALL and GM3 in T-ALL. We found that this antibody was reactive with non-T-ALL blasts, although fluorescence was dim; the antibody reacted poorly with T-ALL blasts. Trypsin treatment enhanced the staining to the non-T-ALL cells, but had no effect on the T-ALL blasts. Since GM3 is a major ganglioside in T-ALL and non-T-ALL leukemic lymphoblasts, as determined by resorcinol detection or by immunostaining with M2590, the low immunoreactivity of M2590 to the samples of T-ALL blasts studied to date was surprising. Recent studies of M2590 reactivity with cell surfaces show a dependence on density of GM3, with a high threshold concentration required for immunoreactivity (13). T-ALL and non-T-ALL blasts may not contain threshold concentrations of GM3, whereas the concentration and/or conformation of SPG in non-T-ALL blasts may result in an antigenic species recognizable by M2590 antibody. Further studies are required to assess the specific reactivity of M2590 in leukemic lymphoblasts.

Although the exact ganglioside specificity of M2590 reactivity is unclear, this antibody is a useful antibody to react with gangliosides of non-T-ALL. The ratio of R24/M2590 <1.0 is due to the absence of GD3 in non-T-ALL. With respect to T-ALL, we initially chose 10 % positive cells as a cut-off % to distinguish the positive from negative GD3 population, an arbitrary figure. Since the assignment of a patient to GD3⁺ or GD3⁻ may have prognostic significance (see below), a more reliable assessment of the GD3⁺ vs. GD3⁻ population is required. Since the ratio of R24/M2590 is <1.0 in patients studied to date with low GD3 content, similar to non-T-ALL, we propose that the ratios of these antibodies may provide a more definitive cut-off to distinguish these populations.

The ganglioside GD3 was detected by Macher and colleagues in acute myelogenous leukemias but not in chronic myelogenous leukemias, and in both chronic and acute lymphoid leukemias (14). The possible immunoreactivity of R24 antibody to GD3 on the cell surface of these blasts by immunofluorescence techniques was not shown. Our studies extend analysis of GD3 in the acute lymphoid leukemias to show the restriction to the T-cell subclass of this disease. In a recent study by Kyogashima et al. (15), the lipid extracts from blasts from a T-All patient contained 52 % GD3 and 45 % GM3 while the ganglioside content of the cells from a second patient was 100 % GM3. The non-T-ALL patient cells studied contained only GM3. GD3 was not found in any of the myeloid leukemia cells studied. GD3 has also been found in cell lines established from adult T-cell leukemic lymphoblasts, although the ganglioside pattern in these lines is much more complex than that found in blasts from 2 patients with adult T-ALL (16) or that found in blasts from childhood T-ALL patients that we have studied.

In contrast to the generally high percentage of T-ALL lymphoblasts which express GD3 as shown by this report, only a small percentage of the peripheral blood T-lymphocytes express this ganglioside (17). The expression of this ganglioside is increased by the anti-GD3 antibodies or non specific lectins (17, 18); this appears to be due to expansion of the GD3⁺ pool (17). The fact that all T lymphocytes do not express GD3 upon lectin stimulation suggests that this ganglioside may not be a lymphocyte proliferation antigen but rather in T-All reflects the malignant transformation of early T lymphocytes. That GD3 is expressed on a large number of fetal thymocytes (17) supports this hypothesis. Since GD3 is expressed in T-ALL blasts and not in non-T-ALL strongly suggests that GD3 is not passively absorbed to the cell surface from serum of T-ALL patients, although the enzymatic basis for enhanced GD3 in these T-ALL blasts has not been investigated to date. Due to the absence of higher gangliosides in these blasts, precursor accumulation due to blocked synthesis is possible, as has been suggested for melanoma (18), although enhanced synthesis due to increased GD3 sialyltransferase in these blasts relative to resting normal T cells is also likely. The possible association of this disease with a derepressed sialyltransferase is particularly exciting and is under study in our laboratory.

The detection of GD3 at the cell surface in a large subclass of childhood ALL with a monoclonal anti-GD3 antibody indicates a clear diagnostic and possible therapeutic potential for anti-GD3 antibodies in T-ALL. Preliminary assessment of R24 reactivity by lymphoblasts among T-cell ALL patients suggests that duration of remission is longer in these patients whose leukemic blasts expressed GD3 compared to those whose cells failed to express GD3. Well-controlled prospective studies will be required to fully assess whether GD3 expression will be a useful prognostic indicator in T-cell ALL. The immunotherapeutic potential of R24 in T-ALL is suggested by the ability of R24 to mediate cytolysis in *in vitro* cytotoxicity assays. The antibody is reactive with T-lymphoblasts at a concentration similar to that reactive in human melanoma (11). Phase I trials of R24 in melanoma have demonstrated its potential as an immunotherapeutic agent (11). Due to the heterogeneous expression of GD3 in a single population of lymphoblasts, clearly a mixture of antibodies will be required in an immunotherapeutic approach to T-cell ALL, although current studies are aimed at enhancing the GD3 expression in those T-lymphoblast populations that express low to moderate levels of GD3.

Summary

Analysis of the gangliosides of lymphoblasts from children with acute lymphoblastic leukemia (ALL) showed that disialolactosylceramide (GD3) was increased in cells from T-cell ALL relative to normal thymocytes from children. Blasts from children with non T-ALL contained hematoside (GM3) and sialosylparagloboside (SPG) and lacked detectable GD3. The distribution of these gangliosides was confirmed by TLC immunostaining using a monoclonal anti-GD3 antibody (R24) and a monoclonal antibody reactive with GM3 and SPG (M2590). R24 was then utilized to assess the cell surface expression of GD3 on T-ALL and non-T-ALL blasts. Immunofluorescence microscopy (IF) with R24 showed that whereas blasts from none of 33 non-T-ALL samples were reactive, 37 out of 50 (74%) of T-ALL samples were positive. R24 reactivity most closely paralleled expression of the sheep erythrocyte receptor antigen (CD2) and could not be enhanced by pretreatment with trypsin. Studies of complement-mediated and antibody-dependent cellular cytotoxicity showed that anti-GD3 antibodies were cytotoxic to T-ALL, and cytotoxicity (% cell lysis) correlated with cellular IF. Anti-GM3/SPG (M2590) was also found to stain leukemic lymphoblasts although staining was dim. The ratio of R24/M2590 staining in non-T-ALL was <1.0 and in T-ALL appeared to distinguish two subpopulations, a GD3$^+$ population (R24/M2590 >1.0) and a GD3$^-$ population (R24/M2590 <1.0). These results show that a large subclass of T-ALL is distinguished by high anti-GD3 binding and low anti-GM3/SPG binding, and suggests that anti-GD3 antibodies may be useful agents for the immunodiagnosis and immunotherapy of T-ALL.

References

1. Harden, E. A., and B. F. Haynes. Phenotypic and functional characteristics of human malignant T cells. Seminars in Hematology, 22, 13, 1985.
2. Nadler, L. M., S. J. Korsmeyer, K.C. Anderson, A.W. Boyd, B. Slaughenhoupt, E. Park, J. Jensen, F. Coral, R. J. Meyer, S. E. Sallan, J. Riza, and S. F. Scholossman. B cell origin of non-T cell acute lymphoblastic leukemia. A model for discrete stages of neoplastic and normal pre-B cell differentiation. J. Clin. Invest., 74, 332, 1984.
3. Merritt, W. D., J.T. Casper, S. J. Lauer, and G. H. Reaman. Expression of GD3 ganglioside in childhood T-cell lymphoblastic malignancies. Cancer Res., 47, 1724, 1987.
4. Merritt, W. D., M. B. Sztein, and G. H. Reaman. Detection of GD3 ganglioside in childhood acute lymphoblastic leukemia with monoclonal antibody to GD3: restriction to immunophenotypically-defined T-cell disease. J. Cell Biochem., 37, 11, 1988.
5. Hirabayashi, Y., A. Hamaoka, M. Matsumoto, T. Matsubara, M. Tagawa, S. Wakaboyashi, and M. Taniguchi. Syngeneic monoclonal antibody against melanoma antigen with interspecies cross-reactivity recognizes GM3, a prominent ganglioside of B16 melanoma. J. Biol. Chem., 260, 13328, 1985.
6. Reaman, G. H., B. H. Taylor, and W. D. Merritt. Selective expression of disialosylceramide (GD3) by lymphoblasts of T-cell lineage in acute lymphoblastic leukemia of childhood. Manuscript, submitted for publication.
7. Vogel, C.W., S.W. Welt, E. A. Carswell, L. J. Old, and H. J. Muller-Eberhard. A murine IgG monoclonal antibody to a melanoma antigen that activates human complement *in vitro* and *in vivo*. Immunobiology, 164, 309, 1983.
8. Knuth, A., W. G. Dippold, A. N. Houghton, K. Meyer zum Büschenfelde. H. F. Oettgen, and L. J. Old. ADCC reactivity of human melanoma cells with mouse monoclonal antibodies. Proc. Am. Assoc. Cancer Res., 25, 1005, 1984.
9. Cheresh, D., C. J. Honsik, L. K. Staffileno, G. Jung, and R. A. Reisfeld. Disialoganglioside GD3 on human melanoma serves as a relevant targe antigen for monoclonal antibody-mediated tumor cytolysis. Proc. Natl. Acad. Sci. USA, 82, 5155, 1985.
10. Hellstrom, I., V. Brankovan, and K. E. Hellstrom. Strong anti-tumor activities of IgG3 antibodies to a human melanoma-associated ganglioside. Proc. Natl. Acad. Sci. USA, 82, 1499, 1985.
11. Houghton, A. N., D. Mintzer, L. Cordon-Cardo, S. Welt, B. Fliegel, S. Vadhan, E. Carswell, M. R. Melamed, H. F. Oettgen, and L. J. Old. Mouse monoclonal IgG3 antibody detecting GD3 ganglioside: a phase I trial in patients with malignant melanoma. Proc. Natl. Acad. Sci. USA, 82, 1242, 1985.
12. Vadham-Raj, S., C. Cordon-Cardo, E. Carswell, D. Mintzer, L. Dantis, M. A. Templeton, H. F. Oettgen, L. J. Old, and A. N. Houghton. Phase I trial of a mouse monoclonal antibody against GD3 ganglioside in patients with melanoma: induction of inflammatory responses of tumor sites. J. Clin. Oncol. In press, 1988.
13. Nores, G. A., D. Taeko, M. Taniguchi, and S. Hakomori. Densitydependent recognition of cell surface GM3 by a certain anti-melanoma antibody, and GM3 lactone as a possible immunogen: requirements for tumor-associated antigen and immunogen. J. Immunol., 139, 317, 1987.
14. Siddiqui, B., J. Buehler, M.W. DeGregorio, and B. A. Macher. Differential expression of ganglioside GD3 by human leukocytes and leukemia cells. Cancer Res., 44, 5262, 1984.
15. Kyogashima, M., T. Killemura, and T. Taketomi. Comparison of glycolipids in various human leukemia cells. Jpn. J. Cancer Res. (GANN), 78, 1229, 1987.

16. Suzuki, Y., Y. Hirabayashi, N. Matsumoto, H. Kato, K. Hidari, K. M. Tsuchiya, M. Matsumoto, H. Hoshimo, A. Tozawa, and M. Miwa. Aberrant expression of ganglioside and asialoglycophingolipid antigens in adult T-ALL leukemia cells. Jpn. J. Cancer Res. (GANN), 78, 1112, 1987.
17. Welte, K., G. Miller, P. B. Chapman, H. Yuasa, E. Natoli, J. E. Kunicka, C. Cordon-Cardo, C. Buchrer, L. J. Old, and A. N. Houghton. Stimulation of T lymphocyte proliferation by monoclonal antibodies against GD3 ganglioside. J. Immunol., 139, 1763, 1987.
18. Hershey, P., S. D. Schibechi, S. Townsend, C. Burns, and D. A. Cheresh. Potentiation of lymphocyte responses by monoclonal antibodies to the ganglioside GD3. Cancer Res., 46, 6083, 1986.
19. Hakomori, S. Tumor-associated glycolipid antigens, their metabolism, and organization. Chem. Phys. Lipids, 42, 209, 1986.
20. Foon, K. A., and R. F. Todd. Immunologic classification of leukemia and lymphoma. Blood, 68, 1, 1986.

15. Mouse Monoclonal Antibodies to Ganglioside GD2: Characterization of the Fine Structural Specificities

T. Tai, I. Kawashima, N. Tada, and T. Fujimori

Abstract

The fine structural specificities of six monoclonal antibodies (MAbs) to ganglioside GD2 were studied. These MAbs were produced by hybridomas obtained from A/J mice immunized with EL4 (C57BL/6 derived/T lymphoma). The binding specificities of these MAbs differed from each other by virtue of their binding to structurally related authentic standard glycosphingolipids as revealed by three different assay systems. The MAbs examined could be devided into three binding types. Three MAbs A1-201, A1-410, and A1-425 bound specifically to ganglioside GD2 and none of the other gangliosides tested. Two other MAbs A1-245 and A1-267 reacted not only with GD2, but also several other gangliosides having the sequence NeuAcα2→8NeuAcα2→3Gal. In addition, these MAbs distinguished between different N-acetyl- and N-glycolyl-neuraminic acid derivatives of ganglioside GD3. The last MAb A1-287 reacted with several other gangliosides but with lower avidity than A1-245 and A1-267. All of these MAbs, furthermore, reacted with ganglioside GD2 lactones. However, the reactivities of these antibodies to various gangliosides lactones also differed from each other. Four MAbs A1-201, A1-287, A1-410, and A1-425 reacted with only GD2 lactones, whereas the other two MAbs A1-245 and A1-267 cross-reacted with the lactones of other gangliosides such as GD1b and GT1b.

Introduction

Many tissue-specific and tumor-specific mouse and human monoclonal antibodies (MAbs) have been described that recognize carbohydrate determinants of glycolipids, glycoproteins or mucins (1–4). The antibodies that react preferentially with tumors of neuroectodermal origin such as melanoma, neuroblastoma, and glioma, but not with normal cells have been shown to be directed to gangliosides. It is of importance to study the fine binding specificity of a MAb. If the precise epitope specificity of the MAb has not been determined, there is no way to judge whether the antibody binds to the authentic antigen or to structurally related substances. Recently, determination of the fine epitope specificity of the MAb has proven useful for studying precise interactions between anti-carbohydrate antibodies and antigenic determinants (5–7). However, there have been few reports on precise binding specificities of MAbs to gangliosides. We recently produces six MAbs to ganglioside GD2 by immunizing mice with a mouse T-cell lymphoma (8). In the present report we determined the fine structural specificities of the MAbs by several assay systems. All of these MAbs also reacted with ganglioside GD2 lactones which are inner esters formed between the carboxyl group of the sialic acids and a hydroxyl group of the ganglioside.

Materials and Methods

Monoclonal Antibodies. Six murine hybrid cell lines, designated A1-201, A1-245, A1-267, A1-287, A1-410, and A1-425, were established as previously described (8). The immunoglobulin classes of these MAbs were as follows. Two MAbs, A1-201 and A1-245, are of the IgM (k) class. The other four MAbs, A1-267, A1-287, A1-410, and A1-425, are of the IgG3 (k) class.

Thin-Layer Chromatography (TLC). Merck precoated TLC-plastic sheets (Merck, Darmstadt, F.R.G.) were used for fractionation of gangliosides. The solvent system used for developing chromatograms was chloroform/methanol/0.22 % CaCl2 in water (55/45/10, v/v). Gangliosides were visualized with resorcinol stain and neutral glycolipids were visualized with orcinol stain.

Glycolipids. Standard gangliosides and neutral glycolipids were prepared as previously described (9). Gangliosides lactones were prepared from purified gangliosides (10). Ganglioside (1 mg) was dissolved in glacial acetic acid (1.0 ml) and incubated at 25°C for four days in the dark. After lyophilization, the products were used as ganglioside lactones. Mild base treatment was performed with 0.05N NaOH in methanol at 37°C for 2 h.

Enzyme Immunostaining on Thin-Layer Plates, Enzyme-Linked Immunosorbent Assay (ELISA), and Immune Adherence (IA) Inhibition Assay: Immunostaining on TLC plates (11), the solid-phase ELISA (12), and the IA inhibition assay (13) were performed as described previously.

Results and Discussions

Immunostaining on TLC of Various Authentic Gangliosides with the Six MAbs: Using six MAbs, we have found that mouse and human T lymphoma-associated antigen is ganglioside GD2 (8). We tested the binding reactivities of the MAbs to various authentic gangliosides. The results of enzyme immunostainings on TLC of di-, tri-, and tetra-sialosylgangliosides and all other glycolipids tested are summarized in Table 1.

Monosialogangliosides (GM4, GM3, GM2, and GM1) and neutral glycolipids (GlcCer, LacCer, GbOs3Cer, GbOs4Cer, GgOs3Cer, and GgOs4Cer) were negative. The MAbs were classified into at least three binding types according to their cross-reactivities with some authentic gangliosides. Since various standard gangliosides having NeuAc and/or NeuGc are not available, four ganglioside GD3 variants including (NeuAc-NeuAc-)GD3, (NeuGc-NeuAc-)GD3, (NeuAc-NeuGc-)GD3, and (NeuGc-NeuGc-)GD3 were tested with the six MAbs (Table 1). Only MAbs of the second type reacted with some of these GD3. MAbs of the first and the third types did not react with any GD3 isomers. The second type reacted with (NeuAc-NeuAc-)GD3 and (NeuGc-NeuAc-)GD3, but not with (NeuAc-NeuGc-)GD3 or (NeuGc-NeuGc-)-GD3. These results clearly indicate that the inner sialic acid of GD3 must be a NeuAc residue and it is very crucial for the reactivity with the MAbs, and that the requirement

Table 1. Summary of enzyme immunostaining on TLC of various authentic gangliosides with six monoclonal antibodies.

Ganglioside[a]	Type I A1-201[b], A1-410, A1-425	Type II A1-245, A1-267	Type III A1-287
(NeuAc-NeuAc-)GD3	−[c]	++	−
(NeuGc-NeuAc-)GD3	−	++	−
(NeuAc-NeuGc-)GD3	−	−	−
(NeuGc-NeuGc-)GD3	−	−	−
GD2	+++	+++	+++
GD1a	−	−	−
GD1b	−	++	−
GT1a	−	++	++
GT1b	−	+	−
GQ1b	−	++	++
GT3	−	−	−
GT2	−	−	−

[a] All of the gangliosides used contains NeuAc as a sialic acid moiety except four GD3 isomers. None of neutral glycolipids (GlcCer, LacCer, GbOs$_3$Cer, GbOs$_4$Cer, GgOs$_3$Cer and GgOs$_4$Cer) or monosialogangliosides (GM4, GM3, GM2 and GM1) tested were detected.
[b] Two MAbs, A1-201 and A1-245, are of the IgM (k) class. The other four MAbs, A1-267, A1-287, A1-410, and A1-425 are of the IgG3 (k) class.
[c] +++, strong; ++, moderate; +, weak or trace; −, negative.

of NeuAc for the terminal sialic acid residue seems to be less important, because ganglioside GD3 with external NeuGc was also reactive.

We recently studied the reactivity of MAb R24 with the four NeuAc/NeuGc-containing isomers of GD3 (14). In contrast to the MAbs A1-245 and A1-267, MAb R24 reacted with (NeuAc-NeuAc-)GD3 and (NeuAc-NeuGc-)GD3 but not with (NeuGc-NeuAc-)GD3 or (NeuGc-NeuGc-)GD3. These data suggest that each anti-ganglioside MAb may have its own individual characteristics in terms of binding and avidity for minor features of its carbohydrate epitope.

Enzyme-Linked Immunosorbent Assay (ELISA) and Immune Adherence (IA) Inhibition Assay with Various Authentic Glycolipids. The ELISA and the IA inhibition assay results using these MAbs agreed well with those obtained by immunostaining on TLC of gangliosides and neutral glycolipids (data not shown). However, several discrepancies were found among these assay systems. It was found that the ELISA is the most sensitive assay among them. There was no significant difference between the enzyme immunostaining on TLC and the IA inhibition test.

TLC Immunostaining of Various Gangliosides Lactones with the MAbs. Purified GD2 showed one clear band, while GD2 lactones revealed several bands (Figure 1A). A major component (90 mol%) migrated in the region between GM2 and GM1 on the TLC. After the GD2 lactones were treated with base, they changed their chromatographic behaviors and migrated exactly as the purified GD2, indicating that these components are simply lactones of GD2. TLC immunostaining showed that MAb A1-201 reacted with GD2 lactones as well as the purified GD2 (Figure 1B). GD2 lactones revealed several bands, probably due to the potential for lactone formation in either or

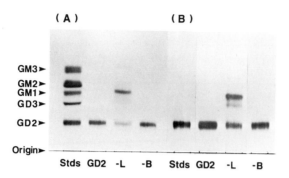

Figure 1. TLC immunostaining of ganglioside GD2 lactones. (A), Ganglioside GD2 lactones (10 nmol as sialic acid content) and the same amount of each standard ganglioside were chromatographed with chloroform/methanol/0.22 % CaCl$_2$ in water (55/45/10, v/v) and visualized with resorcinol. Stds, mixture of standard gangliosides GM3, GM2, GM1, GD3, and GD2; GD2, purified GD2; -L, GD2 lactones; -B, GD2 after base treatment of the GD2 lactones. (B), The same fraction as in (A), 1 nmol/lane was developed similarly and immunostained with MAb A1-201. GD2 lactones were prepared from purified ganglioside GD2 as described in "Materials and Methods". The reactivities of the other three MAbs (A1-287, A1-410, and A1-425) were identical to that of A1-201.

both of the two sialic acids. Reactivity of the major ganglioside GD2 lactone appeared to be similar to that of the purified GD2. None of other ganglioside lactones tested were detected by MAb A1-201. The pattern using the other three MAbs (A1-410, A1-425, and A1-287) was identical to that of A1-201. In contrast, MAb A1-245 reacted with three gangliosides lactones (GD2, GD1b, and GT1b), but not with the other three (GD3, GT1a, and GQ1b) among the six gangliosides tested (Figure 2). The major components of the three ganglioside lactones (GD2, GD1b, and GT1b) appeared to retain their reactivities compared to these purified gangliosides, while those of the other three ganglioside lactones (GD3, GT1a, and GQ1b) lost their binding activities completely. Identical reactivity was obtained by A1-267. Effects of sialidase on major components of ganglioside lactones were tested. None of the major components of ganglioside lactones prepared from the six gangliosides were sensitive with the sialidase, while all of these purified gangliosides were sensitive, demonstrating that at least the outher sialic acid moieties of these gangliosides were involved in lactone formation (15).

A major component of GD3 lactones lost its binding reactivities compared to the purified GD3. The fastest moving band on TLC appeared to be GD3 lactone in which both of two carboxyl residues made ester formation, since this band behaved like neutral glycolipid on TLC and ion-exchange column chromatography and was not sensitive with sialidase treatment. In contrast, major bands of two gangliosides lactones (GD2 and GD1b) that comigrated with GM1 and GD3, respectively, retained their binding activities. These bands would be gangliosides lactones in which the carboxyl group of the two sialic acids in the NeuAcα2→8NeuAcα2→3Gal sequence formed an innerester. Precise structural studies on a major GD1b lactone have been described by Acquotti *et al.* (16). The GD1b lactone contains a single ester linkage involving the external sialic acid carboxyl group and the C-9 hydroxyl group of the internal sialic acid

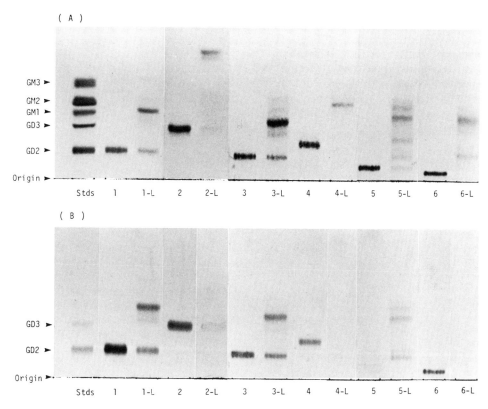

Figure 2. TLC immunostaining of various ganglioside lactones. (A), Each of six purified gangliosides and lactones (10 nmol as sialic acid content/lane) and the same amount of each standard ganglioside were chromatographed as described in Figure 1 and visualized with resorcinol. Stds, mixture of standard gangliosides GM3, GM2, GM1, GD3, and GD2; GD1, GD2, GD3; 3, GD1b; 4, GT1a; 5, GT1b; 6, GQ1b; -L, lactone of the ganglioside. (B), The same fraction as in (A), 1 nmol/lane was developed similarly and immunostained with MAb A1-245. The reactivity of MAb A1-267 was identical to that of A1-245.

unit. These findings suggested that the carboxyl group in the inner sialic acid moiety of these gangliosides may be crucial for the epitope of the two MAbs.

Taken together the results, it was suggested that both the carboxyl group and the acetamido group in the inner sialic acid moiety of these gangliosides are essential for the epitope of the MAbs, whereas neither the carboxyl group nor the acetamido group in the outer sialic acid is important. However, a part of the outer sialic acid moiety must be essential, since the MAbs did not react with any monosialogangliosides. NMR study should be powerful for further characterization of precise interaction between anti-ganglioside antibody and carbohydrate antigenic determinant.

Acknowledgements

The authors thank Drs. T. Yamakawa and A. Hiragun (The Tokyo Metropolitan Institute of Medical Science), for their valuable suggestions and support.

This work was supported in part by a grant from the Science and Technology Agency of Japan and a Grant-in-aid for scientific research from the Ministry of Education, Science and Culture of Japan.

References

1. Hakomori, S. Tumor associated carbohydrate antigens. Annu. Rev. Immunol. 2, 103, 1984.
2. Marcus, D. A review of the immunogenic and immunomodulatory properties of glycosphingolipids. Mol. Immunol. 21, 1083, 1984.
3. Feizi, T. Demonstration by monoclonal antibodies that carbohydrate structures of glycoproteins and glycolipids are oncodevelopmental antigens. Natur London 314, 53, 1985.
4. Reisfeld, R. A. and D. A. Cheresh. Human tumor antigens. Adv. Immunol. 40. 323, 1987.
5. Young, W.W., Jr., H. S. Johnson, Y. Tamura, K. A. Karlsson, G. Larson, J. M. R. Parker, D. P. Khare, U. Spohr, D. A. Baker, O. Hindsgaul, and R. U. Lemieux. Characterization of monoclonal antibodies specific for the Lewis a human blood group determinant. J. Biol. Chem. 258, 4890, 1983.
6. Kaizu, T., S. B. Levery, E. Nudelman, R. E. Stenkamp, and S. Hakomori. Nobel fucolipids of human adenocarcinoma: monoclonal antibody specific for trifucosyl Le^Y (III^3FucV^3 $FucIV^2FucnLc_6$) and a possible three-dimensional epitope structure. J. Biol. Chem. 261, 11254, 1986.
7. Blaszczyk-Thurin, M., J. Thurin, O. Hindsgaul, K.-A. Karlsson, Z. Steplewski, and H. Koprowski. Y and blood group B type 2 glycolipid antigens accumulate in a human gastric carcinoma cell line as detected by monoclonal antibody. J. Biol. Chem. 262, 372, 1987.
8. Kawashima, I., N. Tada, S. Ikegami, S. Nakamura, R. Ueda, and T. Tai. Mouse monoclonal antibodies detecting disialogangliosides on mouse and human T-lymphomas. Int. J. Cancer 41, 267, 1988.
9. Tai, T., I. Kawashima, N. Tada, and K. Dairiki. Different fine binding specificities of monoclonal antibodies to disialosylganglioside GD2. J. Biochem. Tokyo 103, 313, 1988.
10. Tai, T., I. Kawashima, N. Tada, and S. Ikegami. Different reactivities of monoclonal antibodies to ganglioside lactones. Biochim. Biophys. Acta. 958, 134, 1988.
11. Tai, T., L. Sze, I. Kawashima, R. E. Saxton, and R. F. Irie. Monoclonal antibody detects monosialogangliosides having a sialic acidδ2→3galactosyl residue. J. Biol. Chem. 262, 6803, 1987.
12. Tai, T., L. D. Cahan, J. C. Paulson, R. E. Saxton, and R. F. Irie. Human monoclonal antibody against ganglioside GD2: Use in development of enzyme-linked immunosorbent assay for the monitoring of anti-GD2 in cancer patients. J. Natl. Cancer Inst. 73, 627, 1984.
13. Tai, T., J. C. Paulson, L. D. Cahan, and R. F. Irie. Ganglioside GM2 as a human tumor antigen (OFA-I-1). Proc. Natl. Acad. Sci. USA 80, 5392, 1983.
14. Tai, T., I. Kawashima, K. Furukawa, and K. O. Lloyd. Monoclonal antibody R24 distinguishes between different N-acetyl- and N-glycolyl-neuraminic acid derivatives of ganglioside GD3. Arch. Biochem. Biophys. 260, 51, 1988.

15. Riboni, L., S. Sonnino, D. Acquotti, A. Maesci, R. Ghidoni, H. Egge, S. Mingrino, and G. Tettamanti. Natural occurrence of ganglioside lactones: isolation and characterization of GD1B inner ester from adult human brain. J. Biol. Chem. 261, 8514, 1986.
16. Acquotti, D., G. Fronza, L. Riboni, S. Sonnino, and G. Tettamanti. Ganglioside lactones: H-NMR determination of the inner ester position of GD1b-ganglioside lactone naturally occuring in human brain or produced by chemical synthesis. Glycoconjugate J. 4, 119, 1987.

16. Tissue Blood Group Carbohydrate Expression and Self: a Hypothesis

J. Thurin and B. Bechtel

Rigidity and flexibility in antigen recognition. In the field of immunology related to blood group type carbohydrate antigens and melanoma-associated ganglioside antigens, several observations form the basis for a hypothesis that might serve as an appropriate starting point in improving immunotherapy of solid tumors by exploiting carbohydrate antigens: 1) despite the presence of highly tumor-associated antigens of human blood group carbohydrate type on tumor cells, the immune system seems largely to ignore these antigens, even if they are blood group incompatible; 2) blood group incompatible human kidney transplantations (blood group A_2 to O) have a success rate of 10 out of 17 (1); 3) monoclonal antibodies produced to carbohydrate epitopes are, with few exceptions, of mouse isotypes IgM and IgG3, and IgM in rats, all indicative of T cell independence (2); and 4) the majority of human blood group ABO, Pp, Ii specific antisera as well as myeloma proteins and human antibacterial polysaccharide immunoglobulins are also of IgM isotype (3), also demonstrating T cell independence. Finally, it is difficult to imagine how a branched and rigid blood group active oligosaccharide would meet the requirements necessary for binding to MHC molecules (4–6), thus enabling T cell help and/or recognition.

Based on these observations, we hypothesize that the carbohydrate part of glycoprotein and glycolipid antigens cannot be recognized as non-self, since the carbohydrate itself only can act as hapten (T cell independence) and that T cell recognition of carbohydrate haptens requires the co-presence of a carrier or peptide component (Figure 1).

The implication of this hypothesis for transplantation and tumor rejection is that glycolipid-bound blood group type carbohydrates cannot function as rejection targets and that glycoprotein-bound carbohydrates only can serve as targets for rejection if accompanied by changes in the protein, i.e., polymorphisms. Thus, changes in carbohydrate expression alone can not induce an immune response, because these changes do not evoke a non-self response (even if blood group incompatible) and require simultaneous changes in the protein carrier for T cell recognition, since self is the property of the peptide carrier recognized by the T cell. Indeed, T cell independence of glycolipid recognition might be the reason for the abundance of blood group type glycolipids and gangliosides that accumulate on tumor cells.

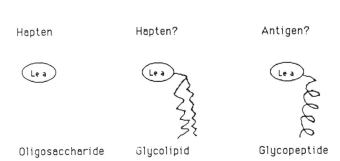

Figure 1. A cartoon illustrates the different forms of carbohydrate "antigens". The carbohydrate part, an oval with (Lewis[a]) assumed to be relatively rigid.

From this hypothesis it follows that optimization of carbohydrate antigen immuno-genicity involves both the "hapten", or carbohydrate part, as well as the "carrier", or protein part. Evidence for the concept of B cell epitopes being more rigid than, for example, the MHC binding sites on antigens stems from the demonstration that bran-ched blood group active saccharides are rigid and that increased rigidity of a saccharide correlates with increased immunogenicity (7, 8). Further evidence for the conclusion that antigenic carbohydrate epitopes generally have branched structures comes from a descriptive study of the carbohydrate specificity for monoclonal antibodies (2), and from a discussion of problems in "epitope mapping" due to conformational properties of a hapten (9). The rigidity concept was also used to propose a likely model for anti-body-carbohydrate hapten interaction (7). This model predicts an initial polar inter-action conferring directional information followed by a stabilizing amphipathic com-plementarity. A similar model for molecular interaction was recently described for T cell antigenic sites (5). Peptidic T cell epitopes, however, seem to be selected for "inhe-rent" flexibility, at least in the part necessary for MHC interaction, since it has been argued that flexibility is necessary in order for all proteins to be "presentable", i.e., to obtain high enough frequencies of MHC binding peptides for enabling a few functional T cell epitopes per protein molecule so that all antigens to be self-non-self screened by T cells (6). These assumptions are summarized in Table 1.

Requirement for the haptenic part and epitope-mapping of carbohydrate haptens. Monoclonal antibodies directed to carbohydrate haptens are generally tested for specificity on a panel of purified and characterized glycolipids or oligosaccharides of related origin to that of the assumed haptens. From the conformation of the hapten the surface topography of a carbohydrate hapten can be approximated if a sufficient num-ber of structurally related analogues is used. Two criteria must be met if this procedure is to be useful: 1) rigidity; and 2) conformational stability upon derivatization. At pre-sent there are no clearly stated guidelines for meaningfully evaluating the absolute degree of rigidity necessary for "good" antigenicity and such guidelines are needed for more investigation of antibody binding specificity using oligosaccharide solution con-formations. However, it is possible to probe for dynamic components in epitope

Table 1. Rigidity vs. flexibility in antigen recognition.

Immune receptor origin	Molecular character of binding site (functional level)	Type of molecular interaction (biophysical level)	Possible function
B cell	rigidity	amphipathic complementarity	conferring specificity
APC	flexibility*	amphipathic complementarity	self-non-self discrimination
T cell	rigidity of complex	amphipathic complementarity	conferring specificity

* Strictly meaning the part of the immunogenic peptide that interacts with MHC, i. e. the carrier. In our model, the part of the molecule recognized by antibody is assumed to have the same properties as the carbohydrate hapten, i. e., rigidity.

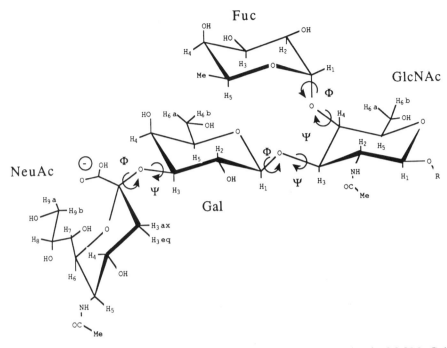

Figure 2. A drawing illustrating the 19-9 tetrasaccharide hapten. R=(Ch$_2$)$_7$-COOMe Galβ1 → 3GlcNAc(4 ← 1αFuc)β1 → R=Cocre Le^a trisaccharide. Φ and Ψ are the torsional angles around which most of the dynamics in the hapten take place. Gal, galactose; Fuc, fucose; GlcNAc, glucosamine; and NeuAc, neuraminic acid.

mapping of carbohydrate haptens and obtain conformational information provided the regidity is below a certain empirical level. For example, monoclonal antibody CO19-9 recognizes the 19-9 hapten, i.e., sialylated Le^a (Figure 2), but does not bind the Le^a hapten (9). Thus, if the Le^a core of 19-9 is rigid, the sialic acid component would form part of the epitope. However, if the conformation of the Le^a core changes upon addition of the sialic acid, then this changed core could serve as the epitope for antibody CO19-9 with no further direct involvement of the sialic acid. To distinguish between these possibilities, we compared the structures of the synthetic, tumor-associated 19-9 tetrasaccharide, NeuACα2→3Galβ1→3βGlcNAc(4←1αFuc)-O(CH$_2$)$_8$-CO$_2$CH$_3$ and its Le^a blood group antigen precursor, Galβ1→3βGlcNAc(4←1αFuc)-O(CH$_2$)$_8$CO$_2$CH$_3$ by two-dimensional 500-MHz ^{1}H-NMR spectroscopy and hard-sphere energy calculations. These two molecules differed significantly only in the protons at or near the linkage site of NeuAc to the Le^a trisaccharide core. Local conformational information is obtained from the coupling constants for the ring protons of both molecules, which did not suggest major deviation from the ^{4}C$_1$ chair conformation for Gal and GlcNAc, the ^{1}C$_4$ conformation for Fuc, or the (2) C$_5$ conformation for NeuAc. Two-dimensional nuclear Overhauser enhancement experiments revealed through-space, interproton interactions that corresponded well with those predicted by the hard-sphere energy minimization programs for both saccharides. These data suggest that the Le^a trisaccharide core in the 19-9 tetrasaccharide is conformationally and dynamically invariant to NeuAcα2→3Gal linkage. The NeuAcα2→3Gal linkage, however, seems to be more flexible than Fucα1→4GlcNAc and the Galβ1→3GlcNAc linkages in the Le^a core, although the degree of this flexibility is less than that discussed earlier for MHC binding peptides. The nonreactivity of monoclonal antibody CO19-9 with Le^a, together with the regidity observed in the Le^a core trisaccharide of the 19-9 antigen, therefore provide strong evidence that the NeuAc unit is directly involved in forming the epitope as an epitope-creating unit involved directly at the antibody binding site.

In conclusion, the functional significance of varying dynamics within a carbohydrate hapten is not known, but it seems likely that rigidity vs. flexibility of carbohydrate haptenic chains does have functional importance. The best evidence comes from the demonstrated rigidity of branched blood group type oligosaccharides which are highly antigenic in most species, and from the abrogation of the immunogenicity of proteins by N-linked glycans, clearly described as being flexible (10). The perhaps best example being the stalk of the influenza hemagglutinin (11, 12). Antigen dynamics might therefore play a crucial role in the nature of the haptenic carbohydrate epitope, such as that of CO19-9, because although the 19-9 antigen in solution might exist in its lowest energy state (9), it might be converted to one of its higher energy minima upon antibody binding. The maximum energy difference between different states is 16 kcal/mol and at least part of this energy could be provided by the antibody for conformational change of the hapten. The enzyme lysozyme, for example, uses 16 kcal/mol to bind and distort its saccharide substrate at the cost of 5 kcal/mol. A question could be raised as to the problem of exemplifying immune interactions with those of enzymes. However, the carbohydrate antigen is relatively small compared to proteins, and therefore a cleft-like antibody paratope would be expected rather than the flat interaction surface demonstrated for the antibody-lysozym interaction recently described (13) which would justify this assumtion. Although factors other than differences in energy are involved in determining conformation, these data indicate the need to incorporate the actual antibody-antigen interaction into the epitope concept, i.e., to study "virtual" rather than "real" epitopes. If our hypothesis will be proven to be correct it will also be necessary to clearly define the properties needed for the haptenic part or epitopic part as well as for the presenting, or agretopic part of a carbohydrate "antigen".

Acknowledgements

We would like to acknowledge Drs. H. Koprowski and A. J. Wand for their most valuable discussions.

This work was supported by the following grants from the National Institutes of Health: #CA-25874, CA-10815, CA-21124, T32-CA-09171, RR-05415, and RR-07083. Address correspondence to Jan Thurin, M. D., The Wistar Institute of Anatomy and Biology, 3601 Spruce Street, Philadelphia, PA 19104.

References

1. Breimer, M. E., H. Brynger, L. Rydberg, and B. E. Samuelsson. Transplantation of blood group A₂ kidneys to O recipients. Biochemical and immunological studies of blood group A antigens in human kidneys. Transplantation Proc. 17, 2640, 1985.
2. Thurin, J. Binding sites of monoclonal anti-carbohydrate antibodies. In: Current Topics in Microbiol. and Immunol. Vol. 139. I. Wilson and A. Clarke, editors. Springer Verlag, Berlin-Heidelberg-New York 59–64, 1988.
3. Spitalnik, S. L. Human monoclonal antibodies directed against carbohydrates. Meth. Enzymol. 138, 492, 1987.
4. Bjorkman, P. J., M. A. Saper, B. Samraoui, W. S. Bennett, J. L. Strominger, and D. C. Wiley. Structure of the human class I histocompatibility antigen, HLA-A2. Nature 329, 506, 1987.
5. DeLisi, C. and J. A. Berzofsky. T-cell antigenic sites tend to be amphipathic structures. Proc. Natl. Acad. Sci. USA 82, 7048, 1985.
6. Buus, S., A. Sette, and H. M. Grey. The interaction between protein-derived immunogenic peptides and Ia. Immunol. Rev. 98, 15, 1987.
7. Lemieux, R. U. The binding of carbohydrate structures by antibodies and lectins. In: IUPAC Frontiers of Chemistry. K. J. Laidler, editor. Pergamon Press, Oxford 3–25, 1982.
8. Jennings, H. J., R. Roy, and A. Gamian. Induction of meningococcal group B polysaccharide-specific IgG antibodies in mice by using an N-propionylated B polusaccharide-tetanus toxoid conjugate vaccine. J. Immunol. 137, 1708, 1986.
9. Bechtel, B., J. Thurin, A. J. Wand, and H. Koprowski. Conformational analysis of the tumor-associated carbohydrate antigen, 19-9 and its Leᵃ blood group antigen component as related to the specificity of monoclonal antibody CO19-9. J. Biol. Chem. submitted. 1988.
10. Homans. S.W., A. Pastore, R. A. Dwek, and T.W. Rademacher. Structure and dynamics in oligomannose-type oligosaccharides. Biochemistry 26, 6649, 1987.
11. Wilson, I. A., J. J. Skehel, and D. C. Wiley. Structure of the haemagglutinin membrane glycoprotein of influenza virus at 3 Å resolution. Nature 289, 366, 1981.
12. Caton, A. J., G. G. Brownlee, J.W. Yewdell, and W. Gerhard. The antigenic structure of the influenza virus A/PR/8/34 hemagglutinin (Hl subtype). Cell 31, 417, 1982.
13. Amit, A. G., Mariuzza, R. A., Phillips, S. E.V., and Poljak, R. J. Three-dimensional structure of an antigen-antibody complex at 2.8 Å resolution. Science 233, 747, 1986.

17. Immunoblotting Detection of Carbohydrate Epitopes in Glycolipids and Glycoproteins of Tumoral Origin

S. Miotti, F. Leoni, S. Canevari,
S. Sonnino, and M. I. Colnaghi

Introduction

The advent of monoclonal antibodies (mAbs)* technology has allowed the development of reagents which have been found to be useful for the characterization of structures present on cancer cell membranes. In particular, in the case of cancer of epithelial origin, the peculiar pattern of mAb reactivity on normal, fetal and cancer tissues led to the identification of several of the recognized molecules as oncodevelopmental antigens (1–3). The biochemical analysis of the latter indicated that they were different kinds of glycoconjugates i.e. mucins, glycoproteins or glycolipids, whose saccharide chains carried epitopes which were identical or related to the haptens of blood group antigens (4). However, as regards the possible biological significance of the simultaneous versus the mutual presence of these carbohydrate epitopes on different kinds of glycoconjugates, our knowledge is still very limited.

In our laboratory a number of different mAbs have been produced against human carcinomas and several of them were found to be directed against carbohydrate antigens (5–12).

In this paper we report results concerning the expression of MBr1, MOv2, and MLuC1 defined structures on breast carcinoma and normal breast cells in different functional conditions.

Materials and Methods

mAbs. MBr1 (IgM), MOv2 (IgM) and MLuC1 (Ig2a) were produced as previously described (5, 8, 12). Their reactivity is summarized in table 1 and described in detail elsewhere for MBr1 (13, 14) for MOv2 (15) and for MLuC1 (12). The biochemical characterization of the target antigens was previously reported for MBr1 (6, 7) and MOv2 (9, 11, 16); as regards MLuC1 the results are still unpublished. The main features of the epitopes and their relationship with blood group determinants are summarized in Table 2.

Immunoblotting analysis. Samples from frozen surgical specimens were obtained by solubilizing for each one 6 tissue slices of 20 μm in 100 μl of Laemmli final sample buffer (17) for 1 hr at room temperature under shaking. Each sample was then boiled for 10 min. at 100°C, centrifuged for 10 min. at 10,000 g and the supernatant was then recovered and subjected to immunoblotting as described (16).

Abbreviations used in this paper. mAb, monoclonal antibody; CaMBr1, epitope recognized by MBr1 mAb; CaMOv2, epitope recognized by MOv2 mAb; CaMLuC1, epitope recognized by MLuC1 mAb; HPTLC, high performance thin layer chromatography; HMWGP, high molecular weight glycoproteins; IMWGP, intermediate molecular weight glycoproteins; GL, glycolipids.

Results

The mAbs used in the present study were raised against human carcinomas and their reactivity is summarized in Table 1. Whichever immunogen was used, none of the mAbs could be considered specific for a certain tumor since, as determined by immunohistochemistry, they all react with breast, ovary and lung carcinomas. When the reactivity on normal epithelial tissues was considered, the three mAbs were consistently positive on breast epithelium and negative on ovary epithelium. Normal epithelial cells of the lung were only positive with MLuC1. These and previously reported data (12–15) clearly show that the three mAbs recognize antigens not specifically expressed on tumor cells.

Table 1. Reactivity of the mAbs used.

Reactivity on:		MBr1	MOv2	MLuC1
		(percentage of positive cases)		
Carcinomas	breast	80	70	70
	ovary	50	70	60
	lung	65	25	85
Normal epithelium	breast	+	+	+
	ovary	−	−	−
	lung	−	−	+

As reported in Table 2, the biochemical characterization of the recognized epitopes (CaMBr1, CaMOv2, and CaMLuC1) demonstrates their saccharidic nature. Studies aimed at elucidating the structure of the epitopes were carried out using different approaches. In the case of CaMBr1, the purified antigen extracted from the immunogen was examined by methylation analysis, NMR spectroscopy, direct probe mass spectrometry and enzymatic degradation (7). As regards CaMOv2 and CaMLuC1, the epitope structures were identified by immunoreaction on purified glycolipids separated by high performance thin layer chromatography (HPTLC), cross-competition experiments using mAbs with defined specificities and binding-inhibition experiments with oligosaccharides (ref. 11 for MOv2 and manuscript in preparation for MLuC1).

Table 2. Characteristics of the target antigens.

	Antigens definded by:		MLuC1
	MBr1	MOv2	
Epitope	saccharidic (CaMBr1)	saccharadic (CaMOv2)	saccharidic (CaMLuC1)
Glycoconjugate on the immunogen	neutral glycolipid	mucins, glycoproteins and a neutral glycolipid	glycoproteins and a glycolipid
Blood group related determinant	Globo-H (GL6)	Lewis[a]	Lewis[y]

The results obtained, as indicated in Table 2, demonstrate that CaMBr1 is carried by the globo-H antigen GL6, CaMOv2 is the Lewis[a] hapten and CaMLuC1 is the Lewis [y] hapten.

We previously described by using MOv2 and samples from ovarian carcinomas that the immunoblotting technique was suitable to simultaneously detect the presence of glycolipid and glycoprotein molecules (16). Since both normal and cancerous breast epithelium were found to be positive with the three selected mAbs (Table 1), the reactivity of the latters was further analyzed by immunoblotting to verify whether a parti-

Table 3. Immunoblotting reactivity of mAbs MBr1, MOv2 and MLuC1 on breast tissues*.

Breast tissues	No. of positive specimens/total no of examined cases		
	MBr1	MOv2	MLuCl
Normal resting	6/8	5/8	1/2
Normal hormone-stimulated**	5/8	6/8	2/2
Benign tumor	3/5	5/5	2/5
Carcinoma (primary + metastasis)	21/34	19/34	11/30

* Soluble extracts from frozen sections of normal and tumor specimens were analyzed as described in materials and methods.
** Including tissues from pregnant and lactating breast.

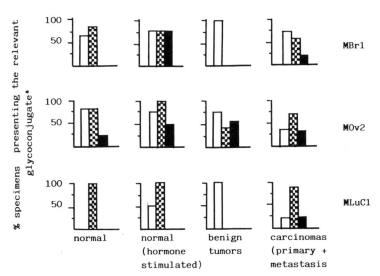

Figure 1. Distribution of the different kinds of glycoconjugates detected by mAbs MBr1, MOv2, and MLuC1 as determined by immunoblotting on breast tissues. Immunostained molecules were operationally defined as: high molecular weight glycoproteins (HMWGP) which do not enter the separation gel (□); intermediate molecular weight glycoproteins (IMWGP) separated by the separation gel (▨); glycolipids (GL) which migrate with the ions boundary (■). *The % of specimens expressing each kind of glycoconjugate was only evaluated on the positive cases reported in Table 3.

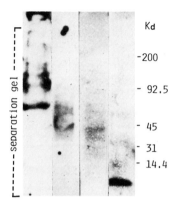

Figure 2. Pattern of CaMLuC1 carrying glycoconjugates as determined by immunoblotting on
breast carcinomas.

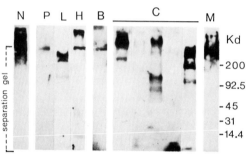

Figure 3. Pattern of CaMBr1 carrying
glycoconjugates as determined by
immunoblotting on breast tissues.
Samples were obtained from: normal
resting (N); normal pregnant (P);
normal lactating (L); human milk fat
globules (H); benign tumors (B);
primary carcinomas (C); metastatic
carcinomas (M).

cular type of glycoconjugate, rather than the single epitope, could be associated with
cell transformation. The relevant results are reported in Table 3 as the number of positive cases on total number of examined cases and in Figure 1 as the distribution of the
different kinds of glycoconjugates. In the legend of this figure the operational criteria
to define the different kinds of glycoconjugates have also been described. Examples of
the pattern of reactivity of MLuC1 and MBr1 are reported in Figure 2 and 3 respectively.

MOv2 reactivity was assayed on 16 samples of normal breast tissues and 11 of them
resulted positive (Table 3). Immunostaining of every kind of molecule was observed
both in resting and in hormone-stimulated breast samples, but the expression of the
MOv2-defined determinant was more commonly associated with HMWGP and
IMWGP than with GL (Figure 1). All the 5 benign tumors tested resulted positive with
a fairly homogeneous distribution of the immunostained molecules, whereas 50 %
only of the 34 breast carcinomas studied were found MOv2 reactive. On the positive
samples CaMOv2 was found to be carried in 70 % of cases by IMWGP and in 35 % by
HMWGP or GL.

As far as MLuC1 is concerned, a limited number of samples from normal tissues
(including both resting and hormones-stimulated) were analyzed and IMWGP were
the more frequently immunostained molecules as far as the 3 positive samples are
concerned. On the contrary, in the case of the 5 benign tumors tested, 2 were possitive
and expressed the epitope on HMWGP only. Thirty samples from carcinomas were
examined and on the 11 MLuC1-positive cases the majority of the immunoreactive

molecules were IMWGP. In a few cases (about 20 % of the positive samples) a GL band was found to express CaMLuC1 (Figure 1 and Figure 2).

The MBr1 epitope was originally described on the MCF7 tumor cell line as carried by GL6 (7). In this study we had evidence that it could also be present on glycoproteins (Figure 1 and Figure 3). The 6 positive cases of normal resting breast only exhibited glycoprotein bands. On the contrary, in the 5 positive cases of hormone-stimulated breast CaMBr1 was also expressed by GL (Figure 3). No MBr1-positive GL were observed on the benign tumors where HMWGP were predominant. The GL appeared on mammary carcinomas in about 20 % of the positive cases, whereas glycoproteins are expressed in 60–70 % of the cases (Figure 1).

From the results described above CaMOv2, i.e. the Lewis^a hapten, appears to be homogeneously expressed on normal and tumor breast by all kinds of glycoconjugates. As regards CaMLuC1, i.e. the Lewis^y hapten, the number of normal samples examined was too low to make any possible suggestions regarding its biological significance. More interesting was the distribution of the CaMBr1 glycoconjugates. In fact, the expression of the GL seemed to be restricted to hormone-stimulated normal breast and to a limited number of carcinomas, thus suggesting a possible physiological role of the CaMBr1 GL.

Discussion

It has been reported that glycoconjugates play a specific role in regulating normal cell behaviour. The appearance of specific glycosilated molecules has been observed in a temporal sequence during embryonal development and a variation in the glycosilation degree has been described during cell differentiation. Moreover, changes in the glycosilation pattern are a well-documented phenomenon in both experimental and human cancers (1–3, 18). In this study, within the limits of the applied technology, we observed general changes in the glycosilation pattern on breast tissues using mAbs which recognize carbohydrate determinants. CaMOv2 was found to be present on the various types of glycoconjugates without any correlation with the normal or transformed status of the breast gland. In the case of CaMLuC1 the number of normal samples was too limited to evaluate possible correlations. However the GL form was found only on carcinomas. It is interesting to note that the same pattern of distribution was observed in a similar study carried out on lung tissues (unreported data). We might therefore speculate that the synthesis of a Lewis^y GL molecule could be associated with transformation of epithelial cells.

As regards CaMBr1, unpublished immunohistochemical studies from our laboratory indicated that its expression on the breast gland was associated with the proliferative and secretory phase of the menstrual cycle (from the 8th to the 22nd day). Moreover, a high antigen expression was also detectable in the breast gland during pregnancy as well as in the lactating mammary gland. Immunoblotting analysis further supported these data and also revealed a peculiar pattern of glycoconjugates distribution. In particular the CaMBr1-GL molecule, which never was observed in the normal resting breast gland, seems to be associated with functional changes related to hormonal stimuli. It is also noteworthy that CaMBr1 expression on breast carcinomas was found to be correlated with the disease progression. In fact patients with MBr1 positive tumors had a worse prognosis in comparison to patients with MBr1 negative tumors (19). In the same retrospective study both MOv2 and MLuCl did not reveal any predicative capability. It would be of great interest to determine whether a correlation exists between the expression of CaMBr1 on a particular glycoconjugate form and the tumor aggressiveness.

Summary

Three monoclonal antibodies (mAbs) MBr1, MOv2, and MLuC1, raised against human carcinomas, were found to be directed against saccharide epitopes related to blood group antigens since they recognize the globo-H (GL6) structure, the Lewis[a] hapten and the Lewis[y] hapten, respectively. To characterize the recognized glycoconjugates, soluble extracts from resting or hormone-stimulated normal breast and benign or malignant mammary tumors were analyzed by immunoblotting. This procedure was in fact found to be suitable to simultaneously identify the presence of different kinds of glycoconjugates, i.e. glycoproteins and glycolipids. CaMOv2 was found to be present on the various types of glycoconjugates without any correlation with the normal or the transformed status of the breast gland. The expression of the glycolipid molecule defined by MLuC1, seemed to be associated to neoplastic conditions. Moreover, the presence of MBr1 defined glycolipid seemed to be related to the functional status of the breast. These results suggest that it is more likely the kind of antigenic glycoconjugate, rather than the presence of the defined determinant, which is associated with differentiation and/or transformation of epithelial breast cells.

Acknowledgements

We thank Mrs. L. Cozzi and Mr. G. DiCarlo for excellent technical assistance, Ms. P. Rocchi and Ms. M. Hutton for manuscript preparation and Mr. M. Azzini for photographic reproduction.

This research was supported in part by grants from the Italian National Research Council, Special Project "Oncology", contract number 87.01509.44 and from the Associazione Italiana per la Ricerca sul Cancro.

References

1. Feizi, T. Demonstration by monoclonal antibodies that carbohydrate structures of glycoproteins and glycolipids are onco-developmental antigens. Nature 314, 53, 1985.
2. Feizi, T. and R. A. Childs. Carbohydrates as antigenic determinants of glycoproteins. Biochem. J. 245, 1, 1987.
3. Hakomori, S. Aberrant glycosilation in cancer cell membranes as focussed on glycolipids: overview and perspectives. Cancer Res. 45, 2405, 1985.
4. Magnani, J. L. Mouse and rat monoclonal antibodies directed against carbohydrates. Methods Enzymol 138, 484, 1987.
5. Ménard, S., E. Tagliabue, S. Canevari, G. Fossati, and M. I. Colnaghi. Generation of monoclonal antibodies reacting with normal and cancer cells of human breast. Cancer Res. 43, 1295, 1983.
6. Canevari, S., G. Fossati, A. Balsari, S. Sonnino, and M. I. Colnaghi. Immunochemical analysis of the determinant recognized by a monoclonal antibody (MBr1) which specifically binds to human mammary epithelial cells. Cancer Res. 43, 1301, 1983.
7. Bremer, E. G., S. B. Levery, S. Sonnino, R. Ghidoni, S. Canevari, R. Kannagi, and S. I. Hakomori. Characterization of a glycolipid antigen defined by the monoclonal antibody MBr1 expressed in normal and neoplastic epithelial cells of human mammary gland. J. of Biological Chemistry 23, 14773, 1984.
8. Tagliabue, E., S. Ménard, G. Della Torre, P. Barbanti, R. Mariani-Costantini, G. Porro, and M. I. Colnaghi. Generation of monoclonal antibodies reacting with human epithelial ovarian cancer. Cancer Res. 45, 379, 1985.
9. Miotti, S., S. Aguanno, S. Canevari, A. Diotti, R. Orlandi, S. Sonnino, and M. I. Colnaghi. Biochemical analysis of human ovarian cancer-associated antigens defined by murine monoclonal antibodies. Cancer Res. 45, 826, 1985.
10. Miotti, S., S. Canevari, S. Ménard, D. Mezzanzanica, G. Porro, S. M. Pupa, M. Regazzoni, E. Tagliabue, M. I. Colnaghi. Characterization of human ovarian carcinoma-associated antigens defined by novel monoclonal antibodies with tumor-restricted specificity. Int. J. Cancer 39, 297, 1987.
11. Leoni, F., J. L. Magnani, S. Miotti, S. Canevari, M. Pasquali, S. Sonnino, M. I. Colnaghi. The antitumor monoclonal antibody MOv2 recognizes the Lewis A hapten. Hybridoma 7, 129, 1988.
12. Agresti, R., R. Alzani, S. Andreola, V. Bedini, S. Giani, S. Ménard, F. Rilke, M. I. Colnaghi. Histopathological characterization of a novel monoclonal antibody, MLuC1, reacting with lung carcinomas. Tumori, in press.
13. Mariani-Costantini, R., M. I. Colnaghi, F. Leoni, S. Ménard, S. Cerasoli, and F. Rilke. Immunohistochemical reactivities of a monoclonal antibody prepared against human breast carcinoma. Virchows Archiv. A. Pathol. Anat. 402, 389, 1984.
14. Mariani-Costantini, R., P. Barbanti, M. I. Colnaghi, S. Ménard, C. Clemente, and F. Rilke. Reactivity of a monoclonal antibody with tissues and tumors from the human breast: Immunohistochemical localization of a new antigen and clinico-pathologic correlations. Am. J. Pathol. 115, 47, 1984.
15. Mariani-Costantini, R., R. Agresti, M. I. Colnaghi, and S. Ménard. Characterization of the specificity by immunohistology of a monoclonal antibody to a novel epithelial antigen of ovarian carcinomas. Pathol Res. Pract. 180, 169, 1985.
16. Leoni, F., S. Miotti, S. Canevari, S. Sonnino, M. Ripamonti, and M. I. Colnaghi. Carbohydrate epitope defined by an antitumor monoclonal antibody detected on glycoproteins and a glycolipid by immunoblotting. Hybridoma 5, 289, 1986.

17. Laemmli, U. K. Cleavage of structural proteins during the assembly of the head of bacterio-phage T4. Nature 227, 680, 1970.
18. Hakomori, S., M. Fukuda, and E. Nudelman. Role of cell surface carbohydrates in differentiation: Behavior of lactosaminoglycan in glycolipids and glycoproteins. In: Teratocarcinoma and Embryonic Cell Interactions. T. Muramatsu, G. Gachelin, A. A. Moscona, and Y. Ikawa (eds). Japan Scientific Societies Press, Tokio 179–200, 1982.
19. Colnaghi, M. I. Monoclonal antibodies in breast cancer studies. In: Bailliere's Clinical Oncology. Baxter L., ed. B. J. Harcourt, London, in press; vol. 2, no. 1, 1988.

18. Fine Specificity Analysis of Human Monoclonal Antibodies Detecting Gangliosides

K. O. Lloyd and K. Furukawa

Recent improvements in techniques for producing monoclonal antibodies (mAbs) from human lymphocytes have resulted in the production of a substantial number of human monoclonal antibodies that react with gangliosides. All of the reported human mAbs to gangliosides have been developed from lymphocytes of patients with melanoma. The basic procedure employed is the transformation of lymphocytes with Epstein-Barr virus (EBV) to produce antibody secreting cells. However, since such cultures are difficult to subclone some investigators have subsequently fused the resulting cells with a mouse myeloma cell line to produce heterohybridomas. These cell lines are difficult to produce initially, but once isolated have the advantage of being easy to subclone and have the property of secreting appreciable amounts of immunoglobulin. When the specificities of these antibodies derived from melanoma patients was analyzed it was found that a surprising number of them were directed towards gangliosides.

Irie and coworkers (1–3) were the first to develop human monoclonal antibodies to gangliosides using the EBV-transformation technique. They produced two such antibodies, designated OFA-I-1 and OFA-I-2 that reacted selectively with melanoma and a few other cell types. Subsequently, these mAbs were shown to detect GM2 and GD2, respectively (2, 3). Each antibody was very selective in its pattern of reactivity and within the sensitivity of the method reacted only with the designated ganglioside. N-Glycolylneuraminic acid-containing gangliosides were not tested for their reactivities with these antibodies.

More recently, Yamaguchi et al. (4) produced a series of antiganglioside mAbs using mainly the EBV/hybridoma technique. The specificity of these antibodies was tested with a large series of gangliosides including those of the ganglio and paragloboside (neolacto) series and with species containing NeuGc. Although each antibody reacted preferentially with a particular ganglioside it also showed a considerable range of cross-reactivity with related species (5, 6). Of the four mAbs isolated in an initial study, two reacted preferentially with NeuAc-containing gangliosides and two with NeuGc-containing gangliosides. The first two antibodies (FCM1 and HJM1) selectively recognized human melanoma cells whereas the latter two mAbs (2-39M and 32-27M) did not react with any human cells.

In serological tests against cell lines Ab FCM1 reacted most strongly with cultures melanoma cell lines and with normal melanocytes. Most other cell types, with the exception of kidney cancer cell lines, were unreactive. In analyses using ELISA and TLC-immunostaining this mAb was found to react with NeuAc-type GM3, GD1a, SPG, and GT1b in decreasing order of reactivity. This antibody also reacted with (NeuAc-NeuGc-)GD3 and -diSPG, but did not react with NeuGc-type GM3, GM2, SPG, GD3 or diSPG. The epitopes recognized by mAb FCM1 are, therefore, NeuAcα2$\rightarrow$3Gal- and NeuAcα2$\rightarrow$8NeuGcα2$\rightarrow$3Gal- as shown in Figure 1. The specificity of this monoclonal antibody is very similar to that of the mouse monoclonal antibody M2590 (7, 5).

AbHJM1 was even more restricted in its pattern of cell surface reactivity with cell lines; it reacted only with melanoma cells. It was interesting to note that, as with AbFCM1, this mAb was absorbed by all cell lines tested when the cells had been broken open by scraping. This result indicates that all cells contain the antigens detected by these antibodies, albeit in a cryptic or intracellular state. When the specificity of AbHJM1 was tested, it was found to react with NeuAc-type GD3, diSPG, GD2,

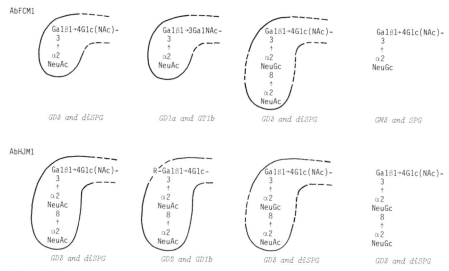

Figure 1. Proposed antigenic determinants recognized by Abs FCM1 and HJM1. The full line indicates sites of maximal interactions with antibody. The gangliosides in which these structures occur are also indicated.

GD1b, GM3, and GT1b, in decreasing order of intensity. Among NeuGc-containing gangliosides, this antibody reacted with (NeuAc-NeuGc-)-GD3 and -diSPG but did not react with gangliosides containing only NeuGc. It was concluded that the epitope structure recognized by AbHJM1 is R-(NeuAcα2a→8Sialic acidα2→3)Galβ1- (Figure 1). The specificity of this human monoclonal antibody is less restricted than that of mouse monoclonal antibody R24 which requires the disialo group to be in a terminal position for maximal reactivity (8, 5).

The main gangliosides recognized by these two antibodies, GM3 and GD3, are the major gangliosides of most human melanoma cells. Given, however, the wide distribution of GM3 in the body it is interesting that AbFCM1 has such a high degree of specificity for melanoma and a few other related cell types. The most likely explanation for this phenomenon is that only these cells have sufficiently high density of GM3 to show positive binding with the antibody (df. 9). Thus, even though these two antibodies are not a specific as some of the mouse anti-ganglioside mAbs, their specificity for antigens that are preferentially expressed on melanoma make them attractive candidates for use in the immunodiagnosis and therapy of this disease.

As mentioned above, the other two antibodies from this study (2-39M and 32-27M) reacted only with gangliosides containing NeuGc. Ab2-39M reacted with (NeuGc)-GM3, -SPG, and -sialyl-hexaglycosylceramide; no reactivity was observed with gangliosides containing only NeuAc or with disialylgangliosides. These reactive species have NeuGcα2→3Gal- terminal sequences in common (Figure 2). Ab32-27M reacted strongly with (NeuGc)₂GD3 and (NeuGc)₂diSPG, and moderately with (NeuAc-NeuGc-)-GD3 and -diSPG. The reactive species have Sialic acidα2→8NeuGcα2→3Gal- sequences in common (Figure 2). These two antibodies, although they are not highly specific for individual structures, may serve as useful reagents for the detection of NeuGc-containing gangliosides in cells and tissues.

Ab2-39M

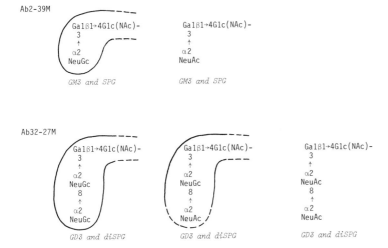

GM3 and SPG   GM3 and SPG

Ab32-27M

GD3 and diSPG   GD3 and diSPG   GD3 and diSPG

Figure 2. Proposed antigenic determinants recognized by Abs 2-39M and 32-27M. The full line indicates sites of maximal interactions with antibody. The gangliosides in which these structures occur are also indicated.

Using these antibodies it has been shown that the detected gangliosides are typical heterophile antigens in that they are absent from human tissues but present in the tissues of other animal species. Thus, Ab2-39 agglutinated horse, sheep, cat and bovine erythrocytes (Table 1). TLC-immunostaining demonstrated that this antibody reacted with (NeuGc)GM3 in all these samples and with two other components, probably (NeuGc)-SPG and hexaglycosylceramide in bovine erythrocytes. Ab32-27 agglutinated cat and sheep erythrocytes but not erythrocytes from other species. TLC-immunostaining demonstrated that two major, but different, gangliosides were reactive in each species. These were identified as (NeuGc)$_2$GD3 and (NeuAc-NeuGc-)GD3 from cat erythrocytes and (NeuGc)$_2$diSPG and (NeuAc-NeuGc-)diSPG from sheep erythrocytes (10).

An interesting aspect of the properties of Ab32-27M was its ability to react with some human cells when they were cultured in the presence of fetal bovine serum (FBS) but not when they were grown in synthetic medium (ITS: insulin : transferrin : sele-

Table 1. Hemagglutination of erythrocytes from various species by human monoclonal antibodies.

Monoclonal antibody	Human	Sheep	Bovine	Dog	Cat	Chicken	Rabbit	Rat	Guinea pig	Mouse	Horse
2-39M	0	128[a]	128	0	512	0	0	0	0	0	512
32-27M	0	512	0	0	1024	0	0	0	0	0	0
FCM1	0	0	0	512	0	0	0	0	0	0	0
HJM1	0	0	0	0	0	0	0	0	0	0	0

[a] Highest dilution of culture supernatant giving positive agglutination.

nium). This reactivity was confined to melanoma and astrycytoma cells. Epithelial and hematopoietic cells were unreactive even when culture in FBS. This effect has been shown not to be due to the simple adsorption of gangliosides from FBS on the surface of the melanoma and astrocytoma cells, but to involve a biosynthetic process.

These two antibodies (2-39M and 32-27M) were also used to analyze human tissues for the presence of NeuGc-containing gangliosides. Previous work, particularly by Higashi and coworkers (11) had demonstrated the presence of NeuGc-containing gangliosides (Hanganutziu-Deicher antigen) in a variety of human tumors, including melanoma. Using the two human antibodies, which are highly sensitive for NeuGc-containing structures, we have been unable to confirm these findings. TLC-immuno-staining with Abs 2-39M and 32-27M failed to detect any positive compounds in 9 colon cancer and 10 melanoma samples (6). Furthermore, chemical analysis using a gas chromatographic method failed to demonstrate NeuGc in the ganglioside fraction from fresh melanoma tumors. In contrast, NeuGc was readily detectable in the gangliosides from FBS-cultured melanoma cells. The possibility that human tumors contain NeuGc needs to be studied further.

We have recently extended this work on the development of human monoclonal antibodies to include the analysis of lymphocytes from patients undergoing vaccination with a GM2-containing vaccine (12). This study (13) has resulted in the development of a hybridoma secreting an antibody (3-207) that recognizes the immunizing antigen (NeuAc-GM2). Surprisingly, however, the strongest reactivity was with NeuAc-GD2. The antibody also reacted with NeuGc-GM2.

The significance of the ability to isolate monoclonal antibodies from melanoma patients and immunized individuals that react with gangliosides is uncertain. The fact that mAbs reacting with the major gangliosides of melanoma cells are readily isolated could indicate that this finding has some significance for the immune response of the patients to their tumors or to immunization. The development of anti-globo-series antibodies from lung cancer patients (14) also indicates a tumor-related response and would also support a biological role for these antibodies. On the other hand, the isolation of antibodies detecting NeuGc-containing glycolipids, which in our studies are undetectable in human tumors, could be interpreted to mean that the clones isolated merely represent the immune repertoire of the individual or a response to exogenous agents. Further work, including the development of antibody-producing clones from other patients and from normal individuals, will be necessary to fully understand the significance of these results.

Acknowledgement

This work is supported by grants from the National Cancer Institute (CA47427 and CA08478).

References

1. Irie, R. F., L. L. Sze, and R. E. Saxton. Human antibody to OFA- 1, a human antigen, produced in vitro by Epstein-Barr virus-transformed human B-lymphoid cell line. Proc. Natl.
Acad. Sci. USA 79, 5666, 1982.
2. Cahan, L. D., R. F. Irie, R. Singh, A. Cassidenti, and J. C. Paulson. Identification of a
human neuroectodermal tumor antigen (OFA-I-2) as ganglioside GD2. Proc. Natl. Acad
Sci. USA 79, 7629, 1982.
3. Tai, T., J. C. Paulson, L. D. Cahan, and R. F. Irie. Ganglioside GM2 as a human tumor antigen (OFA-I-1). Proc. Natl. Acad. Sci. USA 80, 5392, 1983.
4. Yamaguchi, H., K. Furukawa, S. R. Fortunato, P. O. Livingston, K. O. Lloyd, H. F.
Oettgen, and L. J. Old. Cell-surface antigens of melanoma recognized by human monoclonal antibodies. Proc. Natl. Acad. Sci. USA 84, 2416, 1987.
5. Furukawa, K., H. Yamaguchi, H. F. Oettgen, L. J. Old, and K. O. Lloyd. Analysis of the
expression of N-glycolylneuraminic acid-containing gangliosides in cells and tissues using
two human monoclonal antibodies. J. Biol. Chem. - submitted for publication, 1988.
6. Furukawa, K., H. Yamaguchi, H. F. Oettgen, L. J. Old, and K. O. Lloyd. Analysis of the
fine specificity of two human monoclonal antibodies reacting with the major gangliosides of
human melanoma and comarison with two corresponding mouse monoclonal antibodies.
Cancer Res. - submitted for publication, 1988.
7. Hirabayashi, S., A. Hamaoka, M. Matsumoto, T. Marsubura, M. Tagawa, S. Wakabayashi,
and M. Taniguchi. Syngeneic monoclonal antibody against melanoma antigen with interspecies cross-reactivity recognizes GM3, a prominent ganglioside of B16 melanoma. J. Biol.
Chem. 260, 13328, 1985.
8. Tai, T., I. Kawashima, K. Furukawa, and K. O. Lloyd. Monoclonal antibody R24 distinguishes between different N-acetyl and N-glycolyl neuraminic acid derivatives of ganglioside
GD3. Arch. Biochem. Biophys. 260, 51, 1988.
9. Nores, G. A., T. Dohi, M. Taniguchi, and S. Hakamori. Density-dependent recognition of
cell surface GM3 by a certain anti-melanoma antibody, and GM3 lactone as a possible
immunogen: requirements for tumor-associated antigen and immunogenicity. J. Immunol.
139, 3171, 1987.
10. Furukawa, K., B. T. Chait, and K. O. Lloyd. Identification of NeuGc-containing gangliosides of cat and sheep erythrocytes. ^{252}CF fission fragment ionization mass spectrometry in the
analysis of glycosphingolipids. J. Biol. Chem. - in press, 1988.
11. Higashi, H., I. Nishi, Y. Fukui, S. Ueda, S. Kato, M. Fujita, Y. Nakano, T. Taguchi, S. Sakai,
M. Sako, and M. Naiki. Tumor-associated expression of glycosphingolipid Hanganutziu-
Deicher antigen in human cancer. Gann. 75, 1025, 1984.
12. Livingston, P. O., E. J. Natoli, M. J. Calves, E. Stockert, H. F. Oettgen, and L. J. Old. Vaccines containing purified GM2 ganglioside elicit GM2 antibodies in melanoma patients. Proc.
Natl. Acad. Sci. USA 84, 2911, 1987.
13. Yamaguchi, H., K. Furukawa, S. R. Fortunato, P. O. Livingston, K. O. Lloyd, H. F.
Oettgen, and L. J. Old. A human monoclonal antibody derived from the lymphocytes of a
melanoma patient vaccinated with GM2 ganglioside and BCG - paper in preparation, 1988.
14. Schrump, D. S., K. Furukawa, H. Yamaguchi, K. O. Lloyd, and L. J. Old. Recognition of
galactosyl-globoside by monoclonal antibodies derived from patients with primary lung cancer. Proc. Natl. Acad. Sci. USA 85, 4441, 1988.

19. Glycosphingolipid Expression in Murine T Cells and Macrophages

P. F. Mühlradt, J. Müthing, and R. v. Kleist

Introduction

Cells of the immune system are fascinating objects, if one wishes to study changes in glycosphingolipid (GSL)* expression during ontogeny, differentiation, and activation. Like other blood cells, they originate from the bone marrow, migrate with the blood stream, and settle in lymphoid and other tissue. T lymphocytes in particular spend some of their lifetime in the thymus where they mature, differentiate to subpopulations with special tasks, and learn to recognize "self", before they emigrate and settle in specific T-dependent areas of the secondary lymphoid organs from where they circulate with the lymph and to where they return with the blood. Macrophages (MPh), on the other hand, circulate only during their early developmental stage as blood monocytes, and, once they settle in the tissue, probably stay there relatively fixed. The mechanism by which immune cells find the appropriate histological site in the primary and secondary lymphoid organs during ontogeny and maturation is still totally obscure. It is possible that cell surface carbohydrates may be involved.

It is with this in mind that we have compared the GSL composition of murine T cells and MPh at various stages of development and activation. We found that, while most of the GSLs are constantly expressed, others change as cells differentiate or become activated. Examples for such GSLs are globoside (1) and a group of gangliosides with the IVNeuAc/GcGgOse$_5$-Cer structure (2).

Materials and Methods

Animals. Female CBA/J inbred mice were purchased from Gl. Bomholtgard Ltd (RY, Denmark), and used at the age of 6 to 8 weeks.

Cell culture, mitogen stimulation, cloned T lymphocytes. Spleen lympocytes were isolated, stimulated with Concanavalin A (Con A), and cultivated as previously described (2). Resulting T blasts were isolated on a one-step gradient on Lymphoprep (Nyegard, Oslo; 1.077 g/l). Larger amounts of T blasts were propagated in the presence of HPLC purified human T cell growth factor interleukin 2 (4) in bioreactors in up to 2 L volumes (5). Cloned T cells were grown as described in (6).

Metabolic labelling of cells, and GSL extraction. These procedures are described in (2) and (7).

Isolation of gangliosides, high performance thin layer chromatography and autoradiography. Gangliosides were isolated as previously described (2). High performance thin layer chromatography and autoradiography was carried out as in (2).

*Abbreviations used in this paper: BCG, Bacillus calmette-Guerin; CP, Corynebacterium parvum; GSL, glycosphingolipids; LPS, lipopolysaccharide, endotoxin; MPh, macrophage. On T cells, and the Forssman GSL antigen on MPh (3). We shall in the following review our earlier findings, adding new data to create a more complete picture.

Neuraminidase treatment and immunostaining of gangliosides on HPTLC plates. These procedures are described in (8).

Enzyme-linked immunostaining procedure for GSLs on HPTLC plates. The detailed procedure is described elsewhere (9).

Mass spectrometric analysis of purified gangliosides. Fast atom bombardment mass spectrometry (FAB-MS) of the native and permethylated gangliosides was done as described by Egge & Peter-Katalinic' (10).

Preparation of poly- and monoclonal antisera. The preparation of polyclonal rabbit antiserum against globoside is described in (1), that of monoclonal antiserum against Forssman GSL in (3).

Complement elimination studies. Immune cells were trated with antibody and complement, and functional studies with the remaining cells were performed as described in (1) and (3).

Immunostaining of tissue sections and glass adherent cells. Spleens from 2 to 3 months old CBA/J mice were removed and snapfrozen in liquid nitrogen. Four μm sections were cut on a cryostat, air dried, dipped for 5 sec in cold acetone, and kept at 4°C until further processed. Sections or glass adherent cells were fixed for 10 min in 3.7% formalin in PBS. Rat Forssman-specific monoclonal antibody IgG_{2c} from clone III E2 (3) was purified over protein A sepharose and used at 4 μg/ml. FITC-labelled goat anti rat second antibody was purchased from Medac (Hamburg, FRG) and used at 1/10 dilution. Peroxidase-labelled second antibodies were used to stain tissue sections as in (11). Antibodies were diluted in PBS, containing 2% FCS and O.O. 2% azide. Incubations were done for 30 min in the cold, followed by 3 washes with cold PBS.

In vivo induction of Forssman positive peritoneal MPh by inflammatory stimuli. Mice were injected i.p. with the following stimulating agents: 170 μg live *bacilli of Calmette and Guerin* (BCG), 1.4 mg *Corynebacterium parvum* (CP) (both from Calbiochem), 1 ml thioglycollate (TG), 1 ml proteose peptone or phenol extracted smooth-type lipopolysaccharide (LPS, endotoxin) from *Salmonella thyphimurium as indicated*. Peritoneal lavage followed after 4 d.

Glass adherent peritoneal macrophages. The content of MPh in the peritoneal cells varied from 35% in controls up to 75% in TG treated animals. MPh were enriched from peritoneal cells by letting them adhere to glass microscope slides for 4 h at 37°C, after which time they were rinsed and allowed to spread overnight. The cells were then immunostained and assayed for the content of Forssman positive ones.

Preparation of Forssman GSL inducing cytokine. A human myeloid cell line, HL 60, grown in RPMI 1640 medium with 5% fetal calf serum, served as source for the cytokine. This was concentrated by precipitation with ammonium sulfate (90% saturation). The precipitate was redissolved in a minimal volume of saline, extensively dialysed against saline in the cold, and the inner dialysate was cleared by 1 h centrifugation at 30.000 x g.

In vitro induction of Forssman GSL antigen on peritoneal macrophages. Glass adherent, proteose peptone elicited macrophages were incubated with RPMI 1640 medium with 5% fetal calf serum and up to 5% (v/v) cytokine for 3 d in a CO_2 incubator. Forssman positive cells were enumerated after immunostaining.

Results and Discussion

Globoside as marker for murine T lymphocytes. We had originally observed globoside in GSLs from alloantigen stimulated T lymphocytes, whereas B cells stimulated with LPS or T blasts stimulated with Con A did not exhibit this GSL (7). A survey of cloned T cells with either helper or cytolytic function showed this GSL to be characteristic of helper and absent from cytolytic clones (4). In continuation of this work we assayed primary T lymphocytes for the presence of globoside, since it was not certain that cloned T cells, in culture for an extended time period, still exhibit the same GSL as freshly isolated cells (see aslo contributions by P. Fredman and R. F. Irie, this volume). Complement elimination studies and functional analysis of globoside depleted primary spleen cells showed that the situation was indeed more complicated as one might have thought from the early data. About half of the precursors of cytolytic T cells, like precursors of helper T cells, exhibit globoside. However, as cytolytic precursors differentiate to killer effector T cells they lose this marker (1). In contrast, helper effector cells, defined as cells synthesizing interleukin 2 within 12 hours after stimulation, still express globoside and can be largely eliminated by anti globoside antibodies and complement (see Figure 1).

When T cells from different lymphoid organs were investigated for the presence of globoside by immunostaining, the following picture emerged: Of thymocytes only 2–4 % were globoside positive. These could be enriched up to 19 % in the medullary

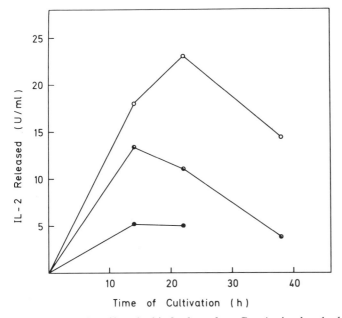

Figure 1. Kinetics of interleukin 2 release from Con A stimulated spleen lymphocytes before and after elimination of globoside positive T cells. Open circles: complement (C) control; half closed circles: anti-globoside antibody (1:80) plus C; closed circles: anti-globoside antibody (1:40) plus C.

fraction which comprises the more mature population, and which can be isolated by differential agglutination with peanut agglutinin (12). Spleen T cells were 30–40 % globoside positive, whereas T cells from lymph nodes were only 3–8 % globoside positive.

The ganglioside IVNeuGc/Ac-GgOse₅ Cer as a T cell marker. We recently elucidated the structures of most gangliosides from T blasts by various methods including mass spectroscopy (2). The separation pattern on high performance thin layer chromatography and the underlying structures are depicted in Figure 2. As shown, the complexity of the separation pattern is mainly caused by heterogeneity in the fatty acid and the sialic acid moiety, the basic structure being GM1b. An extended structure, GalNAc-GM1b

$$GalNAc\beta1,4Gal\beta1,3GalNAc\beta1,4Gal\beta1,4Glc\beta1,1Cer$$
$$|\alpha$$
$$NeuAc(Gc)$$

appears characteristic for T blast gangliosides and does not occur in those from B cells (2). The same ganglioside has recently been characterized as a component of murine spleen gangliosides (13), in the murine tumor MDAY-D2 (14, 15), and, for the first time, as a trace component in human brain gangliosides from Tay-Sachs patients (16).

Gangliosides from Murine T Lymphocytes

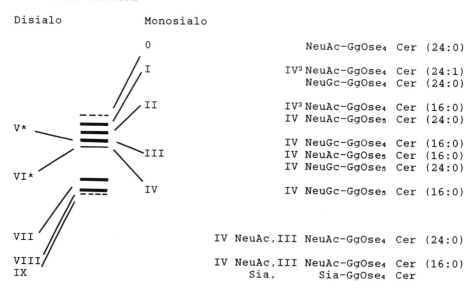

HPTLC Pattern

Disialo   Monosialo

0	NeuAc-GgOse₄ Cer (24:0)
I	IV³ NeuAc-GgOse₄ Cer (24:1) NeuGc-GgOse₄ Cer (24:0)
II	IV³ NeuAc-GgOse₄ Cer (16:0) IV NeuAc-GgOse₅ Cer (24:0)
III	IV NeuGc-GgOse₄ Cer (16:0) IV NeuAc-GgOse₅ Cer (16:0) IV NeuGc-GgOse₅ Cer (24:0)
IV	IV NeuGc-GgOse₅ Cer (16:0)
VII	IV NeuAc,III NeuAc-GgOse₄ Cer (24:0)
VIII	IV NeuAc,III NeuAc-GgOse₄ Cer (16:0)
IX	Sia, Sia-GgOse₄ Cer

* Lactones or O-Acetyl forms of VII and VIII resp.

Figure 2. Separation pattern on thin layer plates, and structures of mono- and disialogangliosides from murine T lymphoblasts.

Within the T cell lineage it is a very interesting marker, detectable only in trace amounts on thymocytes, but distinctly present on two T helper clones, as on Con A blasts. It was found only weakly expressed by one investigated cytolytic T cell clone. These latter data were obtained by specifically immunostaining the gangliosides after neuraminidase treatment on the thin layer plate ([8], and Müthing, Schwinzer, and Mühlradt, unpublished). Although the picture is yet incomplete, and the distribution of GalNAc-GM1b positive T cells in different lymphoid organs is still unclear, it appears that globoside and GalNAc-GM1b are typical differentiation markers for murine T cells, they are subpopulation and partly organ specific, and as far as the thymus goes, are probably restricted to the medulla.

We have tried to correlate the appearance of the above marker GSLs with the maturation pathway of T cells in Figure 3.

Forssman GSL as marker for murine MPh subpopulations. Forssman GSL is another GSL differentiation marker, not only for early embryonic cells (17), but within the immune system for mononuclear phagocytes. We have recently reported that this GSL is neither expressed by blood monocytes nor polymorphonuclear cells, but by 70 % of the macrophages of the spleen and peripheral lymph nodes. It is not expressed by MPh of the liver or lung, nor by resident peritoneal MPh (3).

Anatomical distribution of Forssman positive MPh in spleen tissue. Earlier investigations (18) had shown that Forssman positive MPh reside only in the red pulp of the

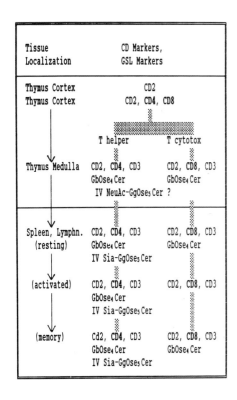

Figure 3. Correlation of expression of glycolipids with differentiation, tissue localization, and activation of T lymphocytes.

spleen (see Figure 4). We know now that other subpopulations of spleen MPh, recognized by the monoclonal antibodies MOMA-1 (11) and ERTR-9 (19), and residing in concentric shells within the white pulp of the spleen (11, 19) do not overlap with Forssman positive MPh (Mühlradt and Dijkstra, in preparation). These findings do not prove, of course, that cell surface carbohydrates such as Forssman GSL specifically direct Forssman positive MPh to the red pulp, but they are compatible with such a notion.

In vivo induction of Forssman GSL on peritoneal MPh. If GSLs were in any way functionally important for immune cells, one would expect that mechanisms exist to modulate their expression. We have shown recently that inflammatory stimuli by CP, TG, or endotoxin applied intraperitoneally, lead to a moderate but significant increase in Forssman positive MPh when compared to resident MPh (18). This was not due to immigration of such cells from the spleen, because Forssman positive MPh appeared in the peritoneum also of splenectomized animals (v. Kleist, Westermann, and Mühlradt, in preparation). Endotoxin in particular is very potent in inducing Forssman GSL, as is shown in a dose response curve in Figure 5. We think that the appearance of Forssman GSL on peritoneal MPh is a very sensitive indicator of an inflammatory process in the peritoneum.

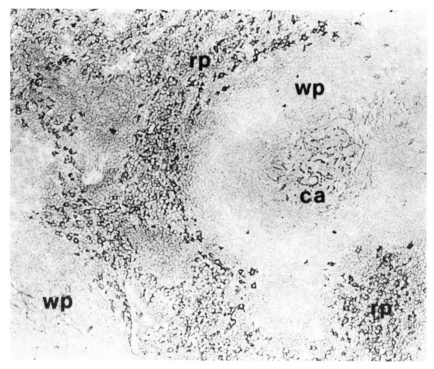

Figure 4. Forssman positive macrophages and reticulum cells in a cryo section of a murine spleen. Peroxidase-labelled second antibodies against Forssman specific monoclonal first antibodies visualize Forssman positive cells. ca = central artery, rp = red pulp, wp = white pulp. Magnification: 97.5 fold.

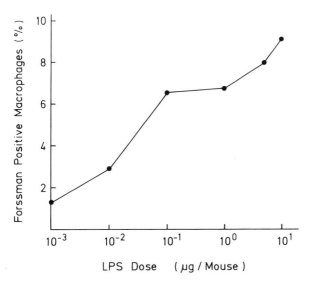

Figure 5. Induction of Forssman GSL *in vivo* on peritoneal macrophages of LPS treated mice. Mice were treated 3 days previous to harvesting the cells by intraperitoneal injections with the indicated doses of S. typhimurium LPS. Forssman positive macrophages were determined in the glass-adherent population by indirect immunofluorescence. Peritoneal macrophages from control animals, receiving mock injections with physiological saline, contained 1.8 % Forssman positive cells.

In vitro induction of Forssman GSL expression in glass adherent peritoneal MPh. The splenectomy experiment does not exclude the possibility that Forssman positive MPh migrated to the peritoneal cavity from elsewhere than the spleen, nor does it give any indication of the mechanism by which the expression of this GSL is brought about. Do formerly negative MPh acquire Forssman GSL, or do a few Forssman positive

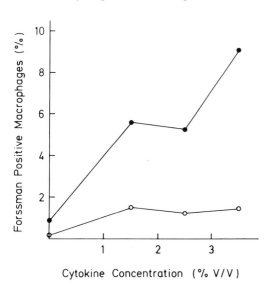

Figure 6. Induction of Forssman GSL expression *in vitro* on peritoneal macrophages by cytokine. Peritoneal macrophages from proteose peptone primed (closed circles) or saline treated (open circles) mice were cultured on microslides for 3 days in the presence of increasing amounts of cytokines from a human myeloid cell line. Forssman positive cells were determined by indirect immunofluorescence.

MPh proliferate in situ? To approach these questions we attempted to induce Forssman GSL in cell culture. In these experiments none of the stimulants that caused in vivo appearance of Forssman positive MPh showed any in vitro activity in this respect. However, we were able to induce Forssman antigen in cell culture on a formerly negative population of glass adherent peritoneal MPh by the addition of a cytokine containing preparation to the culture medium. Induction of Forssman expression was dose dependent (see Figure 6), and worked best with in vivo primed cells. There was no indication of proliferation of formerly Forssman positive MPh. The phenomenon is strongly reminiscent of the induction of class II MHC antigens under similar conditions (20). The nature of the cytokines responsible for Forssman induction is still under investigation.

Conclusions

We think that there is a clear correlation of expression of certain GSLs with the state of differentiation of immune cells. Since expression of GSLs can be modulated in vivo as in vitro, and by a physiologic stimulus such as a cytokine, as exemplified for MPh with the Forssman antigen, it is very likely that these cell surface molecules are in some way functional. So far we were unable to block any in vitro functions by the addition of antibodies against either globoside (1) or Forssman GSL (3). From the contribution of S. Ladisch to this meeting for example it is likely, though, that such functions may exist. It is equally possible that expression of GSL antigens is in some way related to (in the course of differentiation variable), the anatomical distribution of the respective cells. The fact that globoside, within the T cell lineage, is expressed primarily by medullary thymocytes, and spleen T cells, and that Forssman GSL is expressed almost exclusively by MPh in the red pulp of the spleen may suggest such correlation.

Summary

The expression of three GSL differentiation markers, globoside, GalNAc-GM1b, and Forssman GSL, was followed in subpopulations of murine T cells and macrophages, and correlated with anatomical location, functional or developmental stages.

References

1. Mühlradt, P. F., U. Bethke, D. A. Monner, and K. Petzoldt. The glycosphingolipid globoside as a serological marker for cytolytic T lymphocyte precursors and alloantigen responsive proliferating T lymphocytes in murine spleen. Eur. J. Immunol. 14, 852, 1984.

2. Müthing, J., H. Egge, B. Kniep, and P. F. Mühlradt. Structural characterization of gangliosides from murine T lymphocytes. Eur. J. Biochem. 163, 407, 1987.

3. Bethke, U., B. Kniep, and P. F. Mühlradt. Forssman glycolipid, an antigenic marker for a major subpopulation of macrophages from murine spleen and peripheral lymph nodes. J. Immunol. 138, 4329, 1987.

4. Kniep, E.-M., B. Kniep, W. Grote, H. S. Conradt, D. A. Monner, and P. F. Mühlradt. Purification of the T lymphocyte growth factor interleukin-2 from culture media of human peripheral blood leukocytes (buffy coats). Eur. J. Biochem. 143, 199, 1984.

5. Müthing, J. and P. F. Mühlradt. Interleukin-2 (T cell growth factor)-dependent propagation of normal murine lymphocytes in a bioreactor. Biological Chemistry Hoppe-Seyler 365, 1036, 1984.

6. Kniep, B., T. R. Hünig, F.W. Fitch, J. Heuer, E. Kölsch, and P. F. Mühlradt. Neutral glycosphingolipids of murine myeloma cells, and helper, cytolytic and suppressor T lymphocytes. Biochemistry 22, 251, 1983.

7. Gruner, K. R., R.V.W. van Eijk, and P. F. Mühlradt. Structure elucidation of marker glycolipids of alloantigen-activated murine T lymphocytes. Biochemistry 20, 4518, 1981.

8. Müthing J. and P. F. Mühlradt. Detection of gangliosides of the GM1b-type on high-performance thin-layer chromatography plates by immunostaining after neuraminidase treatment. Anal. Biochem. 172, 1988.

9. Bethke, U., J. Müthing, B. Schauder, P. Conradt, and P. F. Mühlradt. An improved semi-quantitative enzyme immunostaining procedure for glycosphingolipid antigens on high performance thin layer chromatograms. J. Immunol. Methods 89, 111, 1986.

10. Egge H. and J. Peter-Katalinic. Fast atom bombardment mass spectrometry for structural elucidation of glycoconjugates. Mass Spectrom. Rev. 6, 331, 1987.

11. Kraal, G. and M. Janse. Marginal metallophilic cells of the mouse spleen identified by a monoclonal antibody. Immunology 58, 665, 1986.

12. Reisner, Y. and N. Sharon. Fractionation of subpopulations of mouse and human lymphocytes by peanut agglutinin or soybean agglutinin. Methods in Enzymol. 108, 168, 1984.

13. Nakamura, K., M. Suzuki, F. Inagaki, T. Yamakawa, and A. Suzuki. A new ganglioside showing choleragenoid-binding activity in mouse spleen. J. Biochem. 101, 825, 1987.

14. Schwartz, R., B. Kniep, J. Müthing, and P. F. Mühlradt. Glycoconjugates of murine tumor lines with different metastatic capacities. II. Diversity of glycolipid composition. Int. J. Cancer 36, 601, 1985.

15. Laferté, S., M. N. Fukuda, M. Fukuda, A. Dell, and J.W. Dennis. Glycosphingolipids of lectin-resistant mutants of the highly metastasic mouse tumor line, MDAY-D2. Cancer Res. 47, 150, 1987.

16. Itoh, T., Y.-T. Li, and R. K. Yu. Isolation and characterization of a novel monosialosylpentahexosyl ceramide from Tay-Sachs brain. J. Biol. Chem. 256, 165, 1981.

17. Willison, K. R., R. A. Karol, A. Suzuki, S. K. Kundu, and D. M. Marcus. Neutral glycolipid antigens as developmental markers of mouse teratocarcinoma and early embryos: an immunologic and chemical analysis. Cell 14, 775, 1982.

18. Conradt, P., R. v. Kleist, and P. F. Mühlradt. Tissue localization and migration of murine spleen macrophages carrying the Forssman glycolipid antigen. In: Proceedings of the Ninth International Conference on Lymphatic Tissues and Germinal Centers. S. Fossum ed. Plenum Press, New York, London, p. in press, 1988.

19. Dijkstra, C. D., E. van Vliet, E. A. Döpp, A. A. van der Lelij, and G. Kraal. Marginal zone macrophages identified by a monoclonal antibody: characterization of immuno- and enzyme-histochemical properties and functional capacities. Immunology 55, 23, 1985.

20. Beller, D. I. and K. Ho. Regulation of macrophage subpopulations. V. Evaluation of the control of macrophage Ia expression in vitro. J. Immunol. 129, 971, 1982.

20. Activation of T Lymphocytes by Binding of Monoclonal Antibodies to Cell Surface GD3

A. N. Houghton, H. Yuasa, P. B. Chapman, and K. Welte

Introduction

There is evidence that gangliosides play a role in cell signaling and recognition (1, 2). In particular, gangliosides and antibodies directed against ganglioside antigens have been found to regulate the growth and activation of cells of the immune system. Gangliosides have been found to inhibit prioliferative responses of immune cells stimulated by mitogens, antigens and interleukin 2, and enhance growth of immunogenic tumors (3–15), although the biological and physiological significance of these findings is still obscure (3).

Direct binding to gangliosides on the cell surface has been found to directly activate lymphoid cells (16) or augment activation by other stimuli (17). Spiegel et al. have demonstrated that binding of the B subunit of cholera toxin to GM1 can directly induce rat thymocyte proliferation (16). Further studies of this phenomenon have shown that B subunit of cholera toxin induces a rapid and sustained increase in cytoplasmic free Ca^{2+}, without an effect on levels of cellular inositol phosphates, intracellular pH, or cellular distribution of protein kinase C (17). These findings suggest that B subunit increases intracellular Ca^{2+} by inducing a net influx of extracellular Ca^{2+}.

Hersey and coworkers first reported that monoclonal antibodies to GD3 (and GD2) could potentiate the proliferative response of mouse natural killer cells to IL-2 and of human peripheral blood lymphocytes to the lectin phytohemagglutinin (PHA) and anti-CD3 monoclonal antibody (18). Based on this initial report, we determined whether cells of the T cell lineage expressed GD3 and explored the possibility that *direct* binding of mAb to GD3 could activate T lymphocytes in addition potentiating mitogenic responses.

Expression of GD3 on Human Thymocytes and Peripheral Blood T Lymphocytes

Using the anti-GD3 monoclonal antibody (mAb) R24, we have found that immature cells in the human T lymphoid lineage express GD3, including subcortical thymocytes and thymocytes located specifically around vessels and Hassal's corpuscles in the medulla (19). The identity of these cells as thymocytes was confirmed by double staining with the thymocyte marker OKT-6. Subcortical thymocytes are presumed to include precursors of mature T cells that reach the periphery, and GD3$^+$ thymocytes that cluster around vessels could represent cells trying to reach the vascular system. On the other hand, GD3$^+$ thymocytes around Hassal's corpuscle presumably include end-stage cells that never reach maturity.

R24 was found to react with peripheral blood mononuclear cells (PBMC) – a mean of $13.9 \pm 5.5\%$ (standard deviation) PBMC were GD3$^+$ (range 7.4–24.3%). mAb 3F8 against GD2 (20) and a control IgG3 mAb (FLOP/c 21) were unreactive with PBMC. Analysis by two-color flow cytometry showed that GD3 was expressed on mainly CD3$^+$ cells ($14.8 \pm 5.7\%$), with approximately an equal proportion of CD4$^+$ and

CD8$^+$ cells. Thus, it appeared that no particular T cell lineage in peripheral blood preferentially expressed GD3. Reactivity of R24 with PBMC was ablated by pre-treatment of target cells with neuraminadase or ethanol (but binding was resist to trypsin and proteases). R24 was found to react with an acidic glycolipid fraction of enriched peripheral blood T cells, and binding was specifically inhibited by GD3 but not GM2, GM3 or GD2. GD3 expression was confirmed by thin layer chromatography. GD3 comprised <3 % of total ganglioside of resting PBMC and 3–5 % of total ganglioside of PBMC stimulated by R24.

Activation of Peripheral Blood T Lymphocytes by mAb against GD3

Monoclonal antibodies against GD3 directly induced T cell proliferation (19), without the addition of mitogens or growth factors (in contrast to previous reports) (18). Maximum proliferation was observed at 5–6 days in culture, and was related to mAb concentration (Figure 1). Proliferation was detected at R24 concentrations of ≥ 1 µg/ml of mAb R24. Proliferation was also induced by F(ab')2 fragments of R24. Two other mAb against GD3, mAb C5 (IgG3) and mAb K9 (IgM) also induced T cell proliferation (Figure 2). It was found that mAb against GD2 (mAb 3F8) did not stimulate, although it has been reported that some anti-GD2 mAb may augment lymphocyte stimulation by mitogens/growth factors (18). One explanation for this discrepancy could be cross-reactivity of some anti-GD2 mAb with GD3. In our studies, no binding of the anti-GD2 mAb 3F8 to T cells was detected, and GD2 was not detected on resting or R24-activated T cells by thin layer chromatography. Other control IgG3 mAb against non-ganglioside antigens and an IgM mAb against GM2 were also inactive

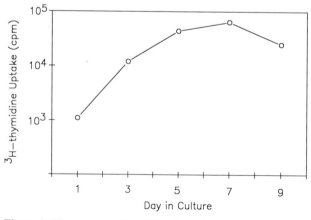

Figure 1. Time course of proliferation of sheep erythrocyte rosette-positive peripheral blood cells (E$^+$ cells) in the presence of mAb R24 100 µg/ml. The results represent the mean of three independent experiments.

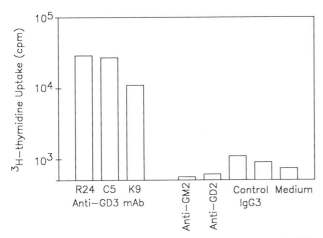

Figure 2. Analysis of specificity of stimulation by mAb. E[+] cells were incubated with mAb 100 μg/ml for 5 days and proliferation measured by incorporation or ^{3}H-thymidine. Anti-GM2 mAb = 10–11; anti-GD2 mAb = 3F8; control IgG3 mAb = F36/22 and FLOP/c 21.

(Figure 2). Increased expression of GD3 appeared to not be simply related to T cell activation since PBMC stimulated by PHA or by anti-CD3 (T3) mAb did not show an increase in GD3-positive cells.

Evidence that mAb R24 Activates a GD3 Subpopulation of T Cells

Activation T cells with R24 led to an increase in the proportion of R24-positive cells over time, from 10–20% of cells at initial culture to approximately 50% by days

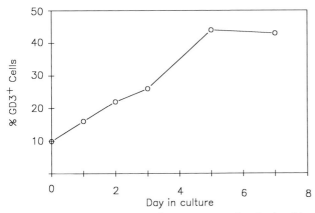

Figure 3. GD3 expression by E[+] cells either preincubation (day 0) or incubated with R24 100 μg/ml for up to 7 days. GD3 expression was determined by measuring R24-positive cells using flow cytometry.

5–7 (Figure 3). Analysis by flow cytometry showed that T cells expressing the highest levels of GD3 were large, blast-like cells, suggesting that it was the GD3-positive population that was proliferating and expanding. Proliferation induced by R24 was dependent on the presence of R24-positive cells in the starting population of T cells. Depletion of GD3-positive cells by complement-mediated lysis with R24 completely abrogated proliferation induced by R24 (Figure 4).

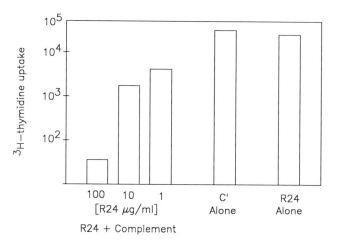

Figure 4. R24-induced proliferation of E⁺ cells after complement-mediated depletion by R24 and human complement. Cells were preincubated with R24 (0, 10, and 100 µg/ml) plus complement, complement alone or R24 (100 µg/ml) alone. The % R24-positive cells was 15 % in untreated, complement alone and R24 alone cells, but decreased with complement to 7 % for R24 1 µg/ml, 3 % for R24 10 µg/ml and <1 % for R24 100 µg/ml. Cells were then incubated with R24 100 µg/ml for 5 days.

Augmentation of R24-induced Proliferation by IL-2

Stimulation of peripheral blood T cells (selected by rosetting with sheep erythrocytes) by R24 led to a marked increase in the proportion of IL-2 receptor positive cells from less than 3 % to approximately 50 % by day 7 (Figure 5). However, only very low levels of IL-2 were detected in culture supernatants of T cells stimulated by R24 – a maximum of only 1–2 U/ml were measured between days one and five stimulation. These results suggested that secretion of IL-2 might not be crucial to activation induced by R24, but any secreted IL-2 might bind to induced IL-2 receptors. The addition of rhIL-2 (100 U/ml) to R24-stimulated cultures markedly augmented proliferation induced by R24 or IL-2 alone (Figure 6). On the other, OKT-11 (anti-CD2) and OKT-3 (anti-CD3) mAb which bind to known activation pathways in T cells were not found to augment activation by R24, and in some experiments substantially inhibited R24-induced proliferation.

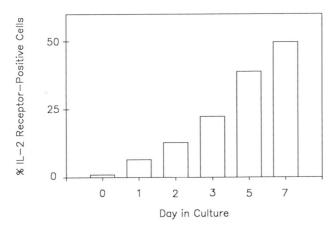

Figure 5. Induction IL-2 receptor expression on E$^+$ cells by incubation with R24 100 μg/ml over 7 days.

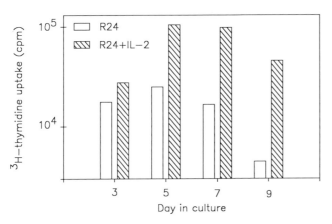

Figure 6. Effect of IL-2 on R24-induced proliferation of E$^+$ cells. Cells were incubated with R24 100 μg/ml alone or R24 100 μg/ml plus IL-2 100 U/ml (Cetus) for up to 9 days. Maximum stimulation by IL-2 100 U/ml alone was 25,361 ± 11,705 cpm at day 7.

Summary

    It is not clear what mechanisms are involved in activation of T cells by R24. There is no evidence that R24 binds to cell surface glycoproteins, including those involved in T cell activation. However, it is possible that GD3 is linked to one of these activation pathways, such as the T cell receptor/CD3 complex of molecules or the CD2 (T11) molecule (these two activation complexes seem to be closely linked in T cell activation). The finding that anti-CD2 mAb can inhibit R24-induced T cell proliferation suggests that this activation pathways might be linked with the R24-induced pathway.

Alternatively, GD3 itself could participate directly as a proximal event in T cell activation, perhaps by regulating net flux of ionized calcium into the cell (not suprisingly, preliminary data suggests that R24 activation is associated with an rapid net increase in cellular calcium) (Yuasa, H., unpublished observation) or by providing messenger molecules. The regulation of T cell activation is one the best characterized cellular phenomenon of humans and higher verterbates, and provides an excellent system to explore the possible role of gangliosides in growth and differentiation of cells.

References

1. Hakomori, S. Glycosphingolipids in cellular interaction, differentiation and oncogenesis. Annu. Rev. Biochem. 50, 733, 1981.
2. Yu, R. K., Kroener, Jr., T. A., Demou, P. C., Scarsdale, J. N., and Prestegard, J. H. Recent advances in structural analysis of gangliosides. Primary and secondary structures. Adv. Exp. Med. Biol. 174, 87, 1984.
3. Marcus, D. M. A review of the immunologic and immunomodulatory properties of glycosphingolipids. Mol. Immunol. 21, 1083, 1984.
4. Agarwal, M. K. and Neter, E. Effect of selected lipids and surfactants in immunogenicity of several bacterial antigens. J. Immunol. 107, 1448, 1971.
5. Miller, H. C. and Esselman, W. J. Modulation of the immune response by antigen reactive lymphocytes after cultivation with gangliosides. J. Immunol. 115, 839, 1975.
6. Esselman, W. J. and Miller, H. C. Modulation of B cell responses by glycolipid released from antigen-stimulated T cells. J. Immunol. 119, 1994, 1977.
7. Ryan, J. L. and Shinitsky, M. Possible role for glycosphingolipids in the control of immune responses. Eur. J. Immunol. 9, 171, 1979.
8. Lengle, E. E., Krishnaraj, R., and Kemp, R. G. Inhibition of the lectin-induced mitogenic response of thymocytes by glycolipids. Cancer Res. 39, 817, 1979.
9. Whisler, R. L. and Yates, A. J. Regulation of lymphocyte responses by human gangliosides. J. Immunol. 125, 2106, 1980.
10. Ladisch, S., Gillard, B., Wong, C., and Ulsh. Shedding and immunosuppressive activity of YAC lymphoma gangliosides. Cancer Res. 43, 3803, 1983.
11. Ladisch, S., Ulsh, L., Gillard, B., and Wong, C. Modulation of immune response by gangliosides: Inhibition of adherent monocyte accessory function in vitro. J. Clin. Investig. 74, 2074, 1984.
12. Gonwa, T. A., Westrick, M. A., and Macher, B. A. Inhibition of mitogen- and antigen-induced lymphocyte activation by human leukemia cell gangliosides. Cancer Res. 44, 3467, 1984.
13. Merritt, W. D., Bailey, M., and Pluznik, D. H. Inhibition of interleukin 2 dependent cytotoxic T lymphocyte growth by gangliosides. Cellular Immunol. 89, 1, 1984.
14. Robb, R. J. The suppressive effect of gangliosides upon IL-2-dependent proliferation as a function of inhibition of IL-2 receptor association. J. Immunol. 136, 971, 1984.
15. Ladisch, S., Kitada, S., and Hays, E. Gangliosides shed by tumor cells enhance tumor formation in mice. J. Clin. Investig. 79, 1879, 1987.
16. Spiegel, S., Fishman, P. H., and Weber, R. J. Direct evidence that endogenous GM1 ganglioside can mediate thymocyte proliferation. Science 230, 1285, 1985.

17. Dixon, S. J., Stewart, D., Grinstein, S., Spiegel, S. Transmembrane signaling by the B subunit of cholera toxin: Increased cytoplasmic free calcium in rat lymphocytes. J. Cell Biol. 105, 1153, 1987.
18. Hersey, P., Schibeci, S. D., Townsend, P., Burns, C., and Cheresh, D. A. Potentiation of lymphocyte response by monoclonal antibodies to the ganglioside GD3. Cancer Res. 46, 6083, 1986.
19. Welte, K., Miller, G., Chapman, P. B., Yuasa, H., Natoli, E., Kunicka, J. E., Cordon-Cardo, C., Buhrer, C., Old, L. J., and Houghton, A. N. Stimulation of T lymphocyte proliferation by monoclonal antibodies against GD3 ganglioside. J. Immunol. 139, 1763, 1987.
20. Saito, M. R., Yu, R. K., and Cheung, N. K. Ganglioside GD2 specificity of monoclonal antibodies to human neuroblastoma cells. Biochem. Biophys. Res. Commun. 127, 1, 1985.

21. Immunoregulatory Activity of Gangliosides Shed by Melanoma Tumors

J. Portoukalian

Introduction

A few years ago, we showed that the plasma and erythrocytes of melanoma tumor-bearing patients are enriched in GM3 and GD3 gangliosides (1) which are the major gangliosides of melanoma tumors (2). After tumor removal, the ganglioside content of both red cells and plasma goes down to the normal values within a few weeks. The finding of high amounts of GD3 in melanoma ascites fluid suggested that GM3 and GD3 were shed from the melanoma cells in proliferation (1). Since gangliosides are known to have an immunomodulatory influence (3, 4, 5), we studied the shedding of gangliosides from malignant melanoma and the effect of such gangliosides on the immune system.

Material and Methods

Melanoma tumors were homogenized in chloroform-methanol 1/1. The tissues were extracted twice with the same solvent. After evaporation, the lipid residue was dissolved in dry chloroform-methanol 2/1, filtered and dried. This operation was repeated twice to remove most peptidic contaminants. Total gangliosides were purified by three successive partitions in chloroform/methanol/phosphate-buffered saline pH 7.2 (1/1/0.7 by volume) and desalting by reverse-phase chromatography on C18-bonded silica gel (6). Gangliosides were then isolated by HPLC on a 25 cm column of silica gel LiChrospher Si 100 (5 μm) (Merck) with an Hitachi L-6200, using a solvent gradient with isopropanol-hexanewater as described by Watanabe and Arao (7). Separation was monitored by HPTLC on silica gel 60 plates (Merck) developed in chloroform-methanol-0.1% $CaCl_2$ 60/35/8. The relative proportion of each ganglioside in the tumors was estimated after resorcinol-HCl by scanning densitometry of the TLC plates on a Shimadzu CS-930 Chromatoscan set at 580 nm.

Tissues and blood samples were obtained from our center and immediately processed. Peripheral blood lymphocytes were purified by Ficoll-Hypaque gradient (Pharmacia). The human melanoma cell lines used in this study were established and characterized in our laboratory.

Results and Discussion

Shedding of gangliosides by melanoma cells and increased ganglioside content of lymphocytes from patients with melanoma. Melanoma cells were metabolically labelled with ^{14}C-galactose in culture conditions and left in serum-free medium for 48 hrs. The gangliosides were then purified from the cells and the ultracentrifuged supernatant, migrated on TLC and exposed to an X-ray film. As can be seen on Figure 1, shedding involves mostly GD3 and GM3. Melanoma gangliosides migrate on TLC as

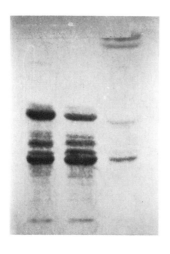

Figure 1. Autoradiogram of gangliosides shed from melanoma cells metabolically labelled. TLC in chloroform-methanol-0.1 % $CaCl_2$ 60/35/8. Left lane: gangliosides of melanoma cell line Beu labelled 24 hrs with ^{14}C-galactose. Center lane: gangliosides of Beu cells kept 48 hrs in culture after labelling. Right lane: gangliosides purified from the ultracentrifuged 48 hrs culture supernatant.

GM3
GM2
O–AcGD3
GD3
GD2

doublets of which the upper band contains gangliosides with mostly long-chain fatty acids (C18 to C24), and the lower band has C16 to C20 constitutive fatty acids. The major long-chain base is C18-sphingosine (Portoukalian, J., unpublished data). Although, in each doublet, the upper band is at a concentration slightly higher than that of the lower one upon visualization with resorcinol-HCl (data not shown), the lower band of each ganglioside is much more labelled and this higher turnover correlates with a higher rate of shedding for lower bands, at least for GM3 and GD3 (Figure 1). This is different from a report on YAC cells-shed gangliosides that have a profile similar to that of the total cellular gangliosides (5). Ascites fluid from several melanoma patients was found to have an increased content of gangliosides with a similar selectivity for GD3 and GM3 and a specificity for short-chain fatty acid species. Figure 2 shows that lymphocytes purified from tumor-bearing patients are enriched in GM3 ganglioside, and especially in its lower band. This is consistent with our finding that patients' erythrocytes are mostly enriched in GM3 (1), and this might be due to some partial hydrolysis of the GD3 taken up by the cells from the sera, since we could not see any specificity in the uptake of gangliosides by lymphocytes (data not shown).

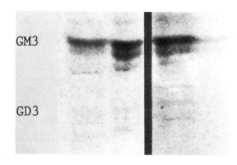

GM3

GD3

Figure 2. Autoradiogram of gangliosides of purified human peripheral blood lymphocytes (PBL) labelled with the Na periodate-K borotritide method. TLC in chloroform-methanol-0.1 % $CaCl_2$ 55/45/10. Left lane: gangliosides of 12 x 10^6 PBL from a normal donor. Center left lane: gangliosides of 7 x 10^6 PBL from a tumor-bearing melanoma patient. Center right lane: gangliosides of 9 x 10^6 PBL from a tumor-bearing melanoma patient. Right lane: standard ^{3}H-labelled GM3.

Immunomodulatory effect of melanoma gangliosides. Since GM3 and GD3 are shed from melanoma cells, the effect of these purified gangliosides was studied on the proliferative response of human lymphocytes to various stimuli. The sample of total

Table 1. Influence of major glycolipids of malignant melanoma on the proliferative response to Con A of lymphocytes from normal donors and melanoma tumor-bearing patients. The lymphocytes (4.10^4 cells/0.2 ml/well) were incubated with Con A (18 μg/ml) and glycolipids (20 nmoles/ml) for 96 hrs. Proliferation was estimated by the uptake of ^{3}H-thymidine added in the last 24 hrs. Results expressed as dpm of ^{3}H-thymidine. Mean ± SD of triplicate measures.

Donor	Culture medium + Con A	+ Total melanoma gangliosides	+ GM3	+ GD3	+ CDH
He (normal)	88 886 ± 7 632	79 184 ± 6 831	62 783 ± 5 497	84 470 ± 8 526	92 851 ± 8 632
Th (normal)	91 599 ± 8 427	69 344 ± 6 450	61 856 ± 7 025	76 851 ± 4 938	83 715 ± 8 144
Po (melanoma)	43 491 ± 5 214	29 346 ± 3 478	22 040 ± 1 858	33 234 ± 3 251	32 908 ± 4 026
Pe (melanoma)	61 439 ± 4 882	32 543 ± 2 826	25 198 ± 2 497	46 865 ± 4 213	40 457 ± 4 120

melanoma gangliosides contained 32 % GM3, 6 % GM2, 58 % GD3, and 4 % GD2 (in % of total sialic acid). The concentration of gangliosides used in these experiments was based on the highest one found in the sera of melanoma patients (20 nmoles/ml of serum, unpublished data). At this concentration, it was possible to obtain a significant inhibition of Con A-induced proliferation (Table 1) and GM3 had the strongest effect. The lymphocytes of melanoma patients seemed to be more sensitive to the influence of exogenous gangliosides than those of healthy controls. The same was true for mixed lymphocyte reactions (Table 2) for which GM3 even lowered on one patient the back-

Table 2. Influence of melanoma gangliosides on mixed lymphocyte reactions using lymphocytes from normal donors and melanoma tumor-bearing patients. $1.5 \cdot 10^5$ peripheral blood lymphocytes were mixed with an equal number of irradiated (5 000 rads) allogeneic lymphocytes in 0.2 ml of serum-containing medium, in the presence of gangliosides (60 nmoles/ml) for a 120 hrs incubation. ^{3}H-thymidine was added in the last 24 hrs to measure proliferation. Results expressed as dpm of thymidine. Mean ± SD of triplicate assays.

Donor	Culture medium	Culture medium + allogen. lymphoc.	+ GM3	+ GD3	+ total melanoma gangliosides
He (normal)	10 090 ± 1 582	65 250 ± 5 432	23 866 ± 2 344	53 822 ± 4 452	62 807 ± 6 149
Mi (normal)	16 485 ± 1 834	110 051 ± 10 244	34 990 ± 4 032	77 153 ± 6 947	59 947 ± 5 835
Po (melanoma)	15 334 ± 1 620	53 385 ± 4 848	26 047 ± 2 456	49 615 ± 4 460	38 048 ± 3 258
Pe (melanoma)	17 509 ± 2 044	39 296 ± 3 456	4 207 ± 355	38 835 ± 3 283	36 236 ± 2 945

ground proliferation due to the culture medium. When compared to other purified gangliosides, GM3 was found to be one of the most inhibitory with GD1a and GM2 (data not shown) on lymphocyte proliferative responses, regardless of the stimuli (Con A, PHA, Pokeweed mitogen, mixed lymphocyte reactions). The effect is nearly dose-dependent, although at low ganglioside concentrations (0.5 to 1 µg/ml) we observed a significant and reproducible enhancement (data not shown). The time of incubation with gangliosides is of importance, and maximal effect is reached after 48 hrs of incubation, as already seen by Whisler and Yates (4). We never experienced any toxic effect of purified gangliosides upon incubation with lymphocytes, and the possibility of the recovery of lymphocyte stimulation was investigated. As seen in Figure 3, the removal of the gangliosides from the culture medium after 48 hrs incubation is not sufficient to block a further increase of the inhibition of lymphocyte proliferation, and it is not before 96 hrs that some recovery is observed. This suggests that the gangliosides are slowly inserted into the plasma membranes of the cells up to a maximal level depending on the concentration of gangliosides used, and when placed in a ganglioside-free medium, the cells are able to release or hydrolyze the incorporated gangliosides to recover their properties.

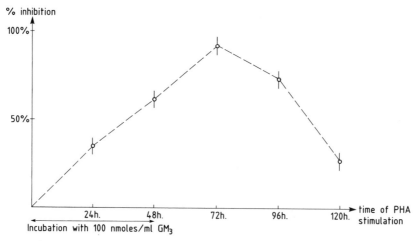

Figure 3. Reversibility of the inhibition by GM3 ganglioside of the mitogenic effect of PHA on human lymphocytes. Peripheral blood lymphocytes were preincubated with or without GM3 ganglioside (100 nmoles/ml) up to 48 hrs, then washed and kept in ganglioside-free medium for up to three more days (total of 5 days incubation). Each day from the beginning, a sample of lymphocytes was taken and stimulated in ganglioside-free medium with PHA (1 µg/ml) for 96 hrs. Proliferation was estimated by ^{3}H-thymidine addition in the last 18 hrs. Results are expressed as the % ratio of thymidine taken up by lymphocytes preincubated with versus without ganglioside.

Influence of melanoma gangliosides on IL 2 induced proliferation, IL 2 production, IL 1 production and IL 1 induced proliferation. Interleukin 2 is involved in most immune reactions and we studied the effect of melanoma-shed gangliosides on the activity of IL 2. Table 3 shows that the proliferation of human lymphocytes induced by low amounts of IL 2 is inhibited by GM3. This is consistent with a recent report by

Table 3. Influence of melanoma GM3 ganglioside on IL 2-induced proliferation of patient's lymphocytes. 4×10^5 peripheral blood lymphocytes were incubated in 0.2 ml RPMI 1640 (Gibco) + 15% AB serum containing 0.05 U of standard IL 2 for 3, 5 or 7 days in the presence of 2.5, 25 or 50 nmole/ml of GM3 purified from melanoma tumors. ^{3}H-thymidine (0.5 μCi) were added for the final 6 hrs. Results as dpm of thymidine. Mean ± SD of quadruplicate experiments.

Incubation	3 days	5 days	7 days
Medium (RPMI 1640 + 15% AB serum)	194 ± 58	216 ± 102	552 ± 258
Medium + IL-2 (0.05 U/ml)	2 215 ± 283	7 469 ± 421	12 546 ± 1 962
+ IL 2 + GM3 2.5 nm/ml	3 216 ± 230	7 685 ± 756	13 307 ± 2 343
+ IL 2 + GM3 25 nm/ml	2 629 ± 598	5 685 ± 664	8 316 ± 2 204
+ IL 2 + GM3 50 nm/ml	2 489 ± 275	4 113 ± 565	5 980 ± 1 384

Hoon et al. (8). However, it can be seen in Table 4 that the activity of preformed IL 2 on IL 2-dependent CTLL2 cells is not sensitive to the presence of gangliosides, although the production of IL 2 by human lymphocytes is blocked. IL 1 is known to be needed for the production of IL 1 and as shown in Table 5, both the production of IL 1 by human monocytes and the activity of the preformed lymphokine are markedly inhibited by melanoma gangliosides. Inhibition does not result from a direct inter-

Table 4. Influence of melanoma gangliosides on the release and activity of human IL 2. In 1 ml of serum-containing medium, 10^6 lymphocytes (irradiated at 1 100 rads) were mixed with 2×10^5 SB cells (irradiated at 5 000 rads) in the presence of PHA (1 μg/ml). After 72 hrs incubation with 60 nmoles/ml of melanoma gangliosides, the supernatant was tested for IL 2 activity. IL 2-dependent CTLL2 cells were incubated at 10^4 cells/0.1 ml/well in culture medium for 48 hrs with 50 μl of diluted supernatants from stimulated lymphocytes, with and without addition of 60 nmoles/ml of gangliosides. ^{3}H-thymidine was added for 6 more hours and the uptaken thymidine was counted. Results expressed as dpm of thymidine per well. Mean ± SD of quadruplicate measures. Three separate experiments gave similar results. IL 2 was quantitated by calculation using computerized standard curves.

Conditions of incubation	IL 2 produced (units/ml)	Dilutions of IL 2-containing supernatants			
		1/2	1/6	1/18	1/54
PHA + SB cells	11.8	80 655 ± 8 452	70 857 ± 2 554	30 127 ± 4 351	11 947 ± 944
Activity after addition of gangliosides		76 233 ± 8 240	65 645 ± 6 238	28 240 ± 3 450	10 817 ± 1 015
PHA + SB cells + gangliosides	4.7	70 189 ± 6 007	33 697 ± 407	14 328 ± 2 373	5 727 ± 743
Activity after addition of gangliosides		68 744 ± 7 211	32 743 ± 2 700	13 334 ± 1 676	4 945 ± 743

action between IL 1 and gangliosides since preincubation of IL 1 with ganglioside-containing liposomes followed by ultracentrifugation did not remove IL 1. Therefore, the effect of melanoma gangliosides on lymphocyte proliferation is not due to an overall effect on the plasma membrane since the signal transduction of IL 2 binding to the specific receptor is not modified whereas the one for IL 1 is blocked. The biochemical mechanism underlying this phenomenon might be related to the production of prostaglandins by macrophages which have been reported to inhibit IL 1 (9). The effects of GM3 ganglioside on the production of IL 1 and arachidonic acid, the direct precursor of prostaglandins, are presented on Table 6. The incubation of monocytes with gangliosides strongly enhanced the release of arachidonic acid whereas it blocked concommitantly the production of IL 1. Prostaglandin E_2 was found to have a similar effect and increasing concentrations of indomethacin, which inhibits the production of prostaglandins, abolished the influence of gangliosides. Thus, ganglioside enrichment of monocytes is likely to lower their lymphokine production by stimulating the release of prostaglandins and arachidonic acid-derived products.

Influence of gangliosides on the cytotoxic activity of lymphocytes. Melanoma gangliosides have very little influence on cytotoxicity of lymphocytes, such as NK and ADCC, in chromium release experiments from labelled targets with 4 hours and even overnight incubation (data not shown). Nevertheless, we were able to obtain some significant modifications of the cytotoxic activity of human lymphocytes after preincubation lasting up to 8 days with melanoma gangliosides. However, as shown in

Table 5. Influence of melanoma gangliosides on the production of interleukin-1 (IL 1) by human monocytes and the activity of IL 1. Plastic-adherent monocytes were stimulated in serum-free RPMI 1640 containing 25 µg/ml of lipopolysaccharide (LPS) from E. Coli 055.B5 and 60 nmoles/ml of melanoma gangliosides. After 24 hrs, the supernatants were dialyzed against RPMI 1640 and tested for IL 1 activity on Balb/C thymocytes during 72 hrs. Dilutions of supernatants were in RPMI 1640 containing 10 % foetal calf serum, 1 % PHA (ref. HA 15 from Wellcome Lab.), with and without 60 nmoles/ml of gangliosides. Proliferation was estimated by the uptake of ^{3}H-thymidine added for the last 4 hrs. Results expressed as dpm of thymidine. Mean ± SD of triplicate measures. The value obtained with thymocytes and PHA only (no supernatant) was 1224 ± 183. Three separate experiments gave similar results.

Conditions of incubation	Dilutions of IL 1-containing supernatants from monocytes		
	1/10	1/50	1/100
Control (monocytes without LPS)	9040 ± 767	4314 ± 544	3343 ± 326
+ gangliosides in the assay of activity	3345 ± 715	1205 ± 249	414 ± 140
Monocytes + LPS	14126 ± 2430	8334 ± 463	6701 ± 873
+ gangliosides in the assay of activity	4966 ± 514	1724 ± 132	781 ± 114
Monocytes + LPS + gangliosides	11102 ± 1821	3273 ± 398	2402 ± 265
+ gangliosides in the assay of activity	3431 ± 498	928 ± 174	852 ± 115

Table 6. Release of IL 1 and arachidonic acid by human monocytes in the presence of melanoma GM3 ganglioside. Human adherent monocytes were labelled for 6 hrs with ^{3}H-arachidonic acid in serumfree RPMI 1640 and washed in the same medium. The monocytes were then stimulated by LPS for IL 1 production, as described on Table 5, in the presence or not of gangliosides (60 nmoles/ml), prostaglandin E_2 (0.5 μg/ml), dibutyryl cyclic AMP (10^{-4} molL^{-1}) and indomethacin (10^{-4} or 10^{-5} molL^{-1}). Aliquots of the supernatants were counted for ^{3}H at 30 mn after addition of LPS. IL 1 assay was performed on mouse thymocytes using ^{14}C-thymidine counted with ^{3}H/^{14}C quenched curves. Results are expressed as dpm of ^{3}H-arachidonic acid released in 30 mn, and as dpm of ^{14}C-thymidine taken up by IL 1 stimulated thymocytes. Mean ± SD of quadruplicate measures. The control value for thymocytes with PHA only was $10\,810 ± 1237$.

Incubation	^{3}H in supern. 30 mn after addition of LPS	Dilutions of IL 1-containing supernatants		
		1/4	1/10	1/40
Monocytes + LPS	$60\,252 ± 4876$	$97\,190 ± 8694$	$83\,703 ± 6597$	$55\,061 ± 6369$
+ gangliosides	$76\,618 ± 6824$	$50\,546 ± 5912$	$48\,882 ± 5367$	$31\,824 ± 4244$
+ PGE$_2$ 0.5 μg/ml	$98\,578 ± 8546$	$41\,450 ± 5127$	$33\,221 ± 3789$	$30\,426 ± 4284$
+ gangliosides + DBcAMP 10^{-4} M	$62\,582 ± 5948$	$49\,081 ± 5637$	$44\,608 ± 5069$	$32\,243 ± 3685$
+ gangliosides + indomethacin 10^{-4} M	$78\,654 ± 6891$	$91\,194 ± 10836$	$76\,034 ± 6945$	$55\,610 ± 5108$
+ gangliosides + indomethacin 10^{-5} M	$87\,264 ± 9673$	$61\,422 ± 6543$	$53\,477 ± 6283$	$43\,601 ± 5280$

Table 7, the effect of GM3 seemed to be different when studied on lymphocytes from healthy donors or melanoma patients. In the latter case, low concentrations of gangliosides had a stimulatory influence on both cytotoxicity to K562 cells, which reflects NK activity, and specific killing of melanoma cells. With a normal donor, low amounts of gangliosides had no effect, and cytotoxicity was close on K562 and Mel 4. Higher concentrations of gangliosides were somewhat inhibitory for the normal lymphocytes and lowered the NK activity of the patient's lymphocytes. IL 2 had an effect only on the non-specific activity of lymphocytes.

Conclusions

Melanoma-shed gangliosides have a modulatory influence on both the humoral and cellular immune system in humans. Low concentrations are stimulatory, whereas increasing concentrations lead to a potent inhibition of all lymphocyte functions, this inhibition being reversible by removing the gangliosides from the extracellular medium. The shed gangliosides might thus be involved in the escape of tumor cells from immune killing.

Table 7. Influence of 8 days incubation with various amounts of Gm3 on the cytotoxic activity of human lymphocytes (PBL) on melanoma Mel 4 cells and K562 cells. Lymphocytes isolated from the peripheral blood of melanoma patients and normal donors were incubated in RPMI 1640 containing 10 % AB serum and melanoma GM3 ganglioside (0, 2 or 20 nmoles/ml). Proliferation was stimulated by PHA (1 µg/ml), or IL 2 (5 U/ml), or PHA+IL 2. Cellular cytotoxicity was tested after 8 days of incubation by a 4 hrs chromium release assay with ^{51}Cr-labelled melanoma Mel 4 cells and K562 cells, at an effector-to-target ratio of 30/1. Results are the mean of triplicate measures.

| Incubation | GM3 µg/ml added | Lymphocytes | | | |
| | | Melanoma patient | | Normal donor | |
		Mel 4	K562	Mel 4	K562
lymphocytes	0	0 %	24 %	31 %	32 %
	2	33 %	42 %	23 %	35 %
	20	10 %	6 %	5 %	8 %
+ PHA (1 µg/ml)	0	0 %	10 %	29 %	52 %
	2	24 %	13 %	25 %	42 %
	20	3 %	17 %	0 %	14 %
+ IL 2 (5 U/ml)	0	0 %	43 %	59 %	69 %
	2	31 %	40 %	71 %	91 %
	20	0 %	55 %	47 %	49 %
+ PHA + IL2	0	3 %	7 %	29 %	50 %
	2	16 %	35 %	27 %	50 %
	20	0 %	21 %	3 %	23 %

References

1. Portoukalian, J., G. Zwingelstein, N. Abdul-Malak, and J. F. Doré. Alteration of gangliosides in plasma and red cells of humans bearing melanoma tumors. Biochem. Biophys. Res. Commun. 85, 916, 1978.
2. Portoukalian, J., G. Zwingelstein, and J. F. Doré. Lipid composition of human malignant tumors at various levels of malignant proliferation. Eur. J. Biochem. 94, 19, 1979.
3. Miller, H. C. and W. J. Esselman. Modulation of the immune response by antigen reactive lymphocytes after cultivation with gangliosides. J. Immunol. 115, 839, 1975.
4. Ladisch, S., B. Gillard, C. Wong, and L. Ulsh. Shedding and immunoregulatory activity of YAC-1 lymphoma cell gangliosides. Cancer Res. 43, 3803, 1983.
5. Whisler, R. L. and A. J. Yates. Regulation of lymphocyte response by human gangliosides. I. Characteristics of inhibitory effects and the induction of impaired activation. J. Immunol. 125, 2106, 1980.
6. Bouchon, B., J. Portoukalian, and H. Bornet. Sex-specific difference of the galabiosylceramide level in the glycosphingolipids of human thyroid. Biochim. Biophys. Acta 836, 143, 1985.
7. Watanabe, K. and Y. Arao. A new solvent system for the separation of neutral glycosphingolipids. J. Lipid Res. 22, 1020, 1981.
8. Hoon, D. S. B., R. F. Irie, and A. J. Cochran. Gangliosides from human melanoma immunomodulate response of T cells to interleukin-2. Cell. Immunol. 111, 410, 1988.
9. Morley, J. Role of prostaglandins secreted by macrophages in the inflammatory process. In: Lymphokines. Vol 4. E. Pick, editor. Academic Press, Inc., New York 335, 1981.

22. Tumor Gangliosides: Shedding, Structural Characterization, and Immunosuppressive Activity

S. Ladisch

Introduction

The purpose of our study of tumor gangliosides is the definition of their potential role in the process of tumor formation. To provide a perspective for this study, some background regarding current concepts of the process of tumor formation must be reviewed. It is generally well recognized that the formation of tumors *in vivo* is a complex and multi-step process. There are, however, two major phenotypic characteristics of cells which have been identified to be necessary for the formation of tumors, and which are under separate genetic control (1). These two characteristics are transformation and tumorigenicity. Transformation, a characteristic defined *in vitro*, indicates that a cell has an autonomous proliferative capability. Tumorigenicity, on the other hand, is a characteristic defined *in vivo,* and is the ability of a transformed cell line to actually form tumors. As such, tumorigenicity heavily reflects the host-tumor cell interaction and the multiple factors which contribute to this interaction. Our interest is in the latter phenotypic characteristic of tumor cells, and we have hypothesized that among the factors which influence tumorigenicity are quantitative aspects of the synthesis and shedding of gangliosides by tumor cells (2). Evidence supporting this view is the subject of this communication.

Hypothesis

The specific hypothesis which underlies the proposed role of gangliosides in tumor formation is that these molecules, shed by the tumor cell into the surrounding environment, enhance tumor formation, possibly by suppressing normal cellular immune responses. Immune suppression by shed tumor gangliosides could contribute to the abrogation of host immune responses which is frequently observed in cancer, and in turn possibly to tumor progression.

Immunoregulation by Shed Gangliosides

Several lines of evidence support the concept that gangliosides modulate immune function. Among the documented immunoregulatory properties of gangliosides are the following: (i) Inhibition of normal human lymphoproliferative responses to mitogens and antigens (2–8), (ii) inhibition of interleukin 2-dependent cell proliferation (9), (iii) preliminary reports of inhibition of cytotoxic effector function (10), (iv) and modulation of the humoral immune response (11, 12).

To be addressed, however, is the question of what requirements underlie a physiologically significant *in vivo* effect of potential immunoregulatory properties of tumor gangliosides. Restated, what are the requisites for *in vivo* modulation of the immune response by gangliosides, in tumor bearing hosts? Two requisites for such an immuno-regulatory role of gangliosides can be postulated. The first is that purified biologically relevant gangliosides, i.e., in this case of tumor origin, modulate immune function. The second is that such gangliosides are prevent *in vivo* in relevant local environments (i.e., the environment of a forming tumor and ultimately in the circulation) and, critically, are present in immunologically active concentrations. This latter requirement can be visualized as being fulfilled by the constant release, or shedding, of gangliosides by the tumor cell *in vivo*.

Shedding, which is a dynamic process of the cell, thus becomes a crucial element contributing to a potential *in vivo* role of gangliosides. This process and its implications are depicted by the model (13) shown in Figure 1. Ganglioside molecules, continuously released from the tumor cell surface, are present in the local environment of these cells. (In this model, low concentrations of structurally unique tumor gangliosides released into the circulation may also act as antigens, resulting in generation of an antibody response [discussed in ref. 14].) In the probably quite high concentrations in the local environment of the tumor, immunologically active cells exposed to shed tumor gangliosides incorporate these molecules into their cell surface. Finally, as a consequence of the incorporation of gangliosides, these immunocytes may become inactivated or suppressed, by mechanisms which remain to be fully elucidated.

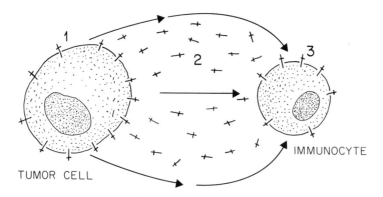

Figure 1. Schematic representation of the dynamic process of ganglioside shedding and its consequences. Tumor cell membrane gangliosides "1" are released into the local environment of the tumor and into the circulation "2" and may subsequently bind to, and inactivate, immunocytes "3". From Ladisch, S. 1987. Tumor cell gangliosides Adv. Ped. 34, 45–58; used by permission.

Tumor Systems

To investigate the above hypothesis regarding the shedding of immunologically active gangliosides, we have been studying two tumor systems. These two systems complement each other with respect to the questions which can be asked. One is the human tumor, neuroblastoma. The use of a human tumor system allows estimation of the quantitative aspects of the process of shedding, in humans, by quantitation of specific circulating tumor-associated gangliosides, i.e., in the plasma of patients bearing a tumor. Furthermore, by using new approaches to ganglioside purification, these gangliosides can be highly purified, allowing their *in vitro* immunoregulatory properties to be defined with confidence. Among human tumors, neuroblastoma was chosen for these initial investigations because it is a clinically very aggressive tumor and a tumor in which our preliminary experiments indicated the ganglioside content (and ganglioside shedding *in vitro,* unpublished results) to be quite high. Thus, study of human neuroblastoma allows study of both the *in vivo* presence and the *in vitro* activity of these molecules.

The other tumor system being studied is a murine lymphoma. Parallel *in vitro* and *in vivo* studies of tumor cell ganglioside metabolism can be undertaken in such a system. The use of an experimental animal tumor has the particular advantage that tumor formation can be experimentally manipulated, allowing direct *in vivo* tests of modulatory activity of tumor gangliosides on this process in a (syngeneic normal) murine tumor system. Thus, the murine system adds to human tumor studies the ability to directly test, *in vivo,* the role of shed tumor gangliosides in tumor formation.

Neuroblastoma Gangliosides – Shedding and Immunoregulatory Activity

Initial studies documented a very high concentration of gangliosides in several neuroblastoma tumor cell lines (13). This was supported by our first study of a small number of neuroblastoma tumors, which also demonstrated the presence of high concentrations of a specific ganglioside, GD2, in several of these tumors (15). We pursued this finding with a systematic investigation of a number of human neuroblastoma tumors, analysed prior to treatment. Quantitative and qualitative aspects of the ganglioside complement were established by a combination of chemical and densitometric methods. These studies demonstrated that high concentrations of gangliosides characterize human neuroblastoma tumors. In a total of 36 neuroblastoma tumors studied, the mean total ganglioside concentration was 402 nmol LBSA/gram tissue (16). GD2 ganglioside was found to be uniformly present in these tumors in concentrations ranging up to almost 200 nmols/gram tissue. This is exemplified in Figure 2, in which high-performance thin layer chromatography (HPTLC) ganglioside patterns of five individual tumors are shown. These thin layer chromatograms demonstrate a heterogeneity of total ganglioside content, but evidence of the uniform presence of GD2.

The high concentrations of total gangliosides, and the uniform presence of a specific ganglioside, GD2, in human neuroblastoma tumors made it of interest to determine whether these molecules have immunoregulatory activity, as suggested by the hypothesis proposed. To answer this question, the total gangliosides of 17 neuroblastoma tumors were purified in quantities sufficient to assess their immunoregulatory activity. These gangliosides were then tested for their modulatory effects on the antigen-

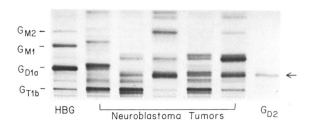

Figure 2. Total ganglioside pattern of five untreated human neuroblastoma tumors (6–8 nmol LBSA/lane). Migration of standard brain gangliosides (HBG) and purified GD2 are shown. All bands are resorcinol-positive. The arrow indicates the migration of GD2, seen to be present in trace quantities (<2 % of total gangliosides) in HBG.

induced normal human lymphoproliferative response, an assay which we had previously used to document an inhibitory effect of gangliosides on monocyte accessory function (7), and a reliable *in vitro* assay of the cellular immune response. The results of this study demonstrated potent immunoregulatory activity by the neuro-blastoma tumor gangliosides; gangliosides of every one of the 17 tumors studied were highly inhibitory, with 43 to >99 % inhibition of the lymphoproliferative response being caused by 30 nmoles gangliosides/ml (17). When these results were analyzed according to the clinical stage of the individual tumors, it was found that the ganglio-sides from clinically more aggressive tumors (stage III and IV) were significantly more immunosuppressive than those of the generally less aggressive (stage I and II) tumors (Table 1). Also shown in Table 1 is evidence that the specific ganglioside GD2, has very potent immunosuppressive activity *in vitro*. For comparison, the predominant normal human circulating (plasma) ganglioside, GM3, is inactive under these experimental conditions. These results provide strong support for one of the conditions for biologic-ally relevant activity – that of potent immunoregulatory activity *in vitro*.

Shedding of gangliosides by tumor cells, thereby causing high concentrations of these molecules in the local environment of the tumor, and possibly in the plasma, is the other requirement of the hypothesis. To assess this, we studied the disialoganglio-side GD2, since in preliminary studies this ganglioside was found to be present in quite high concentrations in the plasma of some patients with neuroblastoma (15, 18), whereas it is not detectable in normal plasma. The quantitation of this ganglioside in the circulation was expected to allow some conclusions to be drawn about tumor ganglioside shedding in humans.

Table 1. Relative immunosuppressive activity of human neuroblastoma tumor gangliosides.

Ganglioside	Inhibitory activity[1]
total neuroblastoma gangliosides	
Stage III-IV (n=12)	72 %
Stage I-II (n=5)	45 %
purified G_{D2}	85 %
purified G_{M3}	<10 %

[1] per cent inhibition of normal human lymphoproliferative responses to tetanus toxoid, as described (17), by gangliosides in a concentration of 4–5 nmol/culture (15–20 nmol/ml).

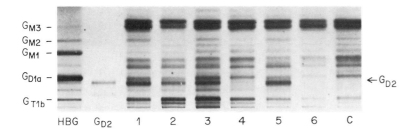

Figure 3. Total plasma ganglioside patterns of six patients with stage IV neuroblastoma. Each lane (1–6, C) contains total gangliosides isolated from 1 ml plasma. C = control plasma; HBG = human brain ganglioside standards. All bands are resorcinol-positive.

To test for the presence of GD2, gangliosides of 1 ml plasma samples were purified by DIPE/butanol partition (19) and analyzed by HPTLC. As seen in Figure 3, GD2 is easily visible in pretreatment plasma of the majority of patients with widespread neuroblastoma (in this figure, 5 of 6 patient samples). In contrast, GD2 is not visible in the normal plasma sample (indicating a concentration of <50 pmol/ml). A comprehensive study of the presence of this ganglioside in neuroblastoma patients was therefore undertaken (20). This study (Table 2) yielded several striking observations. First, the concentration of GD2 in the plasma of all patients (mean concentration of 545 pmol/ml) is very much higher than the detectable limit of ≤50 pmol/ml by direct TLC staining, and several hundred times higher than the most recently documented upper limit of GD2 concentration in normal plasma (<2 pmol/ml, ref. 21). Thus, GD2 is both a tumor tissue marker (for neuroblastoma) and a circulating tumor marker, possibly of clinical value. The second observation is that the circulating concentration of GD2 is highest in patients with the higher stage (III and IV) tumors and lowest in patients with stage I and II tumors. Furthermore, GD2 was not detectable in the plasma of patients having the related but differentiated tumors, ganglioneuroblastoma and ganglioneuroma. It is clear, then, that quantitatively significant ganglioside shedding characterizes human neuroblastoma. The observations also suggest the speculation, which must be tested, that the tendency of the tumor to progress may correlate with the circulating level of GD2.

Table 2. Quantitative aspects of ganglioside shedding by human neuroblastoma tumors: Circulating G_{D2} concentrations.

Plasma sample	G_{D2} concentration (pmol/ml)
normal[1]	≤2
neuroblastoma[2]	545 ± 108
Stage III and IV	603 ± 136
Stage I and II	198 ± 54

[1] from reference # 21
[2] from reference # 20

In summary, we have shown that neuroblastoma tumors have relatively high ganglioside content, that these gangliosides are highly immunosuppressive *in vitro*, and that these gangliosides, and specifically GD2, are shed in substantial concentrations into the peripheral circulation, *in vivo*. Taking all these results together, it is clear that of great importance now is the purification of individual ganglioside species of the total tumor gangliosides, and the study of their biological (including immunologic) activities. In this manner it should be possible to identify what structural characteristics impart the immunosuppressive activity which we observed in testing the total neuroblastoma gangliosides, an activity which may contribute to tumor formation and progression.

Ganglioside Separation, Purification, and Characterization

The purification of human tumor gangliosides is now possible using even only relatively small amounts of tissue. While multiple purification steps are required, the yield of each is relatively high, enabling the recovery of sufficient quantities for structural characterization and functional studies. The sequence of the steps which we are using (manuscript in preparation) in these purifications is summarized below:

total lipid extraction
↓
ganglioside purification by DIPE/1-butanol partition
↓
normal phase high-pressure liquid chromatography
↓
reverse-phase high-pressure liquid chromatography

Briefly, following extraction of tumor tissue with chloroform:methanol, gangliosides are purified by diisopropyl ether/1-butanol/aqueous NaCl partition and gel filtration (22), followed by normal phase high-pressure liquid chromatography (HPLC). The normal phase HPLC separation step yields gangliosides which are homogeneous

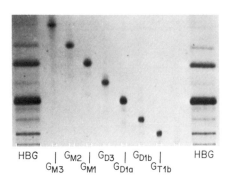

HBG | G_{M2} | G_{D3} | G_{D1b} | HBG
    G_{M3}   G_{M1}   G_{D1a}   G_{T1b}

Figure 4. HPTLC of purified human brain gangliosides, stained with resorcinol. The individual gangliosides spotted in each lane were separated by normal phase HPLC, as decribed by Gazzotti, et al. (23).

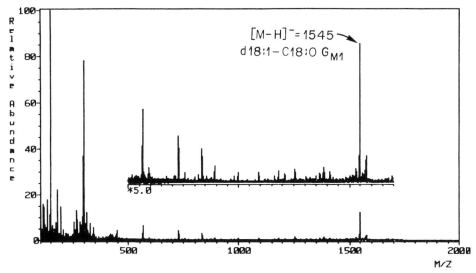

Figure 5. FAB negative ion mass spectrum of GM1 ganglioside from human brain. The HPTLC of this ganglioside is shown in Figure 4.

for the sugar portion of the molecule (23). To exemplify the application of this approach, the HPTLC of total human brain gangliosides well-separated by normal phase HPLC, is shown in Figure 4. These individual gangliosides can then be analyzed by mass spectrometry. This is accomplished by fast atom bombardment (FAB) mass spectrometry of the underivatized gangliosides (24). This is demonstrated in Figure 5 in which the mass spectrum of human brain GM1 ganglioside purified by normal phase HPLC is shown, with the major ceramide isomer (d18:1 C18:0 GM1) shown by the arrow.

The ultimate goal, and a more elusive one, is to obtain molecules also homogeneous (or pure) with respect to the ceramide portion of the glycosphingolipid. This is being accomplished by the last step, reverse phase HPLC (25) of the individual gangliosides isolated by normal phase HPLC. We have applied this method to human brain gangliosides with success, and it is currently being used for human neuroblastoma tumor ganglioside purification. These studies are demonstrating that a much greater heterogeneity exists in the ceramide portion of the human tumor gangliosides, than exists, for example, in normal human brain gangliosides.

Now possible, the complete structural characterization of human neuroblastoma gangliosides, which vary both in the ceramide and sugar portions of the molecules, should ultimately aid in determining possible structure-function relationships among individual gangliosides. These studies should answer the question of the relative importance of specific characteristics of the sugar portion, versus the ceramide portion, of the molecule in imparting biological activity. The high degree of purification which can now be achieved has an additional value, in that we have previously shown, in studies of immunoregulatory activity of mouse lymphoma gangliosides, that a high degree of purity (requiring multiple purification steps) results in maximal immunosuppressive activity by tumor gangliosides (2). These latter observations (2) further support the assignment of immunoregulatory activity to this class of molecules.

Lymphoma Gangliosides – Role in Tumor Formation *in vivo*

The human tumor system (neuroblastoma) permitted documentation of levels of circulating tumor gangliosides *in vivo*. However, this system does not, except by inference, allow conclusions to be drawn about the actual biological role of these molecules *in vivo*. For this reason, we sought to develop a model experimental tumor system in which the modulatory effects of these molecules could be directly tested. In initial studies with a mouse lymphoma, the YAC lymphoma, we had observed (i) significant shedding of the lymphoma gangliosides *in vitro* and *in vivo,* and (ii) highly potent immunosuppressive activity of the tumor cell gangliosides assessed *in vitro* (2). We therefore reasoned that a mouse lymphoma system would allow testing of the *in vivo* effects of gangliosides, on tumor formation.

To examine tumor formation *in vivo,* however, presented a difficulty regarding selection of the tumor to be used in this work. That is, since the hypothesis proposes that the shedding of gangliosides which are biologically active may be a requisite enhancing factor for tumor formation, it would be expected that significant ganglioside shedding might characterize most tumors. In contrast, to be able to demonstrate an enhancement of the process of tumor formation by added gangliosides, a tumor that itself is deficient in gangliosides or ganglioside shedding is required. Finding such a tumor is therefore both necessary but possibly difficult, since the hypothesis predicts that host-tumor interactions might cause such a tumor to be eliminated *in vivo*.

After several unsuccessful attempts to identify an animal tumor defective in ganglioside shedding, the ideal model was found to be a single, heterogeneous spontaneous murine lymphoma (SL 12), from which several different tumor cell sublines had been cloned (26). What suggested the possible utility of this tumor for our work was the observation that the sublines, with almost identical cell proliferation kinetics *in vitro,* had markedly differing tumorigenic potential *in vivo* (26). This would be predicted to allow a test of whether there is a relationship between ganglioside metabolism and tumorgenicity.

Using this tumor system, we first confirmed a previously suggested (e.g., ref. 27) but never directly proven (28) relationship between ganglioside content and tumor formation; the highly tumorigenic line, SL 12.3, contained 71 pmol gangliosides/10^6 cells, compared to only 0.5 pmol/10^6 cells in the case of the poorly tumorigenic SL 12.4 cell line (29). Even more striking, however, was the correlation between ganglioside shedding and tumorigenicity: the SL 12.3 line released 18 pmol/10^6 cells/24 hrs, or almost 100-fold the amount (0.2 pmol/10^6 cells/24 hrs) shed by the SL 12.4 cell line (29). These results established an *in vivo* relationship between ganglioside shedding and tumorigenicity.

The most critical experiments in this study were the testing of the highly purified tumor cell gangliosides for biological activity *in vivo*. The experimental design was based on the hypothesis that the poorly tumorigenic SL 12.4 cells should exhibit enhanced tumor formation when admixed with the gangliosides they were lacking, if ganglioside shedding contributes to the ability of tumor cells to form tumors *in vivo*. To test this hypothesis, gangliosides were isolated and purified from the highly tumorigenic cell line (SL 12.3), co-injected with SL 12.4 cells, and tumor formation monitored. A striking enhancement of tumor formation was observed (29): As little as one to ten picomoles of gangliosides purified from the highly tumorigenic SL 12.3 tumor cell line, co-injected with poorly tumorigenic SL 12.4 cells, increased tumor formation at two weeks from 1/12 (8 %) to 11/12 (88 %) mico injected. These experiments showed for the first time that very minute quantities of tumor gangliosides can in fact modulate tumor formation *in vivo*. These findings have since been corroborated by reports of two other laboratories (30, 31). It is now critical to complete the molecular structural characterization of these highly potent modulators of tumor formation, and then to determine the molecular structural characteristics necessary for biological activity.

In conclusion, the experimental data presented show that gangliosides are shed by tumors in significant quantities, that these tumor-derived gangliosides exhibit potent immunoregulatory activity *in vitro,* and that these molecules enhance tumor formation *in vivo.* While the evidence suggests that tumor enhancement may be directly due to an immunologic mechanism, this requires further study. Establishment of the relationship between ganglioside structure and biological functions (immunosuppressive activity, tumor-enhancing activity) will also be an important future direction in this work.

Acknowledgements

I thank Eileen Schwartz, Grace Floutsis, Heber Becker, and Lisa Ulsh for assistance with various portions of these studies, Douglas Gage (MSU Mass Spectroscopy Facility) for performing the mass spectrum, and Dorothy Ross for preparing the manuscript. This work was supported by grants CA42361 and RCDA CA00821 from the National Cancer Institute, a scholarship of the Leukemia Society of America, American Cancer Society grant PDT-270, and a grant from the Phi Beta Psi Sorority.

References

1. Stanbridge, E. J., C. J. Der, C. Doernsen, R.Y. Nishimi, D. M. Peehl, B. E. Weissman, and J. Wilkinson. Human cell hybrids: Analysis of transformation and tumorigenicity. Science (Wash. DC) 215, 252–259, 1982.
2. Ladisch, S., B. Gillard, C. Wong, and L. Ulsh. Shedding and immunisuppressive activity of YAC lymphoma cell gangliosides. Cancer Res. 43, 3803–3813, 1983.
3. Miller, H. C. and W. J. Esselman. Modulation of the immune response by antigen reactive lymphocytes after cultivation with gangliosides. J. Immunol. 115, 839–843, 1975.
4. Lengle, E. E., R. Krishnaraj, and R. G. Kemp. Inhibition of the lectin-induced mitogenic response of thymoctes by glycolipids. Cancer Res. 39, 817–822, 1979.
5. Ryan, J. L. and M. Shinitzky. Possible role for glycosphingolipids in the control of immune responses. Eur. J. Immun. 9, 171–175, 1979.

6. Whisler, R. L. and A. J. Yates. Regulation of lymphocyte responses by human gangliosides. J. Immunol. 125, 2106–2111, 1980.

7. Ladisch, S., L. Ulsh, B. Gillard, and C. Wong. Modulation of the immune response by gangliosides: Inhibition of adherent monocyte accessory function in vitro. J. Clin. Invest. 74, 2074–2081, 1984.

8. Gonwa, T. A., M. A. Westrick, and B. A. Macher. Inhibition of mitogen- and antigen-induced lymphocyte activation by human leukemia cell gangliosides. Cancer Res. 44, 3467–3470, 1984.

9. Merritt, W. D., M. Bailey, and D. H. Pluznik. Inhibition of interleukin-2 dependent cytotoxic T-lymphocyte growth by gangliosides. Cell. Immunol. 89, 1–10, 1984.

10. Dyatlovitskaya, E.V., E. Klucharevat, V. A. Matveeva, E.V. Sinitsyna, A. S. Akhmed-Zade, A. F. Lemonovskaya, E.V. Fomina-Ageeva, and L. D. Bergleson. Effect of gangliosides on the cytotoxic activity of natural killers from Syrian hamsters. Biokhimika 50, 1514–1516, 1985.

11. Agarwal, M. K. and E. Neter. Effect of selected lipids and surfactants on immunogenicity of several bacterial antigens. J. Immunol. 107, 1448–1456, 1971.

12. Esselman, W. J. and H. C. Miller. Modulation of B cell responses by glycolipid released from antigen-stimulated T cells. J. Immunol. 119, 1994–2000, 1977.

13. Ladisch, S. Tumor cell gangliosides. Adv. Ped. 34, 45–58, 1987.

14. Ladisch, S. and Z.-L. Wu. Circulating gangliosides as tumor markers. Prog. Clin. Biol. Res. 175, 277–284, 1985.

15. Ladisch, S. and Z.-L. Wu. Detection of a tumor-associated ganglioside in plasma of patients with neuroblastoma. Lancet i, 136–138, 1985.

16. Wu, Z.-L., E. Schwartz, R. Seeger, and S. Ladisch. Expression of GD2 ganglioside by untreated primary human neuroblastoma. Cancer Res. 46, 441–443, 1986.

17. Floutsis, G., L. Ulsh, and S. Ladisch. Immunosuppressive activity of human neuroblastoma tumor gangliosides. International J. Cancer, in press, 1988.

18. Schulz, G., D. A. Cheresh, N. M. Varki, A. Yu, L. K. Staffileno, and R. A. Reisfeld. Detection of ganglioside GD2 in tumor tissues and sera of neuroblastoma patients. Cancer Res. 44, 5914–5920, 1984.

19. Ladisch, S. and B. Gillard. Isolation and purification of gangliosides from plasma. Methods Enzymol. 138, 300–306, 1987.

20. Ladisch, S., Z.-L. Wu, S. A. Feig, L. Ulsh, E. Schwartz, G. Floutsis, F. Wiley, C. Lenarsky, and R. Seeger. Shedding of GD2 ganglioside by human neuroblastoma. Int. J. Cancer 39, 73–76, 1987.

21. Yamanaka, T., Y. Hirabayashi, M. Hirota, M. Kaneka, M. Matsumoto, and N. Kobayashi. Detection of gangliotriaose-series glycosphingolipids in serum of cord blood and patients with neuroblastoma by a sensitive TLC/enzyme-immunostaining method. Biochimica et Biophysica Acta 920, 181–184, 1987.

22. Ladisch, S. and B. Gillard. A solvent partition method for micro-scale ganglioside purification. Anal. Biochem. 146, 220–231, 1985.

23. Gazzotti, G., S. Sonnino, and R. Ghidoni. Normal-phase high-performance liquid chromatographic separation of non-derivatized ganglioside mixtures. J. Chromatog. 348, 371–378, 1985.

24. Arita, M., M. Iwamori, T. Higuchi, and Y. Nagai. 1,1,3,3-Tetramethylurea and triethanolamine as a new useful matrix for fast atom bombardment mass spectrometry of gangliosides and neutral glycosphingolipids. J. Biochem. 93, 319, 1983.

25. Gazzotti, G., S. Sonnino, R. Ghidoni, G. Kirschner, and G. Tettamanti. Analytical and preparative high-performance liquid chromatography of gangliosides. J. Neurosci. Res. 12, 179–192, 1984.

26. MacLeod, C. L., S. E. Weinroth, C. Streifinger, S. M. Glaser, and E. F. Hayes. SL 12 murine T-lymphoma: A new model for tumor cell heterogeneity. J. Natl. Cancer Inst. 74, 875–882, 1985.
27. Yogeeswaran, G. and P. L. Salk. Metastatic potential is positively correlated with cell surface sialylation of cultured murine tumor cell lines. Science (Wash. DC) 212, 1514–1516, 1981.
28. Hakomori, S. and R. Kannagi. Glycosphingolipids as tumor-associated and differentiation markers. J. Nat. Cancer Inst. 74, 231–251, 1983.
29. Ladisch, S., S. Kitada, and E. Hays. Gangliosides shed by tumor cells enhance tumor formation in mice. J. Clin. Invest. 79, 1879–1882, 1987.
30. Alessandri, G., S. Filippeschi, P. Sinibaldi, F. Mornet, P. Passera, F. Spreafico, P. M. Cappa, and P. M. Gullino. Influence of gangliosides on primary and metastatic neoplastic growth in human and murine cells. Cancer Res. 47, 4243–4247, 1987.
31. Saha, S. and U. Chattopadhyay. Changes in plasma gangliosides in relation to tumor growth and their tumor-enhancing effect. Int. J. Cancer 41, 432–435, 1988.

23. Clinical Evaluation of Monoclonal Antibody Against GD3 Ganglioside in Patients with Metastatic Melanoma

A. N. Houghton, D. Bajorin,
P. Chapman, J. DiMaggio,
H. F. Oettgen, and L. J. Old

Phase I studies have demonstrated that mouse monoclonal antibodies (mAb) can be safely administered to patients with cancer and that severe toxicity is uncommon. The major challenge now facing the field is to develop effective strategies for therapy. Monoclonal antibodies, either unconjugated or conjugated to radionuclides, toxins, chemotherapeutic drugs and other cytotoxic agents, are being evaluated in clinical trials (1, 2). Three approaches using unconjugated monoclonal antibodies are being explored: 1) activation of components of the immune system (e.g. complement, effector cells), including mediation of cytotoxicity against target tumor cells; 2) induction of active immunity through an idiotype-anti-idiotype network (3); and 3) interference with tumor growth by antibodies directed against molecules critical for proliferation or differentiation (e.g. growth factor receptors) (4). We have focussed our initial clinical studies on biodistribution, pharmacokinetics and tumor localization of ^{131}I-labelled mAb and on evaluation of unconjugated mAb for therapy using the anti-GD3 mAb R24 (26).

Radiolabelled Monoclonal Antibodies

There are indications that radiolabelled monoclonal antibodies may prove useful for tumor diagnosis and possibly therapy (5, 6, 7). However, critical issues remain for the use of immunoconjugates for therapy of solid tumors.

While tumor:normal tissue ratios of radionuclide are typically favorable in patients with solid tumors, the per cent of injected dose that localizes to tumor is almost always <0.1% injected dose/gram of tumor, and typically ≪0.001%/gram. Studies with the anti-GD3 mAb R24 labelled with iodine-131 have shown that GD3-positive tumor can be detected in a proportion of patients (8). After labelling of R24 with iodine-131 by the chloramine T method, greater than 90% of iodine was associated with mAb when determined by SDS polyacrylamide gel electrophoresis. Patients were injected with an intravenous bolus of either 1 mg or 10 mg R24. Pharmacokinetics of 5 patients injected with 10 mg fit a two compartment model. The T1/2 alpha was 4.9 ± 1.2 hrs and T1/2 beta was 50.7 ± 9.0 hrs. Urinary excretion of iodine-131 $25.1 \pm 7.2\%$ at 24 hrs and $60.2 \pm 9.7\%$ at 120 hrs. Biodistribution studies demonstrated that 28% of the injected dose remained in the patient, of which 1.6% injected dose/L remained in the plasma. Biopsies performed 6–7 days after injection demonstrated .0002–.0003% injected dose/gram of tumor in melanomas but only .00006% injected dose/gram in one astrocytoma.

Specificity and affinity of the antibody are almost certainly crucial to tumor localization, but a number of other factors could greatly impact on targeting, including: 1) tumor blood flow; 2) vascular permeability; 3) circulating antigen; 4) human anti-mouse Ig response; 5) tumor size; 6) antigen expression and antigenic heterogeneity in the tumor; and 7) tumor necrosis. Thus, it is possible to observe in some animal models and under some conditions that control monoclonal antibodies show the same tumor localization (or better) compared to a specific mAb (9–12). It is important, therefore, to include a control antibody when assessing tumor localization of a specific mAb. Optimally, evaluation of radiolabelled mAb also should include data derived from biopsies of tumor, bone marrow, and other tissues.

In order to address the role of antibody specificity and affinity in tumor localization, we have isolated variants of R24 that have low or no detectable affinity for the target antigen (13). The Fab portion of the antibody molecule carries the binding region (affinity and specificity) while the Fc portion determines effector functions and binding to Fc receptors. The variant R24 mAb have the same heavy chains as the parental antibodies (and, therefore, nearly identical Fc regions) but have irrelevant light chain on either one arm (V2–R24) or both arms (V1–R24) of the Fab portion. V2– R24 has 1.5 log less binding to GD3 and V1–R24 >4 log less binding (13). Relative functions of the three R24 species are listed in Table 1. Variant antibodies are proving to be useful to investigate the relative role of the Fab versus Fc portion of the antibody molecule in biodistribution, pharmacokinetics and tumor localization.

Table 1. V1-R24 is composed of two R24 heavy chains and two MOPC/21 (irrelevant) light chains. V2-R24 is composed of two R24 heavy chains, one MOPC/21 light chain and one R24 light chain. ADCC was performed at 1 ug/mL concentration of mAb; relative ADCC refers to lytic unit $20/10^7$ cells by each species of mAb. Relative C' (complement-mediated) lysis refers to the relative concentration of mAb mediating 50 % lysis of target cells.

MAb	Relative GD3 Binding	Relative ADCC	Relative C' Lysis	T Cell Prolif.
V1-R24	1	1	Neg	Neg
V2-R24	70	1.7	1	Neg
R24	1 500	9.3	19	Pos

Strategies for Therapy with Unconjugated Monoclonal Antibodies

Therapy with unconjugated monoclonal antibodies, either to induce inflammation or by active immunization, is predicated on the assumption that the immune system is capable of mediating tumor rejection. Although a large number of animal model systems have demonstrated tumor rejection mediated by immunological mechanisms, there is no compelling evidence yet for a major role of immunotherapy in the treatment of human cancer. This statement does not argue against a potential role for immunotherapy. Clearly the immune system is capable of rejecting large tissues, e.g. allogeneic kidneys, lungs and livers in transplantation systems. Thus, given an appropriate target, immunological mechanisms exist for major destruction of tissue.

Although tumor regressions have been observed after immunotherapy with single agents (e.g. interleukin 2, alpha interferon, and monoclonal antibodies), it is unlikely that any one component of the immune system is solely responsible for rejection. Rather, tissue rejection typically requires a coordinated response by multiple components. A number of cytokines have been identified that have potent effects on the growth and activation of cells in the immune system – e.g. IL-2 for lymphocytes, TNF-alpha for neutrophils. Cytokines do not direct specificity of the immune response, however – specificity is directed by antibodies secreted by B cells and the T cell receptor. Thus, one can argue that an effective strategy will require reproducible activation of multiple components of the immune system (e.g. cytokines) and an immune response directed specifically at tumor sites (e.g. mab).

Clinical studies of R24 (anti-GD3) mab (14, 15), 3F8 (anti-GD2) mab (16), and ME-36.1 (anti-GD2/GD3) mab (17) have demonstrated partial and complete response in patients with melanoma and neuroblastoma. In addition, studies by Irie and Morton have shown regression of cutaneous melanoma metastases after intralesional injection of a human monoclonal antibody against GD2 (18). Studies of patients with lymphoid malignancies and colon cancer have demonstrated regression of tumors after treatment with unmodified mabs (19, 20). A common feature of these trials is that virtually all of the mab used for treatment were immunologically active – mab actively mediated antibody-dependent cellular cytotoxicity (ADCC) or complement-mediated cytotoxicity or both. In contrast, several phase I trials in patients with melanoma using mab that were inactive in ADCC and complement killing demonstrated no anti-tumor activity (21, 22). These observations suggest an association between the *in vitro* immunological effects of mab and tumor responses observed in of phase I trials.

Possible Mechanisms for Anti-Tumor Effects of R24

Although direct cytotoxicity is an attractive mechanism for tumor killing, several clinical observations suggest that the anti-tumor effects of R24 are mediated by alternate or additional mechanisms. Tumor regression most frequently begins 4–10 weeks (and as late as 16 weeks) after starting treatment, and tumor sites are characteristically infiltrated by $CD8^+/Ia^+$ T lymphocytes after R24 treatment. The immunological and biological anti-tumor effects of R24 against target melanoma cells including: 1) complement-mediated cytotoxicity, 2) antibody-dependent cellular cytoxicity (R24 can mediate killing of $GD3^+$ target melanoma cells by K cells, macrophages, NK cells and weakly by neutrophils), and 3) direct effects on cell growth and attachment (23–25).

The results suggest that there are several potential mechanisms for the anti-tumor effects of R24. Potential immune mechanisms for R24-mediated anti-tumor effects can be divided into two categories:

Direct Cytotoxicity

1) Complement activation – R24 can directly lyse melanoma cells in the presence of human complement. A potentially important effect may be activation of complement components that increase vascular permeability and trigger inflammatory response mediated by other constituents of the immune system, e.g. C3a and C5a (anaphylatoxin) activating mast cells.

2) Antibody-dependent cellular cytotoxicity (ADCC) – this mechanism involves direct lysis of target cells by effector cells (macrophages, K cells, NL cells or neutrophils).

Immunomodulation and Immunization

1) Specific immunization mediated through anti-idiotype response – based on the network theory of Jerne (3), it has been postulated that generation of an anti-idiotype response to a monoclonal antibody can generate an active immune response (humoral or cellular) against the target antigen recognized by the mAb (27). A prediction of this theory is the development of an active immune response against GD3. Human antibodies against GD3 have not been detected in patients treated with R24, although some patients develop a specific response against the Fab portion of R24 consistent with an anti-idiotype response.

2) Direct activation of $GD3^+$ T lymphocytes by R24 – activation of cytotoxic or regulatory T cells reacting with autologous tumor could generate or augment a cellular immune response.

3) Non-specific activation of cells of the reticuloendothelial system and other immune cells by either mouse immunoglobulin alone or mouse immunoglobulin complexed to antigen. This appears less likely in view of the lack of anti-tumor activity observed with some mouse mab (20, 21).

4) Elicitation of an immune response against mouse immunoglobulin bound to target tumor cells (28) – R24 could elicit an active immune response directed against heterologous mouse immunoglobulin determinants. In this setting, R24 indirectly leads to tumor inflammation and possibly destruction through a by-stander effect.

5) Xenogenization of tumor cells by binding of mouse immunoglobulin elicits an active immune response – several experimental studies have suggested that the expression of foreign determinants on tumor cells (e.g. viral proteins or BCG constituents) can help induce an immune response against endogenous tumor cell antigens (29).

References

1. Mitchell, M. S. and Oettgen, H. F. (editors). Hybridomas in cancer diagnosis and treatment. Prog. Cancer Res. Therapy 21, 1–264, 1982.
2. Houghton, A. N. and Scheinberg, D. A. Monoclonal antibodies: Potential applications to the treatment of cancer. Semin. Oncol. 13, 165–179, 1986.
3. Jerne, N. Towards a network theory of the immune system. Ann. Immunol. (Paris) 125C, 373, 1974.
4. Masui, H., Kawamoto, T., Sato, J. D., et al. Growth inhibition of human tumor cells in athymic nude mice by anti-epidermal growth factor receptor monoclonal antibodies. Cancer Res. 44, 1002–1007, 1984.
5. Larson, S. Radiolabelled antitumor monoclonal antibodies in diagnosis and therapy. J. Nucl. Med. 26, 538, 1985.
6. Mach, J.-P., Chatal, J.-F., Lumbroso, J.-D., et al. Tumor localization in patients by radiolabelled monoclonal antibodies against colon carcinoma. Cancer Res. 43, 5593, 1983.
7. Larson, S. M., Brown, J. P., Wright, P.W., et al. Imaging of melanoma with I-131-labelled monoclonal antibodies. J. Nucl. Med. 24, 123, 1983.
8. Bajorin, D., Yeh, S., Wong, G., Dantis, L., Vadhan, S., Coit, D., Templeton, M., Lloyd, K. O., Oettgen, H. F., Old, L. J., and Houghton, A. N. Pharmacokinetics biodistribution and radiolocalization of 131I-labelled mAb R24. Proc. Am. Assoc. Cancer Res. 28, 384, 1987.

9. Mann, B. D., Cohen, M. B., Saxton, R., et al. Imaging of human tumor xenografts in nude mice with radiolabelled monoclonal antibodies. Limitation of specificity due to non-specific uptake of antibody. Cancer 54, 1318, 1984.

10. Bullard, D. E., Adams, C. J., Coleman, R. E., and Bigner, D. D. *In vivo* imaging of intracranial human glioma xenografts comparing specific with non-specific radiolabelled monoclonal antibodies. J. Neurosurg. 64, 257, 1986.

11. Zalcberg, J. R. Tumor localization using radiolabelled monoclonal antibodies. Am. J. Clin. Oncol. 8, 481, 1985.

12. Sands, H., Jones, P. L., Shah, S. A., et al. Correlation of vascular permeability and blood flow with monoclonal antibody uptake by human clouser and renal cell xenografts. Cancer Res. 48, 188, 1988.

13. Chapman, P. B., Lonberg, M., Duteau, C., et al. Analysis of variants of an anti-GD3 monoclonal antibody. Proc. Am. Assoc. Cancer Res. 29, 1676, 1988.

14. Houghton, A. N., Mintzer, D., Cordon-Cardo, C. et al., Mouse monoclonal IgG3 antibodies detecting GD3 ganglioide: a phase I trial in patients with malignant melanoma. Proc. Natl. Acad. Sci. USA 82, 1242, 1985.

15. Vadhan-Raj, S., Cordon-Cardo, C., Carswell, E., Dantis, L., Templeton, M. A., Duteau, C., Mintzer, D., Oettgen, H. F., Old, L. J., and Houghton, A. N. Phase I trial of a mouse monoclonal antibody against GD3 ganglioside in patients with melanoma. Induction of inflammatory responses at tumor sites. J. Clin. Oncol. (in press).

16. Cheung, N. K.V., Lazarus, H., Miraldi, F., et al. Ganglioside GD2 specific monoclonal antibody 3F8: a phase I study in patient with neuroblastoma and malignant melanoma. J. Clin. Oncol. 5, 1430, 1987.

17. Lichtin, A., Iliopoulos, D., Guerry, D., et al. Therapy of melanoma with an anti-melanoma ganglioside monoclonal antibody: a possible mechanisms of a complete response. Proc. Am. Assoc. Cancer Res. 7, 958, 1988.

18. Irie, R. F., Morton, D. L. Regression of cutaneous metastatic melanoma by intralesional injection with human monoclonal antibody to ganglioside GD2. Proc. Natl. Acad. Sci. USA 83, 8694, 1986.

19. Meeker, T. C., Lowder, J., Maloney, D. G., et al. A clinical trial of anti-idiotype therapy for B cell malignancy. Blood 65, 1349, 1985.

20. Sears, H. F., Herlyn, D., Steplewski, Z., et al. Phase II clinical trial of murine monoclonal antibody cytotoxic for gastrointestinal adenocarcinoma. Cancer Res. 45, 5910, 1985.

21. Oldham, R. K., Foon, K. A., Morgan, C., et al. Monoclonal antibody therapy of malignant melanoma: In vivo localization in cutaneous metastasis after intravenous administration. J. Clin. Oncol. 2, 1235, 1985.

22. Goodman, G. E., Beaumier, P., Hellstrom, I., et al. Pilot trial of murine monoclonal antibodies in patients with advanced melanoma. J. Clin. Oncol. 3, 340, 1985.

23. Vogel, C.W., Welt, S.W., Carswell, E. A., et al. A murine IgG monoclonal antibody to a melanoma antigen that activates human complement *in vitro* and *in vivo*. Immunobiology 164, 309, 1983.

24. Knuth, A., Dippold, W. G., Houghton, A. N., et al. ADCC reactivity of human melanoma cells with mouse monoclonal antibodies. Proc. Am. Assoc. Cancer Res. 25, 1005, 1984.

25. Cheresh, D. A., Pierschbacher, M. D., Herzig, M. A., et al. Disialogangliosides GD2 and GD3 are involved in the attachment of human melanoma and neuroblastoma cells to extracellular matrix proteins. J. Cell Biol. 102, 688, 1986.

26. Dippold, W. G., Lloyd, K. O., Li, L.T. C., et al. Cell surface antigens of human malignant melanoma. Proc. Natl. Acad. Sci. USA 77, 6614, 1980.

27. Koprowski, H., Herlyn, D., Lubeck, M., et al. Human anti-idiotypic antibodies in cancer patients. Is the modulation of the immune response beneficial to the patient. Proc. Natl. Acad. Sci. USA 81, 216, 1984.

28. Lanzavecchia, A. Exploiting the immune system's own strategies for immunotherapy. Immunol. Today 9, 167–168, 1988.
29. Kobayashi, H. Xenogenization of tumor cells. Plenum Press 1976.

24. Immunological Response to Intrathecal GD3-Ganglioside Antibody Treatment in Cerebrospinal Fluid Melanosis

W. G. Dippold, H. Bernhard, and K.-H. Meyer zum Büschenfelde

Introduction

In recent years a large number of antigens on human malignant melanoma cells have been identified by means of monoclonal antibodies (1, 2). The availability of these antibodies has rapidly led to clinical investigations. Experience with monoclonal antibodies in the treatment of patients with melanoma is limited (3–9), because only small groups of patients have been treated so far. According to these studies, treatment with ganglioside antibodies appears most promising.

Recent studies indicate the importance of gangliosides as targets for immunological effector mechanisms in neuroectodermal tumors. Gangliosides GD3 and GD2 represent tumor restricted molecules (9–11). Ganglioside antibodies interfere with cell attachment (12, 13), mediate complement (14) and antibody dependent cellular cytotoxicity (15, 1). Naturally occuring ganglioside antibodies have been found in patients with malignant melanoma (17–19) and we and others (6–9) have demonstrated the efficacy of monoclonal antibodies to gangliosides in inducing inflammatory responses and tumor remissions.

Here we report on the first application of a mouse monoclonal antibody, the GD3-ganglioside antibody R-24, into the cerebrospinal fluid of two patients with meningeosis carcinomatosa. The aim of this study was not only to achieve tumor remission, but also to monitor closely the immunological effects caused by this antibody. This is possible, because cerebrospinal fluid can be obtained repeatedly during and after treatment.

Materials and Methods

Antibody. MAb R-24 was prepared from hybridoma ascites of BALB/c mice as previously described (6) and purified over Protein A sepharose columns (Pharmacia Inc., Freiburg, W.-Germany). Safety testing was checked by standard procedures (Behring-Werke, Marburg, W.-Germany). MAb R-24 was administered intrathecally after lumbar puncture in 5 ml 0.9 % (w/v) NaCl and 0.6 % (w/v) human serum albumin. Before Ab-application 5 ml of cerebrospinal fluid (c.s.f.) were withdrawn each time for cell and Ab-monitoring.

Patient A. received 10 times mAb R-24 (dose 1.: 2 mg, dose 2.–10.: 10 mg) over a period of five weeks, patient B. 8 times 1 mg mAb R-24 (day 1, 3, 5, 7, 9, 33, 36, 41) intrathecally.

Patient characteristics. Patient A. was a 34 year old male, Karnovsky performance status 80 % with no solid tumor mass in CAT-scans. He had been already on dexamethasone (9 mg daily) for the relief of cerebral symptoms (visual disturbances, nausea, vomiting, headache) 3 weeks before starting mAb-treatment.

Patient B., a 44 year old male, Karnovsky performance status 60 %, presented with a malignant melanoma located on the medulla oblongata, infiltrating the routes of the nervi XI and XII and the a. vertebralis. The tumor was removed completely, but black spots of tumor cells remained. As a consequence of the tumor and the surgery performed, hemiplegia of his left side had developed.

The cerebrospinal fluid (c.s.f.) of both patients proved to contain melanoma cells, which were all GD3-ganglioside positive, as shown by immunocytochemical analysis.

Cytochemical analysis. Cerebrospinal fluid (c.s.f.) was cytocentrifuged (Cytospin 2 Shandon) onto glass slides, the cells air-dried and stained by indirect immunoperoxidase as described (11).

Determination of mAb R-24 in serum samples. A double-determinant ELISA was employed, to calculate the concentration of infused mouse mAb in the patients' cerebrospinal fluid (c.s.f.) and serum samples. Rabbit anti-mouse antibody (Dakopatts Z 109, Roskilde, Denmark) was diluted 1 : 100 in 0.1 M phosphate buffered saline (PBS) and 50 µl coated to the wells of flat bottom microfluor "W" plates (Dynatech, Alexandria, VA) at 4 °C for 4 h. After rinsing the plates with 0.1 M PBS, 200 µl 0.1 M PBS + 10 % human serum albumin (HSA) were added and incubated at 4 °C for 24 h to block unspecific reactions. Then the plates were rinsed again in 0.1 M PBS + 0.1 % HSA three times and 50 µl of the patients' sera or c.s.f. samples and as standard, purified mAb R-24 serially diluted in normal human serum were added for 1 h at 4 °C. The plates were rinsed with 0.1 M PBS + 0.1 % HSA for 20 minutes at 4 °C again three times, and as 2nd antibody 100 µl of β-galactosidase-labelled F (ab)$_2$ rabbit anti-mouse antibody (Zymed G1-6321, CA), approximately diluted (1 : 500) in 0.1 PBS + 10 % HSA were added for 45 minutes.

The enzyme reaction was developed with 200 µl 4-methylumbelliferyl-β-D-galactoside (1 mg dissolved in 59 ml 0.1 M PBS, pH 6.9, Sigma, St. Louis, MO) as substrate at 37 °C for ½ h and evaluated by a Dynatech microfluor reader.

Human serum and c.s.f. samples collected at various times after treatment were tested for the presence of human IgG directed against the administered murine mAb. Flat bottom ELISA plates (Immunol. Dynatech M129A) were coated with 50 µl of mAb R-24 (5 µg/ml) for 4 h at room temperature. The plates were rinsed and blocking solution was added as above. Then 50 µl of the test samples, diluted in 100 % foetal bovine serum (FCS) were added for 1 h at 4 °C. The plates were washed again three times for 20 minutes at 4 °C. Finally 50 µl of peroxidase conjugated rabbit anti-human antibody (Dakopatts P212), diluted 1 : 10 in 0.1 M PBS (supplemented with 20 % FCS free; GIBCO, Scotland) were added. The enzyme reaction was developed with 50 µl of 2.2' azinobis (3-ethyl-benzthiazoline-6-sulfonic acid) 2NH$_4$-salt (Serva, Heidelberg, W.-Germany) as substrate for 30 minutes. The values were measured as optical density in a Flow reader. Antibody titers were evaluated as positive, if the corresponding ELISA-values were greater than three times the negative control.

In vitro culture of lymphocytes. Mononuclear cells (PBL) were obtained by density gradient centrifugation of 10 ml heparinized blood in 25 ml RPMI-medium and 15 ml Ficoll-Hypaque (Pharmacia, Munich, d = 1.077, No. 6129) at 3000 g for 15 min. PBLs and lymphocytes obtained from the c.s.f. were counted and cloned by limiting dilution (100, 10, 1 cell/well) in 96 well V-bottom plates (Nunc) in RPMI culture medium + 10 % FCS. Growing cultures from the lowest dilution were cultured and cloned again.

Polyclonal proliferation of lymphocyte growth was achieved by stimulation with 0.5 µg/ml PHA (No. H16 Wellcome, Burgwedel, W.-Germany) for three days on feeder cells (1×10^6 PBL/ml, irradiated with 10.000 rad). Then PHA containing medium was removed from the cultures and replaced by 200 µl IL-2-medium (No. 811030, Biotest, Frankfurt, W.-Germany). IL-2 medium: RPM-1 + 10 % FCS + 2 % L-glutamine + IL-2, diluted 1 : 250. Cultures were fed 2 times/week and every ten days fresh feeder cells were added.

Cellular cytotoxicity. In vitro cultured lymphocytes were added to ^{51}Cr-labelled target cells (0.5×10^6 target cells + 100 µCi ^{51}Cr) (Amersham) at an effector/target ratio of 20 : 1, 10 : 1, 5 : 1 for five hours at 37 °C. Target cells: melanoma cells (SK-Mel 19,29), the corresponding EBV-transformed B-cell line of SK-Mel 29 melanoma, another unrelated EBV-transformed B-cell line (LAZ 509) and the natural killer target cell K-562. Percent cytotoxicity was calculated by the formula A-B/C-B x 100, in which A is cpm in the supernatant of the test sample, B is cpm in the supernatant of target cells + medium, and C is cpm in Nonidet NP40 treated targets for maximum ^{51}Cr-release.

Results

Intrathecal application of GD3-ganglioside antibody to patients with cerebrospinal fluid melanosis. Two patients with melanosis of the meninges received mAb R-24 intrathecally. The first patient obtained 10 doses of mAb R-24 (dose 1: 2 mg; doses 2–10: 10 mg), the second patient, 8 doses of 1 mg mAb R-24 after incomplete removal of a malignant melanoma in the area of the brain system. Tumor cells and inflammatory cells in the cerebrospinal fluid (c.s.f.) were monitored during and after treatment. Antibodies applied intrathecally were also detectable in the serum of both patients. Patient A. developed anti-mouse antibodies (HAMA), patient B. did not. In the case of patient A. they developed 15 days after the first application in the serum, but not until the 25th day in the c.s.f. Shortly after ending treatment HAMA-titers had risen up to 1 : 25.600 in the serum and 1 : 1600 in the c.s.f. of patient A. The reactivity of the HAMA-response was not anti-idiotypic, because they reacted with two unrelated mouse monoclonal antibodies equally well.

The administration of mAb R-24 caused an increase in the number of inflammatory cells in the c.s.f. of both patients. GD3-ganglioside-negative tumor cells were found at high Ab-levels in the c.s.f. of patient A. Besides, the percentage of some cell types changed significantly, for example the number of granulocytes increased at the beginning of therapy and the number of plasma cells at the end, as determined by histochemical analysis.

Regressive changes of tumor cells were observed in the c.s.f. of patient A. 6 weeks after starting mAb-therapy. Treatment was stopped at the point, when routine cytological examination showed no tumor cells at two successive lumbar punctures. Two weeks later tumor cells without regressive features had reappeared. At this time CT-scans of the brain did again not show any solid tumor, but a NMR-image performed for the first time, revealed three up to 1.5 cm large tumor nodules. The patient died 6 weeks later.

No tumor cells were detected in the c.s.f. of patient B. after antibody therapy. Meanwhile, 18 months have passed, and no evidence of tumor has been obtained either by cytologic studies or by CT or NMR-images of this patient. He is working again full-time. Six weeks after the end of his treatment, c.s.f. lymphocytes were cultured by limiting dilution and tested for tumor cell cytotoxicity. In 13 out of 96 wells plated, lymphocytes grew. All 13 different c.s.f. lymphocyte cultures showed a high degree of cytotoxicity for malignant melanoma cells and the natural killer cell (NK) target K-562, but not for the corresponding Epstein-Barr virus transformed B cells. One highly cytotoxic c.s.f. lymphocyte culture grew well enough for FACS (Fluorescence activated cells sorting) analysis to be performed. The cells expressed the antigens CD2 (99.6 %), CD3 (53.5 %), and CD8 (68 %). In contrast, lymphocyte cultures established simultaneously from PBLs of patient B. did not show this cytotoxic activity. Therefore, this treatment approach may induce a cellular response against the tumor.

Discussion

The tumor responses induced by ganglioside antibodies, which have been observed by several investigators in two different tumor systems, melanoma and neuroblastoma, are encouraging. However, experience with this form of therapy is still very limited. For example dose levels or intervals of antibody administration are chosen arbitrarily. Ganglioside antibodies represent good tools for tumor treatment because they are immunologically "armed", being potent activators of human complement and mediators of antibody-dependent cellular cytotoxicity. In addition, GD3-ganglioside antibody R-24 induces an increase in the number of inflammatory cells at the tumor site, as shown in both patients with melanosis of the meninges. The mechanism of tumor regression, which occurs as late as 8 to 10 weeks after ganglioside antibody therapy, however still remains to be elucidated.

The generation of 13 highly cytotoxic lymphocyte cultures which were obtained from the c.s.f. of patient B. 6 weeks after the end of antibody administration is striking. They all efficiently lysed melanoma and K-562 target cells. Similar cytotoxic cells were not obtained from PBL-cultures of this patient, which were established at the same time. The functional properties of these cells, as well as their antigenic phenotype, characterizes these cells as cytotoxic T cells with NK cell activity and without MLC-restriction. This phenotype does not characterize the major human NK effector cell, which is a non-T/non-B CD3$^-$ lymphocyte (20). However, human cells with NK activity are heterogeneous in their antigenic phenotype, and cells, that display a combination of T-cell markers (CD2, CD3, CD7, and CD8) have been described.

Tumor responses could be a sequence of events induced by ganglioside antibodies. Complement is activated during treatment, as evidenced by decreases in serum complement levels and by the deposition of complement components at tumor sites. Complement fixation and antibody dependent cellular cytotoxicity may lead to the release of histamine and other mediators of inflammation. This initial event may cause an increase in blood flow, which in turn may permit better access of infiltrating lymphocytes into tumors. GD3-ganglioside-positive lymphocytes may then preferentially locate at the tumor site, because mAb R-24 may bring together GD3-ganglioside-positive tumor cells and GD3-positive lymphocytes.

The results of the studies applying ganglioside antibodies in the treatment of neuroectodermal tumors do not permit any conclusions about the efficacy of treatment or about factors that predict response. However, it is interesting to note that lower doses of antibody may be at least as effective as higher doses. The challenge now is to optimize doses and schedule and to evaluate methods to augment the antitumor effects of ganglioside antibodies in vivo. An obvious next step in the treatment of patients consists in combining monoclonal antibodies against different ganglioside molecules (GD3, GD2, GM2). An additional way of augmenting the observed responses may be to administrate ganglioside antibodies together with cytostatic drugs or with biological response modifiers. In the long term, well-characterized tumor-restricted monoclonal antibodies will gain more clinical application because selective tumor cell destruction will remain a central goal in cancer therapy. In this regard the development of "humanized" monoclonal antibodies by molecular techniques and of antibody drug conjugates appear very promising.

The other conclusion that may be drawn is, that immunity against a group of ganglioside antigens should be induced by active vaccination (see Livingston et al. this issue). The immunologic status of the individual patient may be the major reason for the unpredictable natural course of patients with malignant melanoma.

Acknowledgements

This work was supported by the Deutsche Forschungsgemeinschaft Di 245/3–4.

References

1. Lloyd, K. O. Human tumor antigens: Detection and characterization with mouse monoclonal antibodies. In: Herberman, R. B. ed. Basic and clinical tumor immunology. Martinus Nijhoff, pp. 160–214, 1983.
2. Sell, S., Reisfeld, R. (eds.). Monoclonal antibodies in cancer. Contemporary Biomedicine Clifton, NJ, Humana 1–485, 1985.
3. Larson, S. M., Carrasquillo, J. A., Krohn, K. A., Brown, J. P., McGruffin, R.W., Ferens, J. M., Graham, M. M., Hill, L. D., Beaumier, P. L., Hellström, K. E. Localization of ^{131}I-labelled p97-specific Fab fragments in human melanoma as a basis for radiotherapy. J. Clin. Invest. 72, 2101, 1983.
4. Oldham, R. K., Foon, K. A., Morgan, A. C., Woodhouse, C. S., Schroff, R.W., Abrahams, P. G., Fer, M., Schoenberger, C. S., Farrell, M., Kimball, E. Monoclonal antibody therapy of malignant melanoma: In vivo localization in cutaneous metastasis after intravenous administration. J. Clin. Oncol. 2, 1235, 1984.

5. Goodman, G. E., Beaumier, A., Fernyhough, B., Hellström, I., Hellström, K. E. Pilot trial of murine monoclonal antibodies in patients with advanced melanoma. J. Clin. Oncol. 3, 340, 1985.

6. Dippold, W. G., Knuth, A., Meyer zum Büschenfelde, K.-H. Inflammatory tumor response to monoclonal antibody infusion. Eur. J. Cancer Clin. Oncol. 21, 907, 1985.

7. Houghton, A. N., Mintzer, D., Cordon-Cardo, C., Welt, S., Fliegel, B., Vadhan, S., Carswell, E., Melamed, M., Oettgen, H. F., Old, L. J. Mouse monoclonal antibody detecting GD3 ganglioside: A phase I trial in patients with malignant melanoma. Proc. Natl. Acad. Sci. USA 82, 1242, 1985.

8. Irie, R. F., Morton, D. L. Regression of cutaneous metastatic melanoma by intralesional injection with human monoclonal antibody to ganglioside GD2. Proc. Natl. Acad. Sci. USA 83, 8694, 1986.

9. Cheung, N. K., Lazarus, H., Miraldi, F. D., Abramowsky, C. R., Kallick, S., Saarinen, U. M., Spitzer, T., Strandjord, S. E., Coccia, P. F., Berger, N. A. Ganglioside GD2 specific monoclonal antibody 3F8: a phase I study in patients with neuroblastoma and malignant melanoma. J. Clin. Oncol. 5, 1430, 1987.

10. Dippold, W., Lloyd, K. O., Li, L.T. C., Ikeda, H., Oettgen, H. F., Old, L. J. Cell surface antigens of human malignant melanoma: definition of six antigenic systems with monoclonal antibodies. Proc. Natl. Acad. Sci. USA 77, 6114, 1980.

11. Dippold, W., Dienes, H. P., Knuth, A., Meyer zum Büschenfelde, K.-H. Immunohistochemical localization of ganglioside GD3 in human malignant melanoma, epithelial tumors, and normal tissues. Cancer Res. 45, 3699, 1985.

12. Dippold, W. G., Knuth, A., Meyer zum Büschenfelde, K.-H. Inhibition of human melanoma cell growth in vitro by monoclonal anti-GD3-ganglioside antibody. Cancer Res. 44, 806, 1984.

13. Cheresh, D. A., Harper, J. R., Schulz, G., Reisfeld, R. A. Localization of the gangliosides GD2 and GD3 in adhesion plaques and on the surface of human melanoma cells. Proc. Natl. Acad. Sci. USA 81, 5767, 1984.

14. Vogel, C.W., Welt, S.W., Carswell, E. A., Old, L. J., Müller-Eberhard, H. J. A murine IgG3 monoclonal antibody to a melanoma antigen that activates complement in vitro and in vivo. Immunobiology 164, 309, 1983.

15. Knuth, A., Dippold, W. G., Meyer zum Büschenfelde, K.-H. Disialoganglioside GD3-specific monoclonal antibody in ADCC for human malignant melanoma. In: Gagnara, J., Klaus, S. N., Paul, E., Schartl, M. (eds.) Biological. Molecular and Clinical Aspects of Pigmentation, University of Tokyo Press, Tokyo, pp. 421, 1985.

16. Cheresh, D. A., Honsik, C. J., Staffileno, L. K., Jung, G., Reisfeld, R. A. Disialoganglioside GD3 on human melanoma serves as a relevant target antigen for monoclonal antibody-mediated tumor cytolysis. Proc. Natl. Acad. Sci. USA 82, 5155, 1985.

17. Watanabe, T., Pukel, C., Takeyama, H., Lloyd, K. O., Shiku, H., Li, L.T. C., Travassos, L. R., Oettgen, H. F., Old, L. J. Human melanoma antigen AH is an autoantigenic ganglioside related to GD2. J. Exp. Med. 155, 1884, 1982.

18. Irie, R. F., Sze, L. L., Saxton, R. E. Human antibody to OFA-1, a tumor antigen, produced in vitro by Epstein-Barr virus-transformed human B-lymphoid cell lines. Proc. Natl. Acad. Sci. USA 79, 5666, 1982.

19. Cahan, L. D., Irie, R. F., Singh, R., Cassidenti, A., Paulson, J. C. Identification of a human neuroectodermal tumor antigen (OFA-12) as ganglioside GD2. Proc. Natl. Acad. Sci. USA 79, 7629, 1982.

20. Reynolds, C.W., Ortaldo, J. R. Natural killer activity: the definition of a function rather than a cell type. Immunol. Today 8, 172, 1987.

25. Gangliosides Recognized by Human Monoclonal Antibody: Targets for Immunotherapy of Cancer

R. F. Irie and P. J. Chandler

Our group utilizes the human melanoma model to assess the potential of ganglioside antigens as targets for immunotherapy with human monoclonal antibody (HuMAb). Ganglioside antigens are desirable targets for immunotherapy because they undergo characteristic changes during malignant transformation and thus act as tumor antigens. These changes are evident in human melanoma; normal melanocytes express predominately GM3 (90 %), with GD3 a minor component (5 %) (1), whereas melanoma cells contain a large quantity of GD3 (48 %) and a variety of other ganglioside molecules including, GM2, GD2, O-acetyl GD3 and N-glycolyl containing gangliosides (2–5). Our group and others have demonstrated that many of these gangliosides are immunogenic in man (6–10). The potential of passive immunotherapy using HuMAb to control human tumors is encouraging in light of the immunogenic nature of ganglioside antigens, their association with the malignant cell and their wide distribution in other cancer systems. Moreover, recent evidence indicating that anti-ganglioside HuMAb can induce active specific immunity via the anti-idiotypic network provides additional support for the potential therapeutic value of HuMAb.

Human Monoclonal Anti-Ganglioside Antibody

While murine monoclonal antibodies have been developed against many melanoma-associated ganglioside antigens, only two groups have reported the production of human monoclonal anti-ganglioside antibodies. In 1982, we first reported the successful establishment of human B-cell lines that produced human monoclonal antibodies to GD2 (L72) and GM2 (L55), respectively (11–13). This was accomplished by the use of EBV-transformation techniques where B lymphocytes from melanoma patients were infected with Epstein-Barr virus (EBV) in vitro and cloned for the selection of antibody producing B-lymphoblasts. More recently we reported the development of our third anti-ganglioside antibody of which the epitope was identified to be gangliosides having the terminal structure, NeuAc-Gal-GlcNAc (L87) (14). Yamaguchi et al. have established stable antibody producing cell lines by fusion of EBV-transformed human lymphoblasts with mouse myeloma cell line NS-1 (15). The antibodies reacted to common epitopes among several gangliosides including: Mab-HJM1 which reacted strongly with GD3, and weakly with GD2 and GD1b; Mab-FCMI reacted strongly with GM3 and GD1a, and weakly with GD3 and GD2; and MAb-32-27 reacted with di and tri-sialogangliosides. All HuMAb anti-ganglioside antibodies produced thus far are IgM class, are effective in complement-dependent cytotoxicity (16), and none have been demonstrated to be capable of mediating antibody-dependent cellular cytotoxicity.

Clinical Trials of Human Monoclonal Antibody

Evaluation of the therapeutic efficacy of our 3 HuMAbs (L72, L55, L87) has been initiated. In 1986 we reported the first clinical trial (8 melanoma patients) of intra-lesionally administered HuMAb L72 (17). Since that time 5 more patients have been added to the L72 protocol and the independent clinical assessment of L55 and L87 is underway.

Table 1. Intralesional injection of L72 HuMAb[a] to cutaneous recurrent melanoma.

# patients treated	13
# patients responded	8
# nodules (0.2–1.9 cm) treated with antibody	35
# nodules responded	28 (80%)
# nodules treated with HSA	7
# nodules responded	0 (0%)
# large size nodules (4.0–5.2 cm) treated with antibody	6
# large-sized nodules responded	1 (17%)

[a] Human monoclonal antibody to GD2.
Responded = 50% or greater reduction in tumor size.

HuMAb L72 reacts with ganglioside GD2 which is found in 70% of melanoma tumors (2). Thus far in the clinical evaluation of this antibody, 8 of 13 patients with cutaneous metastases that received intralesional injection have demonstrated a tumor regression of at least 50% (Table 1). This regression occured within 4 weeks of the initial treatment and in 4 of the 8 patients the injected lesions experienced complete tumor regression. The specificity of L72 is evident in that those tumors not having a significant clinical response were devoid of the GD2 antigen as detected by the immunologic and/or biochemical analysis. A differential clinical response has been observed between small tumors (.2–1.9 cm) and larger tumors (4.0–5.2 cm). Twenty-eight of 35 (80%) small tumors injected have regressed at least 50% while only 1 of 6 (17%) larger tumors have shown a similar response.

The anti-tumor effect and the demonstrated specificity of HuMAbs L55 and L87 appear to be quite similar to that of L72. Thus far, complete regression has been obtained by both HuMAbs independently and again, tumors not sensitive to HuMAb do not express the appropriate cell surface antigen. With the exception of mild erythema around the injection site, no side effects have been observed in any application of our HuMAbs.

Prospects of Human Monoclonal Anti-Ganglioside Antigens

While the clinical trials of HuMAb are still in their early stages it is becoming increasingly clear that ganglioside antigens are a valuable target for passive immunotherapy and all three of our HuMAbs possess a specific cytotoxic effect. While our clinical trials are restricted to melanoma tumors, the successful demonstration of the efficacy of HuMAb has important consequences to many other tumor systems that also express immunogenic ganglioside antigens. The most immediate application of intralesional administration of HuMAb is to recurrent cutaneous malignant melanoma and to non-resectable primary melanoma. Conventional treatment of cutaneous recurrent melanoma in our clinic is the administration of intralesional BCG. While this treatment is relatively successful, it can induce systemic side effects including chills and high fever and can cause severe ulceration at the administration site. Intralesional HuMAb administration has the advantage that it induces no toxic effects other than slight erythema at the tumor. The demonstrated cytotoxic activity of HuMAb together with the lack of toxicity make intralesional therapy with HuMAb a strong alternative to conventional therapy.

One disadvantage of ganglioside antigens as targets for HuMAb is their relatively low density on melanoma. In addition as we described previously, ganglioside expression is widely heterogeneous among individual melanomas (2). To overcome these problems our laboratory is developing new HuMAbs to immunogenic ganglioside antigens such as O-acetyl GD3 and N-glycolyl neuraminic acid containing gangliosides, to use as a "cocktail" which will increase the density of antibody-bound antigen to be attached by complement and/or effector cells.

In light of recent success in the applications of murine monoclonal antibody to systemic melanoma recurrence (18, 19) and the strong anti-tumor effect of our HuMAb on cutaneous melanoma (17, 20), the efficacy of systemic passive immunotherapy with the anti-ganglioside HuMAb is promising. Thus far a major obstacle to systemic application of HuMAb has been the low yield of antibody production by the lymphoblastoid cells compared to their murine hybridoma counterparts. While our HuMAb production is continous, our current production by these lymphoblastoid cell lines ranges between 10 to 20 μg per ml of culture supernatant as compared to murine hybridoma technology which produces up to 10 mg of protein per ml in ascites of syngeneic mice. We have been actively investigating methods to increase the efficiency of HuMAb and have expanded our current production system in order to produce the large quantities needed for a systemic trial.

The efficacy of HuMAb systemic therapy was investigated for HuMAb L72 (anti-GD2) using the nude mouse model (20, 21). While L72 is an IgM class antibody we demonstrated that it has the ability to cross the blood tumor barrier (22). We administered L72 (200 μg/mouse) either i.p. or i.v. to nude mice bearing subcutaneous human melanoma or lung and liver metastases. Control mice included those with a GD2 negative human melanoma cell line or without tumor. We observed a marked reduction in the anti-GD2 titer after 2 hours in mice bearing GD2-positive tumors while reduction was minimal for control mice. In a separate experiment the tumor cells were removed from the mice and surface-bound antibody was tested IA. Up to 86 % of GD2-positive tumor cells rosetted erthrocytes while only 1–3 % of controls were rosette positive. This indicates that HuMAb L72 has the ability to cross the blood tumor barrier and bind to tumor cells. It is important to note that no toxicity was observed in the mice when systemically administered 200 μg of L72 (a foreign protein in this case). This dosage is comparable to 600 mg in a 60 kg human adult (a protein of the same species in this case). While HuMAb was administered in one large dose in these experiments, a clinical administration would be given over many hours. This indicates that large doses may be feasible in human application.

One significant issue associated with the production of HuMAb to ganglioside antigens has been the inability to generate IgG class antibody. In previous studies examining sera from 2,000 non-immunized melanoma patients we have not detected the presence of IgG class autoantibody to ganglioside antigens. Moreover, antibody induced in melanoma patients by melanoma cell vaccine has also been primarily of the IgM class (6). It seems quite possible that we will not be able to produce IgG class antibody in vitro using standard techniques. One potential solution is the use of recombinant DNA technology to develop an IgG class human-human chimeric antibody. Recently investigators have reported the successful production of human-mouse chimeric antibody using mouse myeloma cells transfected with mouse variable region genes and the genes coding a human constant region (23, 24). Because we have already established B cell lines producing HuMAb with ganglioside specificity the same technology could be applied to produce a human-human chimeric antibody using the gene sequence of the antibody variable region with genes coding for the IgG class constant region. The establishment of IgG class anti-ganglioside HuMAb will allow us to switch from the primarily complement-dependent tumor killing of IgM to a cell mediated killing system. In light of the cost inefficiencies for IgM HuMAb production and the inability to produce IgG class antibody to ganglioside antigens, human-human chimeric antibody could be the key to both future large scale clinical trials of HuMAb and more effective intralesional and systemic immunotherapy.

Application of Human Monoclonal Antibody to Active Specific Immunization

Our group and others have demonstrated that production of antibody against certain tumor-associated gangliosides is associated with prolonged survival in melanoma patients (25–27). This observation has been the basis of current clinical investigations of active specific immunization of melanoma using whole tumor and purified ganglioside vaccines. Unfortunately, these trials encountered some major obstacles including, the induction of T-cell suppressors, antigen tolerance and production of large quantities of purified gangliosides. To circumvent these problems we have begun to investigate the application of anti-idiotype technology to human tumor systems. This technology is based on the network theory proposed by Jerne which predicted that idiotype antibody (Ab1) could induce the production of anti-idiotype antibodies (Ab2) of which some possess a conformationally identical determinant to that of the original antigen (Ab2). Ab2 could then stimulate the generation of antibodies to the original antigen (Ab3). The efficacy of Ab2 for vaccination of infectious diseases has been well demonstrated in animal models and the ability of both Ab1 and Ab2 to induce anti-tumor antibodies has been clearly shown (29–33). While the role of anti-idiotype antibody in immune regulation and tumor defense has not been completely elucidated, recent reports have indicated the mechanisms of the anti-idiotype network for tumor systems. Raychaudhuri et al. demonstrated that of two different anti-idiotype antibodies produced against the same idiotype one could induce anti-tumor immunity while the other could not. The ability of anti-idiotype antibody to induce protective immunity was correlated with the presence and/or absence of certain regulatory T cells. Moreover, the same group has demonstrated the existence of anti-idiotype recognizing T-helper cells which exert differential controls on tumor growth (34). One advantage of anti-idiotype active immunization is that the antigen is presented in a new environment and thus it might be possible to avoid T-cell suppressor mechanisms by activating silent clones (35) and by activation of T-helper cells (34). Thus far all of the studies have been done using murine hybridoma Ab1 and Ab2 developed as hybridoma monoclonal or polyclonal antibodies in animals.

In our recent clinical trials with L72 anti-GD2 HuMAb we have demonstrated the induction of antibodies specifically reactive to L72 HuMAb (17). Table 2 shows the results of serum analysis of the first eight patients receiving HuMAb L72 intralesional injection. Five of the eight patients demonstrated an Ab2 response against L72 as detected by the passive hemagglutination assay (PHA). In the PHA, sheep red blood cells were coated with HuMAb L72 and reacted with patients serum which was preabsorbed with sheep erthyrocytes to minimize non-specific binding. The dose of HuMAb needed to induce Ab2 production ranged between 2.6 to 14.7 mg and the onset of Ab2 production averaged approximately 15 days after the first injection of HuMAb L72. Two patients demonstrated Ab2 of which PHA reactivity was specifically blocked by purified GD2. This indicates that these Abs were specific for the antigen binding region of L72.

In our second group of patients receiving intralesional injection with HuMAb L72 we observed the production of IgG class antibody reactive to GD2 on melanoma cells in one patient whose tumor had undergone complete regression (submitted). This patient received a total of 8.0 mg of L72 over a 50 day period. Ab2 was first detected by ELISA 12 days after the initial injection. The Ab2 production peaked after 62 days and maintained an elevated level. Anti-ganglioside antibodies were first detected 137 days after the initial L72 injections by the IgG-membrane immunofluorescence assay. The specificity of the IgG was confirmed by ELISA using purified GD2. Since L72 is of the IgM class, the detection of IgG anti-GD2 antibody indicates the production of Ab3 through the anti-idiotypic network.

The generation of active specific immunity by injection of HuMAb is an exciting advance in tumor immunotherapy. Our current investigation includes the development of anti-idiotype monoclonal antibodies against these HuMAb. Whereas melanoma vaccines using whole tumor or purified antigen induce primarily IgM class antibody, HuMAb or monoclonal antibody to the idiotype would enable us to utilize

Table 2. Anti-L72 HuMAb antibody response in melanoma patients receiving L72 HuMAb treatment. The antibody levels were tested by passive hemagglutination (PHA).

Patient #	L72 injected (mg)	PHA[a] (days)[b]	Inhibition by GD2
1	14.7	++ (14)	No
2	3.0	+/−	NT[c]
3	9.0	+/−	NT
4	2.6	+++ (7)	Yes
5	7.4	−	NT
6	4.8	++ (26)	Yes
7	4.5	++++ (13)	No
8	7.9	++ (10)	No

[a] Serum was tested at 1:40 dilution.
[b] Days after initial L72 injection in which Anti-L72 antibody was detected.
[c] Not Tested.

the anti-idiotypic network to generate a large, sustained IgG anti-ganglioside response. Induction of IgG class antibodies is possible because the antigen is being "converted" from a glycolipid to a protein and thus B-cell activation is transfered from a T-cell independent to a T-cell dependent system. Studies by other investigators and our observations provide the basis for future studies aimed at investigating the efficacy of active specific immunization using HuMAb to ganglioside antigens or monoclonal antibody (murine or human) to the HuMAb in melanoma patients that are at high risk of recurrence.

Our Approach for the Production of Human Monoclonal Antibody for Treatment of Cancer

Since we have clearly demonstrated the specific cytotoxic effect of antiganglioside HuMAb, the ultimate effectiveness of this therapy will depend on our ability to generate a comprehensive panel of antibodies to overcome the heterogeneity of ganglioside expression of human melanoma (2). In light of our previous success at producing HuMAb we are confident that our systematic approach to HuMAb production (Figure 1) will allow us to produce antibody to the remaining immunogenic antigens of melanoma. We believe our success has been largely due to our unique strategy of studying only antigens known to be immunogenic in man. Our method for the detection of such antigens has been to use sera from cancer patients as the antibody

Figure 1. Procedure for development of human monoclonal antibody for treatment of melanoma.

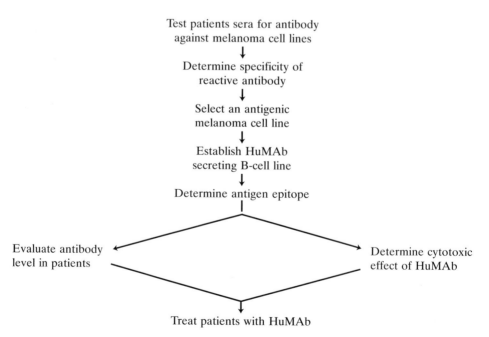

Test patients sera for antibody
against melanoma cell lines
↓
Determine specificity of
reactive antibody
↓
Select an antigenic
melanoma cell line
↓
Establish HuMAb
secreting B-cell line
↓
Determine antigen epitope

Evaluate antibody
level in patients

Determine cytotoxic
effect of HuMAb

Treat patients with HuMAb

source. By using human sera we eliminate the involvement of species-specific and tissue-specific antigens, and increase the likelihood of discovering immunogenic tumor antigens. The melanoma cell line, UCLASO-M14 (36), that contains large quantities of the immunogenic gangliosides GM2 and GD2 (7, 12, 13) has been our target in immunologic assays monitoring the supernatant of human lymphoblastoid cell lines in antibody production. This melanoma cell line was also utilized in subsequent studies as an antigen source to purify and chemically characterize the antigenic epitope, and in several preclinical experiments including the identification of the cytotoxic mechanisms in vitro and in nude mice (16, 20, 21, 22).

References

1. Carubia, J. M., Yu, R. K., Macala, L. J., Kirkwood, J. M., Varga, J. M. Gangliosides of normal and neoplastic human melanocytes. Biochem. Biophys. Res. Commun. 120, 500–504, 1984.
2. Tsuchida, T., Saxton, R. E., Morton, D. L., Irie, R. F. Gangliosides of human melanoma. J. Natl. Cancer Inst. 78, 45–54, 1987.
3. Cherish, D. A., Varki, A. P., Varki, N. M., Stallcup, W. B., Levine, J., Reisfeld, R. A. A monoclonal antibody recognizes an O-acetyl sialic acid in a human melanoma-associated ganglioside. J. Biol. Chem. 259, 7453–7459, 1984.
4. Thurin, J., Herlyn, M., Hindsgaul, O., Stromberg, N., Karlsson, K.-A., Elder, D., Steplewski, Z., Koprowski, H. Proton NMR and fast-atom bombardment mass spectrometry analysis of the melanoma-associated ganglioside 9-O-acetyl GD3. J. Biol. Chem. 260, 14556–14563, 1985.
5. Hirabayashi, Y., Higashi, H., Kato, S., Taniguchi, M., Matsumoto, M. Occurrence of tumor-associated ganglioside antigens with Hanganutziu-Deicher antigenic activity on human melanomas. Jpn. J. Cancer Res. 78, 614–620, 1987.
6. Tai, T., Cahan, L. D., Tsuchida, T., Saxton, R. E., Irie, R. F., Morton, D. L. Immunogenicity of melanoma-associated gangliosides in cancer patients. Int. J. Cancer 35, 607–612, 1985.
7. Irie, R. F., Tai, T., Morton, D. L. Antibodies to tumor-associated gangliosides (GM2 and GD2): Potential for suppression of melanoma occurrence. In: "Basic Mechanisms and Clinical Treatment of Tumor Metastasis" M. Torisu and T. Yoshida (eds.), Academic Press: San Diego, pp. 371–384, 1985.
8. Livingston, P. O., Natoli, E. J., Calves, M. J., Stockert, E., Oettgen, H. F., Old, L. J. Vaccines containing purified GM2 ganglioside elicit GM2 antibodies in melanoma patients. Proc. Natl. Acad. Sci. USA 84, 2911–2915, 1987.
9. Nakarai, H., Saida, T., Shibata, Y., Irie, R. F., Kano, K. Expression of heterophile, Paul-Bunnell and Hanganutziu-Deicher antigens on human melanoma cell lines. Int. Archs. Allergy Appl. Immun. 83, 160–166, 1987.
10. Ravidranath, M. H., Paulson, J. C., Irie, R. F. Human melanoma antigen O-acetylated ganglioside GD3 is recognized by cancer antennarius lectin. J. Biol. Chem. 263, 2079–2086, 1988.
11. Irie, R. F., Sze, L. L., Saxton, R. E. Human antibody to OFA-I, a tumor antigen, produced in vitro by EBV-transformed human B-lymphoblastoid cell lines. Proc. Natl. Acad. Sci. 79, 5666–5670, 1982.

12. Cahan, L. D., Irie, R. F., Singh, R., Cassidenti, A., Paulson, J. C. Identification of a human neuroectodermal tumor antigen (OFA-I-2) as ganglioside GD2. Proc. Natl. Acad. Sci. 79, 7629–7633, 1982.

13. Tai, T., Paulson, J. C., Cahan, L. D., Irie, R. F. Ganglioside GM2 as a human tumor antigen (OFA-I-1). Proc. Natl. Acad. Sci. 80, 5392–5396, 1983.

14. Matsuki, T., Sze, L., Giuliano, A. E., Irie, R. F. Human monoclonal antibody reacting with sialosylneolactotetraosylceramide. Proc. Am. Assoc. Cancer Res. 29, A1694, 1988.

15. Yamaguchi, H., Furukawa, K., Fortunato, S. R., Livingston, P. O., Lloyd, K. O., Oettgen, H. R., Old, L. J. Cell surface antigens of melanoma recognized by human monoclonal antibodies. Proc. Natl. Acad. Sci. USA 84, 2416–2420, 1987.

16. Katano, M., Saxton, R. E., Irie, R. F. Human monoclonal antibody to tumor-associated ganglioside GD2. J. Clin. Lab. Immunol. 15, 119–126, 1984.

17. Irie, R. F., Morton, D. L. Regression of cutaneous metastatic melanoma by intralesional injection with human monoclonal antibody to ganglioside GD2. Proc. Natl. Acad. Sci. USA 83, 8694–8698, 1986.

18. Houghton, A. N., Mintzer, D., Cordon-Cardo, C., Welt, S., Fliegel, B., Vadhan, S., Carswell, E., Melamed, M. R., Oettgen, H. F., Old, L. J. Mouse monoclonal IgG3 antibody detecting GD3 ganglioside: A phase I trial in patients with malignant melanoma. Proc. Natl. Acad. Sci. USA 82, 1242–1246, 1985.

19. Cheung, N. V., Lazarus, H., Miraldi, F. D., Abramowsky, C. R., Kallick, S., Saarinen, U. M., Spitzer, T., Strandjord, S. E., Coccia, P. F., Berger, N. A. Ganglioside GD2 specific monoclonal antibody 3F8: A phase I study in patients with neuroblastoma and malignant melanoma. J. Clin. Oncol. 5, 1430–1440, 1987.

20. Irie, R. F., Chandler, P. J., Morton, D. L. In: "Human antigens and specific tumor therapy". Eds. R. Metzgar and M. Mitchell. Pub. Alan R. Liss Inc., New York, NY.

21. Katano, M., Irie, R. F. Suppressed growth of human melanoma in nude mice by human monoclonal antibody to ganglioside GD2. Immunology Letters 8, 169–174, 1984.

22. Katano, M., Saxton, R. E., Tsuchida, T., Irie, R. F. Human IgM monoclonal anti-GD2 antibody: Reactivity to a human melanoma xenograft. Jpn. J. Cancer Res. (Gann) 77, 584–594, 1986.

23. Liu, A. Y., Robinson, R. R., Murray, D., Ledbetter, J. A., Hellstrom, I., Hellstrom, K. E. Production of mouse-human chimeric monoclonal antibody to CD20 with potent Fc-dependent biologic activity.

24. Nishimura, Y., Yokoyama, M., Araki, K., Ueda, R., Kudo, A., Watanabe, T. Recombinant human-mouse chimeric monoclonal antibody specific for cALLA. Cancer Res. 47, 999–1005, 1987.

25. Morton, D. L., Nizze, J. A., Gupta, R. K., Famatiga, E., Hoon, D. S. B., Irie, R. F. Active specific immunotherapy of malignant melanoma. In: "Current Status of Cancer Control and Immunobiology". Eds. and Pub. J. P. Kim, Kim, J.-G. Park, pp. 152–161, 1987.

26. Jones, P. C., Sze, L. L., Liu, P. I., Morton, D. L., Irie, R. F. Prolonged survival for melanoma patients with elevated IgM antibody to oncofetal antigen. J. Natl. Cancer Inst. 66, 249–254, 1981.

27. Livingston, P. O. Experimental and clinical studies with active specific immunotherapy. In: "Immunity to Cancer II". Eds. M. S. Mitchell. Pub. Alan R. Liss. Inc., New York, NY, in press.

28. Kennedy, R. C., Dreesman, G. R., Kohler, H. Vaccines utilizing internal image anti-idiotypic antibodies that mimic antigens of infectious organism. Biotechniques 3, 404, 1985.

29. Viale, G., Grassi, F., Pelagi, M., Alzani, R., Menard, S., Miotti, S., Buffa, R., Gini, A., Siccardi, A. G. Anti-human tumor antibodies induced in mice and rabbits by "internal image" anti-idiotypic monoclonal immunoglobulins. J. Immunology 138, 4250–4255, 1987.

30. Nepom, G.T., Nelson, K. A., Holbeck, S. L., Hellstrom, I., Hellstrom, K. E. Induction of immunity to a human tumor marker by in vivo administration of anti-idiotypic antibodies in mice. Proc. Natl. Acad. Sci. 81, 2864–2867, 1984.
31. Herlyn, D., Lubeck, M., Sears, H., Koprowski, H. Specific detection of anti-idiotypic immune responses in cancer patients treated with murine monoclonal antibody. J. Immun. Meth. 85, 27–38, 1985.
32. Defreitas, E., Suzuki, D., Herlyn, M., Lubeck, H., Sears, M., Herlyn, M., Koprowski, H. Human antibody induction to the idiotypic and anti-idiotypic determinants of a monoclonal antibody against a gastrointestinal carcinoma antigen. In: Current Topic in Microbiology and Immunology, Vol. 119 pp. 75–89.
33. Bhattacharya-Chatterjee, M., Pride, M.W., Seon, B. K., Kohler, H. Idiotype vaccines against T cell acute lymphoblastic leukemia: I. Generation and characterization of biologically active monoclonal anti-idiotypes. J. Immunology 139, 1354–1360, 1987.
34. Raychaudhuri, S., Saeki, Y., Chen, J.-J., Kohler, H. Tumor specific idiotype vaccines: III. Induction of T helper cells by anti-idiotype and tumor cells. J. of Immunology 139, 2096–2102, 1987.
35. Bona, C. E., Herber-Katz, E., Paul, W. E. Idiotype-antiidiotype regulation. I. Immunization with a levan-binding myeloma protein leads to the appearance of auto-anti-(anti-idiotype) antibodies and to the activation of silent clones. J. Exp. Med. 153, 951–967, 1981.
36. Irie, R. F., Irie, K., Morton, D. L. A membrane antigen common to human cancer and fetal brain tissues. Cancer Res. 36, 3510–3517, 1976.

26. Therapy of Neuroblastoma with GD2 Specific Monoclonal Antibody 3F8

D. H. Munn, C. Cordon-Cardo,
S. D. J. Yeh, B. H. Kushner, and
N.-K. V. Cheung

Abstract

Despite more sophisticated application of chemotherapy, the ultimate obstacle in the treatment of neuroblastoma derives from refractory microscopic disease. A promising treatment alternative is immunotherapy using monoclonal antibodies (MoAb) as targeting vehicles. Neuroblastoma is ideally suited for testing these options because: 1. neuroblastoma cells express with minimal heterogeneity and in high density the ganglioside GD2 which is absent from most normal tissues and does not modulate after antibody binding; 2. they lack decay accelerating factor and therefore cannot interfere with complement activation; 3. they are destroyed by natural killer cells, an effect that is enhanced by lymphokine activation, and by MoAb-armed granulocytes and lymphocytes; 4. they have a limited ability to repair radiation damage. Murine MoAb 3F8 (an IgG3) to the ganglioside GD2 has been selected because: 1. it activates human complement; 2. it promotes target-specific cell-dependent cytotoxicity with both lymphocytes and granulocytes; 3. it binds to neuroblastomas with high avidity and can deliver radioisotopes to the tumors *in vivo* with minimal uptake by the normal liver. Preliminary clinical studies have shown that IgG3 antibodies can be used safely in patients with tolerable side effects (pain, urticaria and hypertension) and major anti-tumor responses. 3F8 may be efficacious as an adjuvant in patients at the time of minimal disease. Radiolabelled 3F8 is useful in the localization of metastatic sites. It has superior sensitivity and selectivity compared to conventional imaging methods. In addition, improved delivery of radioisotopes followed by rescue with autologous marrow may permit targeted radiotherapy of refractory neuroblastoma. Mechanisms of tumor response in patients remain to be defined.

Introduction

Neuroblastoma (NB) is the most common extra-cranial solid tumor of childhood, accounting for 7–10% of pediatric malignancies and 15% of all cancer deaths in children (1). Despite advances in the therapy of this disease (myeloablative chemotherapy followed by autologous or allogeneic bone marrow rescue), the outlook for most children with NB remains grim. Of the 70% of patients who present with unresectable disease at diagnosis, over 50% will die within three years. The overall long term disease free survival for these children is less than 30% in most studies. These statistics illustrate the need for alternative forms of therapy in NB.

One promising possibility is targeted immunotherapy with neuroblastoma-specific monoclonal antibodies. Because of their selectivity for malignant cells, monoclonal antibodies offer potential anti-tumor effect with reduced systemic toxicity. To realize this potential, an antibody must show specificity for antigen(s) expressed on most, if not all of the malignant cells found in a patient (or tumor); and must be capable of significant *in vivo* anti-tumor effects, either by targeting existing immune effector mechanisms, or by delivering cytotoxic agents to the tumor nests both obvious and occult.

We have produced several murine monoclonal antibodies against human NB (2). 3F8, an IgG3, meets the expectations outlined above and has shown potential in the therapy of neuroblastoma. We have recently reported the results of clinical studies using 3F8 in the diagnosis and treatment of NB. We will summarize these, and some of the preclinical experimental data which underlies the design of our clinical trials.

Background

The target antigen for the antibody 3F8 is the glycolipid molecule GD2 (3), a disialo-ganglioside normally found in a restricted distribution on some neurons of the central nervous system, some peripheral nerves, cells of the adrenal medulla and some skin melanocytes. It is strongly expressed on many tumors of neural crest origin – e.g., neuroblastoma (2–4) malignant melanoma and CNS tumors – and on small cell lung carcinoma (5) and osteogenic sarcoma (6). GD2 serves a major role in the attachment of anchorage-dependent human melanoma and neuroblastoma cell lines to tissue-culture substrates (7), but is also expressed on melanoma and neuroblastoma lines that show little or no anchorage dependence (Cheung, unpublished data). Of interest for its potential role as a target of immunotherapy. GD2 is strongly expressed on 98–100 % of cells in virtually all cultured neuroblastic cell lines tested (2). In immuno-fluorescent staining of 31 cryopreserved neuroblastoma tumor samples in our labora-tory, 100 % of tumors stained strongly positive using 3F8. More than 95 % of histologi-cally identifiable tumor cells were stained in each biopsy specimen. In tumors where isolated foci of neuroblasts were scattered among other benign elements, the malignant cells stained clearly with 3F8.

The antigen density of GD2 on the surface of cultured NB cells was determined by radioimmunoassay using ^{125}I-labelled 3F8 antibody. Over 5×10^6 binding sites per cell was found by scatchard analysis, which agrees roughly with the figure of 1×10^7 mole-cules of GD2 per cell determined by Wu, et al., using biochemical analysis (8). The dissociation constant (Kd) for the binding of 3F8 to GD2 was between 1×10^{-9} and 1.7×10^{-8} M. (The latter figure probably representing nonspecific interactions among antibody molecules rather than antigen-antibody binding.) This dissociation constant is consistent with avid binding of 3F8 to its target antigen.

The monoclonal antibody 3F8 is of the murine IgG$_3$ subclass. This subclass, although relatively rare among antibodies produced by conventional hybridoma tech-niques, is gaining increasing attention due to its ability to mediate anti-tumor cytotoxi-city via both complement and cellular effector mechanisms (9, 10), (also see Boslett et al. in this book). We have investigated the ability of 3F8 to activate complement and mediate antibody-dependent cellular cytotoxicity (ADCC), and found it to be efficient in both respects.

Complement Cytotoxicity

Cultured human neuroblastoma cell lines were tested for sensitivity to complement-mediated lysis in the presence of 3F8 using a standard chromiumrelease assay (12). The source of complement was serum from normal volunteers or from various animal species. 3F8 was found to mediate efficient lysis of NB cells using human serum, as well as rabbit and guinea pig sera (although not using mouse serum). Human melanoma cell lines showed a variable pattern of sensitivity to complement lysis. This appears to be related to the presence or absence of the anti-complement protein DAF (decay accelerating factor) on the tumor cell membrane (11). Those melanoma cell lines which express DAF are relatively resistant to complement cytotoxicity even though they may bind the antibody well, and this resistance is abrogated by anti-DAF monoclonal antibody. None of the NB cell lines tested expressed DAF, and all were sensitive to complement. Under optimum conditions, 100 % of cultured NB cells were lysed by 3F8 plus human complement.

Cellular Cytotoxicity

Neuroblastoma cells almost entirely lack the major histocompatibility complex (MHC) surface antigen (13), and are not sensitive to lysis by classical cytotoxic T-cells (14). However, they are sensitive to lysis by natural killer (NK) cells, and to ADCC by peripheral blood lymphocytes (Figure 1). The concentration of 3F8 required to achieve optimal ADCC with peripheral blood lymphocytes varies between 0.4 µg/ml

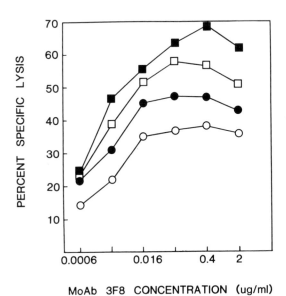

Figure 1. Dose dependence of ADCC mediated by PBMC. ADCC by PBMC from a normal volunteer donor, measured in a 4-hr chromium-release assay against the neuroblastoma cell line NMB7. Solid squares = E:T ratio of 100:1, open squares = 50:1, solid circles = 25:1, open circles = 12.5:1 (from: Cheung, N.-K.V., et al., ref 30).

and 2 μg/ml for the NB cell lines tested. Polymorphonuclear leukocytes (PMN) are also able to lyse NB targets in the presence of 3F8, although there is considerable variation in cytotoxicity between individuals (15).

Biodistribution *in vivo*

In order to test the ability of 3F8 to localize to neuroblastoma following intravenous injection into animals, we used human NB tumors growing subcutaneously in athymic nude mice. Such tumors grown in nude mice retain their characteristic histologic and biologic properties through multiple serial passages (16). We used murine tumors established from fresh patient samples or from human NB cell lines propagated *in vitro* for these experiments. Radiolabelled monoclonal antibody was prepared by a modification of the chloramine T method (17) using ^{131}I or ^{125}I, and had a specific activity of approximately 5 μCi/μg. Fifty μCi of I-131-3F8 was injected intravenously into nude mice bearing human NB xenografts. The animals were sacrificed on day 1, 2 or 4 following injection, and the radioactivity in the tumors and various organs and tissues measured by gamma counting. The tumor to non-tumor (T:NT) ratios of radioactivity varied from 27.6 (for blood) to 130.0 (muscle), (18). The blood-brain barrier efficiently excluded radioactive 3F8 from the central nervous system, with brain showing a

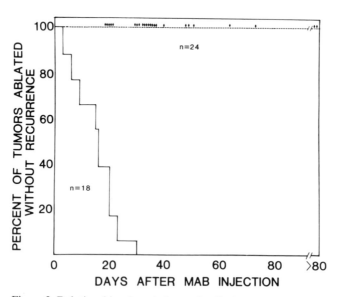

Figure 2. Relationship of remission and radiation dose delivered. Y-axis is the percent of tumors in remission. X-axis is the number of days after ^{131}I-3F8 injection. Eighteen tumor xenografts with radiation dose of <3900 rad recurred within 30 days of treatment; 24 tumors with radiation dose of >4200 rad had no detectable tumor recurrence. Each diamond represents each individual treated tumor at the time of necropsy or autopsy. MAB = monoclonal antibody 3F8 (from: Cheung, N.-K.V., et al., ref 17).

T:NT ratio of >400. Binding of radiolabelled monoclonal antibody to the tumors was between 8–50 % of injected dose per gram of tumor tissue (depending on tumor size) at 24 hours after injection.

When ^{131}I-labelled 3F8 (I-131-3F8) was injected into nude mice bearing human NB xenografts at doses from 125 µCi to 1 mCi, a clear anti-tumor effect was seen (17). Dosimetry calculations showed that when the injected dose of radioactive antibody reached 1.0 mCi/gram of tumor, the total dose of radiation delivered to the tumor exceeded 5000 rads. Of the animals receiving >4200 rads of calculated radiation dose to their tumors, 100 % had complete ablation of their xenografts without recurrence after 30–80 days. In those animals receiving less than 4200 rads, 100 % of tumors had recurred by 30 days (Figure 2).

Clinical Trials

Bone marrow purging. On the basis of the above *in vitro* and *in vivo* experiments, we have begun several phase I clinical trials using 3F8 (or 3G6, a murine monoclonal of the IgM class, also directed against GD2 and able to mediate efficient complement cytotoxicity *in vitro*). We have shown that immunofluorescent staining using mono-clonal antibodies against neuroblastoma can sensitively detect small numbers of tumor cells (1/10,000 normal cells) artificially seeded in normal bone marrow (19). We have also shown that complement lysis using human serum and the 3G6 monoclonal anti-body is able to effect a >99.9 % reduction in NB cells seeded in normal bone marrow, while allowing better than 95 % recovery of bone marrow nucleated cells (12). Bone marrow cells thus treated show normal hematopoietic colony growth in soft agar, suggesting that the stem cells are not damaged by monoclonal antibody. On the basis of these experiments, we have carried out a pilot study of *in vitro* purging of bone marrow prior to cryopreservation for use in autologous bone marrow transplantation.

Of the three patients treated in our pilot study to assess toxicity (20), all three successfully engrafted. Times required to reach an absolute neutrophil count of >500/mm^2 were 23, 45, and 86 days. This is longer than is seen with most autologous transplant regimens, but comparable to other patients treated with the high-dose thiotepa regimen used in this study. No overt toxicity was attributable to the mono-clonal antibody purging. Two of the three patients underwent a second transplant with purged autologous marrow. Both required injection of their unpurged back-up marrow because of poor marrow engraftment. Both were subsequently treated with intravenous 3F8 for *in vivo* purging but no further chemotherapy and both patients have long progression free survivals (16 months, 16 + months).

Imaging with radiolabelled antibody. The staging of neuroblastoma, and detection of occult metastases, is important for the proper management of this disease. On the basis of preclinical studies showing good localization of ^{131}I-labelled 3F8 in nude mice with human NB xenografts, we are using radiolabelled 3F8 for diagnostic imaging in patients with metastatic disease.

We have reported our initial experience with six NB patients (21), each of whom received 3–5 mCi of [131]I-3F8 (specific activity 5 µCi/µg). Localization of radiolabelled antibody was demonstrated as focal uptake of isotope by gamma scintigraphy. Many of these areas of focal uptake correlated with known areas of disease as demonstrated by conventional studies, but there were sites detectable with antibody that were previously not suspected to have disease (Figure 2). In our cumulative experience to date with >50 patients, [131]I-3F8 scans have successfully detected 100 % of active neuro-blastoma lesions demonstrable by any combination of CT scan, bone scan, MRI or MIBG scan, while adding other focal lesions whose existence was unsuspected by other techniques. (Many of these lesions have on follow-up become evident clinically or by conventional techniques.) A comparative study between 3F8 and MIBG in 21 patients with neuroblastoma has recently been reported (22) (Figure 3). In patients with limited extent of disease, agreement between the two imaging techniques was generally found. In patients with widely metastatic disease bone scan detected about 40 %, while MIBG traced two thirds of all abnormal areas (bones plus soft tissues) indicated by 3F8.

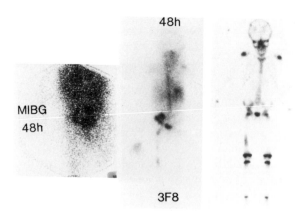

Figure 3. Comparison of ^{131}I-MIBG, [131]I-3F8, and bone scans in a patient with metastatic neuro-blastoma. MIBG (metaiodobenzylguanidine) is selectively taken up by neuroectodermal tumors including neuroblastoma. Both ^{131}I scans were done 48 hours after intravenous injection. A right pelvic mass, as well as metastatic disease in the vertebral column, right femur and left shoulder were evident on the 3F8 scan. Although the right pelvic mass was also seen on MIBG scan and suggested by bone scan, the other sites of disease were less obvious.

Dosimetry calculations were performed based on planar scintigraphic scans. In patients whose tumors were removed at surgery within 5 days of antibody injection, the calculated retained dose of radioactivity correlated closely with the actual measured dose. Estimates of the total radiation dose delivered per mCi of injected iodine were made, based on surgical specimens and gamma camera images. Tumor tissue was estimated to receive 36.6 rads/mCi of injected dose; blood received 3.4–5.2 rads/mCi; other tissues received between 0.6–3.3 rads/mCi. On the basis of these studies it was concluded that a dose of 100 mCi of I-131-3F8 could provide significant and potentially therapeutic doses of radiation to tumors, but with potentially toxic irradiation of blood (and hence bone marrow). This dose of radioactive 3F8 was selected for use in further therapeutic trials on the basis of these considerations.

Therapy with radiolabelled 3F8. Three patients with disseminated NB were treated in a pilot study using ^{131}I-labelled 3F8 (23). All three had advanced, progressive disease involving bone and bone marrow; two had bulky disease in the chest or abdomen. Each received a single injection of 100 mCi ^{131}I-3F8. All three patients showed measurable response of the tumors in the bone marrow following a single dose of therapy, and all reported subjective improvement (sense of well-being and diminution of bone pain). Acute toxicity related to the antibody infusion was minimal, in contrast to unlabelled antibody (see below), but delayed pancytopenia was marked. None of the patients required hospitalization for complications of low counts, but all required transfusion support. Since extensive bone marrow involvement was present in all patients, it is possible that some of the observed pancytopenia was a result of "by-stander" irradiation received by normal marrow elements. Whether patients with less marrow disease will experience less bone marrow toxicity remains to be seen.

Myelosuppression constitutes the dose-limiting toxicity for this form of therapy, and 100 mCi/dose appears close to this limit. However, the calculated radiation dose delivered to the tumor (approximately 3600 rads for a 100 mCi injection of ^{131}I-3F8) is close to the ablative dose seen in animal studies (4200 rads) (17). For these reasons we are pursuing means of reducing bone marrow toxicity so as in order to permit escalation of the radioactivity dose. Preliminary results in the nude-mouse xenograft model suggest that the injection of a second antibody, directed against 3F8 itself, increases the clearance of unbound radioactive antibody from the blood, and thus potentially increases the tumor to non-tumor ratio of radioactivity (24). Alternatively, the use of purged autologous bone marrow rescue or colony-stimulating factors to hasten marrow recovery following therapy may be of benefit.

Phase I trials with unlabelled antibody. We have treated 17 patients (eight with NB and nine with malignant melanoma) using 3F8 antibody (not conjugated to ^{131}I) in a phase I clinical trial (25). All patients had progressive disease and most had failed prior intensive chemotherapy and radiation therapy. After enrollment but prior to treatment, each patient's tumor was studied *in vitro* by immunofluorescent staining, and/or *in vivo* by ^{131}I-3F8 imaging, for the presence of the target antigen GD2. All 17 patients showed binding of 3F8 antibody to the tumor by one or both methods. In the NB patients, 7/8 patients had tumor specimens available for immunostaining, and all were strongly positive (3 to 4 + on a scale of 0–4, 100 % of cells positive). Of the six NB patients who underwent radioimaging all were positive. The melanoma specimens showed greater heterogeneity in immunostaining (2 to 4 +, 10–100 % positive), and 3/8 patients had radiologically demonstrable disease which failed to image with ^{131}I-3F8.

The study design was that of a phase I dose-escalation trial. Two patients received 5 mg/m^2 of 3F8, five received 20 mg/m^2, four received 50 mg/m^2, and six received 100 mg/m^2. The antibody was given as a continuous infusion at 1–10 mg/hr over 8 hrs per day for 2 to 4 days. Measured peak serum concentration of 3F8 varied linearly with the dose of 3F8 infused, and reached a maximum of 22.4 ± 7.6 µg/ml in the patients receiving 100 mg/m^2 of antibody.

The principal toxicities related to antibody therapy were pain, hypertension and urticaria. Severe pain requiring narcotic analgesics developed in all patients during the infusion of 3F8. This pain typically involved the abdomen, lower back and extremities. It usually started within the first hour of antibody infusion, and resolved after the infusion ended. Since 3F8 is known to bind to histologic sections of peripheral nerve pain fibers (26), we presume that this is the mechanism of the pain experienced by our patients. Patients who have received radiolabelled 3F8 have not had pain, and radio-labelled 3F8 has been shown not to activate complement or mediate ADCC (unpublished data). It is thus not unreasonable to conclude that pain is due to stimulation of pain fibers mediated by the biologic activity of the intact 3F8 molecule, rather than by binding of antibody *per se*.

Besides the acute toxicities, some delayed side effects may be attributable to 3F8. Some patients have had mild diffuse arthralgias for 1–2 months after treatment. Two patients described mild decreases in sensitivity to heat and cold for a month after therapy. No significant neurologic deficits have been detectable following 3F8 treatment in patients followed for as long as 2½ years.

Other acute toxicities observed were urticaria, which responded well to diphenhydramine in most cases, and hypertension. Hypertension has limited further dose escalation, with 6/6 patients experiencing a >40% elevation in diastolic blood pressure at the dose of 100 mg/m^2. In most patients hypertension resolved promptly at the end of the infusion, although two children with NB required oral antihypertensive medication for several weeks. We also observed a 6–28% decrease in complement activity (CH_{50}, C_3, C_4) without clinical sequelae.

Inflammation around cutaneous lesions were observed in 2 patients after 3F8 treatment. Inflammation was followed by tumor regression in one of these patients. Tumor necrosis was noted after 3F8 treatment in biopsies of the bone marrow as well as cutaneous metastatic tumor. One patient with neuroblastoma had cutaneous tumor biopsy done before 3F8 therapy and it showed no significant cellular infiltrate. After 3F8, diffuse infiltration by lymphocytes, monocytes, and mast cells were seen. Three melanoma patients showed similar increases in tumor infiltration by lymphocytes, monocytes, and mast cells after 3F8 treatment. There was deposition of complement C3, C5, and C9 in these post therapy tumors. Most of the patients have decreases (average of 25%) in their serum complement levels, independent of the dose of 3F8. These preliminary results suggest that complement activation and infiltration of tumors by effector cells may be related to the necrosis noted in histological analyses, and to the clinical inflammation and regression of tumors that were observed.

Significant antitumor effects were seen in 4/17 patients. Two patients with NB had complete responses of bone and bone-marrow disease lasting 28 and 64 weeks, respectively. Two patients with malignant melanoma had partial responses (resolution of visceral adenopathy and resolution of liver disease) lasting 22 and 56+ weeks respectively. Two patients showed mixed responses. Since the completion of the phase I trial we have continued to see a similar response rate of approximately 30% (complete responders plus partial responders) in our on-going phase II study.

Future directions. The ideal time for immunotherapy is during a period when disease is minimal (preferably microscopic) and the immune system is competent. Children who have malignancies, and those who have received extensive chemotherapy, often have depressed natural killer cell function and other measures of cellular immunity. With the availability of recombinant biological response modifiers such as interleukin-2 and other cytokines, it is reasonable to ask whether these factors are able to stimulate the effector cells to obtain maximum advantage of monoclonal antibody.

We and others have shown (27, 29) that interleukin-2 is able to augment ADCC against neuroblastoma and malignant melanoma *in vitro* using monoclonal antibodies against GD2 and GD3 (Figure 4). The effector cells for interleukin-2 activated ADCC are peripheral blood lymphocytes which bear the CD-16 (Leu11) antigen. It has also been demonstrated that granulocyte-macrophage stimulating factor (GMCSF) is able to augment ADCC by polymorphonuclear leukocytes against human leukemia cells (29). We have shown that GMCSF also augments granulocyte ADCC against neuroblastoma using 3F8 (15). These two factors, and others which may have an ability to boost the effector cell response to monoclonal antibody *in vivo*, may have a place in future clinical trials for combination immunotherapy.

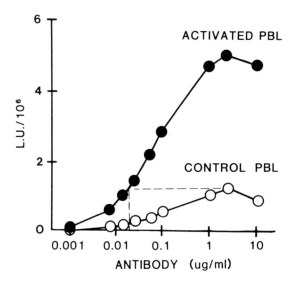

Figure 4. Enhancement of peripheral blood lymphocyte ADCC by interleukin-2. PBMC from normal volunteer donors were used either immediately or after incubation for 2 days with 6 μ/ml of interleukin-2. ADCC at various concentrations of 3F8 was determined as in Figure 1. Cytotoxicity is expressed in lytic units (50 % lysis of 10^4 target cells) per 10^6 effective cells. The dashed line shows the antibody concentration at which interleukin-2 activated cells mediate ADCC comparable to fresh PBL at 2 μg/ml of 3F8 (from: Munn, D. and Cheung, N.-K.V., ref 28).

References

1. Kushner, B. H., N.-K.V. Cheung. Treatment of neuroblastoma. In: DeVita, V.T., Hellman, S., Rosenberg, S. A., eds. Cancer Updates, Vol 2., Philadelphia, Lippincott, 1988.
2. Cheung, N.-K.V., U. M. Saarinen, J. E. Neely, B. Landmeier, D. Donovan, P. F. Coccia. Monoclonal antibody to a glycolipid antigen on human neuroblastoma cells. Cancer Res. 45, 2642, 1985.
3. Saito, M., R. K. Yu, N.-K.V. Cheung. Ganglioside GD2 specificity of monoclonal antibodies to human neuroblastoma cell. Biochem. Biophys. Res. Comm. 127, 1, 1985.
4. Shultz, G., D. A. Cheresh, N. M. Varki, A. Yu, L. K. Staffileno, R. A. Reisfeld. Detection of ganglioside GD2 in tumor tissues and sera of neuroblastoma patients. Cancer Res. 44, 5914, 1984.
5. Cheresh, D. A., J. Rosenberg, K. Mujoo, L. Hirschowitz, R. A. Reisfeld. Biosynthesis and expression of the disialoganglioside GD2, a relevant target antigen in small cell lung carcinoma for monoclonal antibody-mediated cytolysis. Cancer Res. 46, 5112, 1986.
6. Heiner, J. P., F. Miradli, S. Kahick, J. Makley, W. H. Smith-Mensah, N.-K.V. Cheung. Localization of GD2-specific monoclonal antibody 3F8 in human osteosarcoma. Cancer Res. 47, 5377, 1987.
7. Cheresh, D. A., M. D. Pierschbacher, M. A. Herzig, K. Mujoo. Disialogangliosides GD2 and GD3 are involved in the attachment of human melanoma and neuroblastoma cells to extracellular matrix proteins. J. Cell Biol. 102, 688, 1986.
8. Wu, Z. L., E. Schwartz, R. Seeger, S. Ladisch. Expression of GD2 ganglioside by untreated primary human neuroblastomas. Cancer Res. 46, 440, 1986.
9. Kawashima, I., N. Tada, S. Ikegami, S. Nakamara, R. Ueda, T. Tai. Mouse monoclonal antibodies detecting disialogangliosides on mouse and human T lymphomas. Int. J. Cancer 41, 267, 1988.
10. Anasetti, C., P. J. Martin, Y. Morishita, C. C. Badger, I. D. Bernstein, J. A. Hansen. Human large granular lymphocytes express high affinity receptors for murine monoclonal antibodies of the IgG3 subclass. J. Immunol. 138, 2979, 1987.
11. Cheung, N.-K.V., E. I. Walter, W. H. Smith-Mensah, W. S. Ratnoff, M. L. Tykocinski, M. E. Medof. Decay-accelerating factor protects human tumor cells from complement-mediated cytotoxicity *in vitro*. J. Clin. Invest. 81, 1122, 1988.
12. Saarinen, U. M., P. F. Coccia, S. L. Gerson, R. Pelley, N.-K.V. Cheung. Eradication of neuroblastoma cells *in vitro* by monoclonal antibody and complement: method for purging autologous bone marrow. Cancer Res. 45, 5969, 1985.
13. Lampson, L. A., C. A. Fisher, J. P. Whelan. Striking paucity of HLA-A, B, C, and B2-microglobulin on human neuroblastoma cell lines. J. Immunol. 130, 2471, 1983.
14. Main, E. K., L. A. Lampson, M. K. Hart, J. Kornbluth, D. B. Wilson. Human neuroblastoma cell lines are susceptible to lysis by natural killer cells but not by cytotoxic T lymphocytes. J. Immunol. 135, 242, 1985.
15. Kushner, B. H., N.-K.V. Cheung. GM-CSF enhances granulocyte mediated monoclonal antibody-dependent cellular cytotoxicity against human neuroblastoma and melanoma *in vitro*. Proc. AACR 29, 1470, 1988.
16. Neely, J. E., E.T. Ballard, A. L. Britt, et al. Characteristics of 85 pediatric tumors heterotransplanted into nude mice. Exp. Cell Biol. 51, 217, 1983.
17. Cheung, N.-K.V., B. Landmeier, J. Neely, et al. Complete tumor ablation with Iodine 131-radiolabelled diasialoganglioside GD2-specific monoclonal antibody against human neuroblastoma xenografted in nude mice. J. Natl. Cancer Inst. 77, 739, 1986.

18. Cheung, N.-K.V., J. Neely, B. Landmeier, D. Nelson, F. Miraldi. Targeting of ganglioside GD2 monoclonal antibody to neuroblastoma. J. Nucl. Med. 28, 1577, 1987.

19. Cheung, N.-K.V., D.D. Van Hoff, S.E. Strandjord, P.F. Coccia. Detection of neuro-blastoma cells in bone marrow using GD2 specific monoclonal antibodies. J. Clin. Oncol. 4, 363, 1986.

20. Stein, J., S. Strandjord, U.M. Saarinen, et. al. In vitro treatment of autologous bone marrow from neuroblastoma patients with anti-GD2 monoclonal antibody and comple-ment: a pilot study. In: Advances in neuroblastoma Research 2, Evans A.-E., et al. (Ed), Alan R. Liss, Inc., New York, p. 233, 1988.

21. Miraldi, F.D., A.D. Nelson, C. Kraly, et al. Diagnostic imaging of human neuroblastoma with radiolabelled antibody. Radiology 161, 413, 1986.

22. Yeh, S., B.H. Kushner, M. Sullivan, N.-K.V. Cheung. Radioimaging of human neuro-blastoma: a comparison between ^{131}I-3F8 and ^{131}I-MIBG. J. Nucl. Med. 29, 846, 1986.

23. Cheung, N.-K.V., F.D. Miraldi. Iodine 131 labelled GD2 monoclonal antibody in the dia-gnosis and therapy of human neuroblastoma. In: Advances in neuroblastoma Research 2, Evans A.E., et al. (Ed), Alan R. Liss, Inc., New York, p. 595, 1988.

24. Cheung, N.-K.V., D.H. Munn, B.H. Kushner, N. Usmani, S.D. Yeh. Targeted radio-therapy and immunotherapy of human neuroblastoma with GD2 specific monoclonal anti-bodies. In: In vivo diagnosis and therapy of human tumor with monoclonal antibodies. Eckelman, W.C., et al. (Ed), Pergammon Press, London, in press, 1988.

25. Cheung, N.-K.V., H. Lazarus, F.D. Miraldi, et al. Ganglioside GD2 specific monoclonal antibody 3F8: a phase I study in patients with neuroblastoma and malignant melanoma. J. Clin. Oncl. 5, 1430, 1987.

26. Cordon-Cardo, C., N.J. Anderson, A.N. Houghton, N.-K.V. Cheung. Distribution of GD2 ganglioside in the human nervous system detected by mouse monoclonal antibody 3F8, submitted 1988.

27. Honsik, C.J., G. Jung, R.A. Reisfeld. Lymphokine activated killer cells targeted by monoclonal antibodies to the disialogangliosides GD2 and GD3 specifically lyse human tumor cells of neuroectodermal origin. Pool. Natl. Acad. Sci. 83, 7893, 1986.

28. Munn, D.H., N.-K.V. Cheung. Interleukin-2 enhancement of monoclonal antibody-mediated cellular cytotoxicity against human melanoma. Ca. Res. 47, 6600, 1987.

29. Fabian, I., G.D. Baldwin, D.W. Golde. Biosynthetic granulocyte-macrophage colon-stimu-lating factor enchances neutrophil cytotoxicity toward human leukemia cells. Leukemia 1, 613, 1987.

30. Cheung, N.-K.V., M.E. Medof, D.H. Munn. Immunotherapy with GD2 specific mono-clonal antibodies. In: Advances in neuroblastoma Research 2. Evans, A.E., et al. (Ed), Alan R. Liss, Inc., New York, p. 619, 1988.

27. GM3 Lactone as an Immunogen Associated with Melanoma: Effect of Immunization with GM3 Lactone on Melanoma Growth *in vivo*

T. Dohi, G. A. Nores, H. Oguchi, H. Inufusa, and S. Hakomori

Introduction

A specific organization of GM3 at the melanoma cell surface creates an unique antigenicity recognized by MoAbs* established after immunization with B16 melanoma cells in syngeneic C57/BL6 mice. Murine MoAb M2590, established by Taniguchi and Wakabayashi (1), has the ability to recognize GM3 ganglioside (2) having higher density than 5–10 mole % at the liposome surface, or on plastic surfaces (3). The antibody may also recognize a specific high density of GM3 at the surface of melanoma cells, as well as other types of cells. Since the majority of mouse, human, and hamster melanomas have been characterized by high GM3 densities, the antibody showed preferential reactivity with melanoma over other cell types (3). Subsequently, the antibody was found to have much higher affinity with GM3 lactone (KD 0.3–0,5 μg/ml) than with GM3 (KD 7–18 μg/ml). It was suspected, therefore, that the real melanoma-associated immunogen was GM3 lactone, or GM3 having lactone-like conformation. A series of experiments was directed toward: i) detection of GM3 lactone in melanoma cells; ii) comparison of immunogenicity of GM3 vs. GM3 lactone in mice; iii) effect of immunization with GM3 lactone vs. GM3 on melanoma growth *in vivo*. The results clearly indicate that: a) GM3 lactone showed much higher immunogenicity than GM3 in BALB/c and C57/BL6 mice; b) extensive immunization with GM3 lactone in C57/BL6 mice resulted in greatly enhanced tumor-promoting effect; c) in contrast, weak immunization with GM3 lactone resulted in clear reduction of melanoma deposits in lung.

Chemical Detection of GM3 Lactone in B16 Melanoma

TLC of the total lipid fraction extracted from B16 melanoma cells followed by immunostaining with MoAb M2590 showed a clear and intense band corresponding to GM3 lactone. The bands were multiple above the position of GM3, one of the major bands corresponding to GM3 lactone as described by Yu et al. (4). Alkaline treatment of the sample, e.g., exposure of TLC to ammonia vapor, abolished the reactivity of the lactone bands with M2590. The quantity of the lactones in B16 melanoma lipid extract was too small to be detectable by chemical reaction if starting from chemically manageable amounts of B16 cells (e.g., 50–100 mg cellular protein sample per extraction, followed by TLC analysis of lipids derived therefrom). Although the probable presence of lactones in ganglioside fractions has been repeatedly described (5, 6), it was difficult to assess their natural occurrence since lactones can be readily formed from native gangliosides at slightly acidic pH during preparation of cell culture,

---

Abbreviations: EDTA, ethylenediaminetetraacetic acid; MoAb, monoclonal antibody; PBS, phosphate-buffered saline (140 mM NaCl, 15 mM phosphate buffer, pH 7.0); TLC, thin-layer chromatography.

extraction followed by chromatography, and other isolation procedures. In order to avoid such possible artifacts, reductive cleavage of lactones was performed directly on the cell pellet. Aliquots of 0.2 ml of packed cells were suspended in 0.2 ml of PBS supplemented by 50 μl of KB[^{3}H]$_4$ (1 mCi activity) dissolved in 0.01 N NaOH and allowed to stand for 2 hrs at 4°C, followed by addition of another 50 μl of KB[^{3}H]$_4$. After 1 h at 4°C, the cell suspension was supplemented with 50 μl of cold 1% NaBH$_4$ in 0.01 N NaOH. After 1 h at 4°C, pellets were washed in PBS, extracted with chloroform-methanol 2:1, and the glycolipid fraction was prepared. The fraction contained significant [^{3}H]-labelled gangliosidol which showed TLC behavior identical to that of standard gangliosidol preparation from reductive cleavage of GM3 lactone as previously described (5, 7) (see Figure 1).

R   F

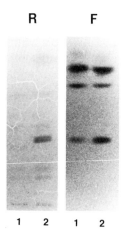

1   2   1   2

Figure 1. [^{3}H]-labelled GM3 gangliosidol detected in B16 melanoma cells treated with KB[^{3}H]$_4$.
B16 melanoma cells were treated with KB[^{3}H]$_4$, and the lipids were extracted and purified as described. Lane 1, neutral glycolipid fraction of the labelled B16 melanoma cells; lane 2, GM3 gangliosidol, prepared from lactones of GM3 of B16 melanoma cells added to the neutral glycolipid fraction of B16 melanoma cells. Panel R is the chromatogram reacted with resorcinol reagent. Gangliosidol added to lane 2 appeared as an orange spot. Panel F is fluorography of the same chromatogram as shown in panel R.

Immunogenicity of GM3 and GM3 Lactone to BALB/c Mice

Immunization of mice with GM3 lactone coated on *Salmonella minnesotae* was compared to that with lactone-free GM3. Repeated immunization was followed by fusion of spleen cells with mouse myeloma NS/1, counting of antibody-producing hybridoma wells, and determination of antibody activity. As shown in Table 1, immunogenicity of GM3 was essentially negative in contrast to that of GM3 lactone, which produced a significant number of wells showing weak or strong reactivity with GM3 or GM3 lactone. The antibody produced after immunization with GM3 lactone showed reactivity to both GM3 lactones and GM3. Some hybridomas (e.g., DH2) established after immunization with GM3 lactone showed, however, a preferential reactivity to GM3 lactone (8).

Table 1. Immunogenicity of GM3 and GM3 lactone to BALB/c mice as expressed by the number of positive hybridomas resulting from one fusion distributed over two 96-well plates by limited dilution[a].

| | Immunization with: | | | |
| | GM3 lactone | | GM3 | |
Reactivity with:	Strong positive (2000 cpm)	Weak positive (800–1500 cpm)	Strong positive (>2000 cpm)	Weak positive (800–1500 cpm)
GM3 lactone	1/192 5/288[b] 2/288[b]	23/192	0/192	5/192
GM3	0/192	9/192	0/192	0/192

[a] Forty μg of GM3 or GM3 lactone dissolved in water were incubated with a 1 mg suspension of S. minnesotae in water and lyophilized. The residue was suspended in 4 ml of PBS. Aliquots of 200 μl were injected i.v. every week and repeated 8 times. Spleen cells (10^8) were fused with 5×10^7 SP/2 myeloma cells, and hybridomas were grown in 96-well polyvinyl plastic plates (Costar Laboratories, Cambridge, MA). The supernatants on the 7th day after fusion were assayed on flexible 96-well plates coated with 0.1% gelatin and 0.2 μmol/ml glycolipid solution. The antibody bound was determined by second antibody (anti-mouse IgM + IgG) and ^{125}I-protein A. Each well excised was counted in a gamma counter. Only strongly active wells (>2000 cpm) were regarded as positive.
[b] Separate experiments based on three 96-well plates. Antibodies from these hybridomas react with both GM3 and GM3 lactone after their establishment (Dohi T, Nores GA, Hakomori S, unpublished data).

Effect of Intensive Immunization with GM3 Lactone on B16 Melanoma Growth in C57/BL6 Mice

Under the same conditions as described in Table 1 for immunization of BALB/c mice, C57/BL6 mice were immunized with GM3 lactone coated on S. minnesotae by intravenous injection, once a week and repeated eight times during eight weeks. GM3 lactone preparation from chloroform-methanol-12 N HCl (60:30:4.5 v/v/v) was dissolved in water, thoroughly mixed with acid-treated S. minnesotae, incubated for 1 h with occasional agitation, lyophilized, and suspended in PBS. 2 μg of GM3 lactone coated on 50 μg of S. minnesotae was injected (8x) in female C57/BL6 mice via tail vein. The control group was treated in the same way with the same amount of GM3-coated S. minnesotae or S. minnesotae alone in PBS. Three days after the last injection, 1×10^7 B16 melanoma cells in 200 μl PBS were inoculated subcutaneously (day 0). On days 8, 10, 13, and 15, the three diameters of tumors were measured and tumor volume was calculated as $\pi(D_1 D_2 D_3)/2$. Tumor growth was significantly enhanced in the animals intensively immunized with GM3 lactone. In order to observe the effect of such immunization on lung metastatic deposits of B16 melanoma cells, 10 female C57/BL6 mice were immunized with 2 μg GM3 lactone and 50 μg *S. minnesotae* 8x weekly as described above. Three days after the last injection, 5 x 10⁴ B16/BL6 cells were detached from cultures with EDTA, washed with PBS, suspended in 200 μl PBS, and injected intravenously. The animals were killed after 17 days by cervical dislocation, lungs were removed and fixed with 10 % formaldehyde in PBS, and number of tumor colonies in lung was determined by counting under a dissecting microscope. The number of lung colonies was unchanged or slightly higher in the group intensively immunized with GM3 lactone compared with the control group (Figure 2).

FIGURE 2. Effect of active
immunization with GM3 lactone.

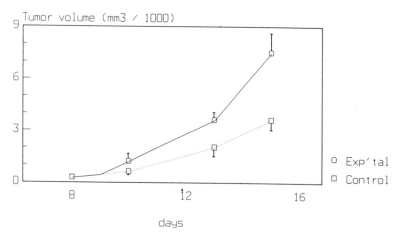

Figure 2. Effect of active immunization with GM3 lactone on B16 melanoma growth in C57/BL6 mice. GM3 lactone was prepared when GM3 solution in chloroform:methanol: 12 N HCl 60:30:4.5 was allowed to stand for 18 hrs at room temperature. GM3 lactone solution was mixed with acid-treated *S. minnesotae,* incubated, lyophilized and suspended in PBS as decribed previously. Two μg of GM3 lactone and 50 μg of *S. minnesotae* were injected into female C57/BL6 mice via tail vein once a week, and injection was repeated 6 times. For the control group, the same amount of *S. minnesotae* in PBS was injected. Each group contained 10 mice. Three days after the last injection, 1 x 10⁷ B16 melanoma cells in 200 μl of PBS were inoculated subcutaneously (day 0). On days 8, 10, 13, and 15, tumor volume was calculated as described in the text.

Effect of Weak Immunization with GM3 Lactone on B16 Melanoma Growth in C57/BL6 Mice

In another set of experiments, weak immunization with GM3 lactone was performed as described below and compared with not only GM3 but also several other GM3 species used as immunogens, i.e., lactones derived from NeuAcGM3 (GM3 containing *N*-acetylneuraminic acid), lactones derived from NeuGcGM3 (GM3 containing *N*-glycolylneuraminic acid), native NeuAcGM3 and NeuGcGM3, and 4-*O*-acetyl-NeuGcGM3 (9). An aqueous solution of each ganglioside was mixed with *S. minnesotae,* lyophilized, resuspended, and injected intravenously as described above. 2 µg of each ganglioside species coated on 50 µg *S. minnesotae* in 200 µl PBS was intravenously injected twice with a 10-day interval. Three days after the second injection, 5×10^4 B16/BL6 cells in 200 µl PBS were injected via the tail vein. 17 days after this tumor cell challenge, lungs were removed and fixed with 10 % formaldehyde in PBS, and number of tumor colonies in lung was determined by counting under a dissecting microscope. Results are shown in Table 2, section A. Clearly, the group injected with NeuAcGM3 lactone and 4-*O*-acetyl-NeuGcGM3 showed a significantly smaller number of lung colonies. These results were further confirmed by a third set of experiments carried out under the same conditions, in which a group of animals injected with NeuAcGM3 lactone showed a clearly reduced lung colony number. In separate experiments, immunization with subcutaneous injection of the same dosage of GM3 analogues together with *S. minnesotae* did not have any effect on tumor cell growth *in vivo* (data not shown).

Table 2. The effect of active immunization with GM3 and its derivatives on experimental lung metastasis of B16/BL6 melanoma in C57/BL6 mice.

A. Two µg of each ganglioside and 50 µg of *S. minnesotae* in 200 µl of PBS were injected intrave-nously *twice* with a 10-day interval. Three days after the second injection, 5×10^4 B16BL6 cells in 200 µl PBS were injected. 17 days after this tumor cell challenge, lungs were removed and numbers of tumor colonies were counted, after fixation in 10 % formaldehyde, under a dissecting microscope.

Immunogen	No of lung colonies/mouse (No. of colonies with diameter >1 mm)				
NeuAcGM3	30(13)	26(13)	12(6)	10(5)	9(5)
NeuAcGM3 lactone	8(6)	6(3)	6(3)	2(0)	0(0)
NeuGcGM3	16(8)	14(6)	10(7)	8(7)	2(2)
NeuGcGM3 lactone	20(11)	20(11)	16(11)	5(4)	0(0)
4-O-acetyl-NeuGcGM3	8(7)	6(2)	4(3)	1(1)	0(0)
control (*S. minnesotae* only)	17(4)	15(5)	10(3)	6(3)	2(0)

B. In a separate experiment, GM3 and GM3 lactone were injected 8 times. No significant difference in number of colonies was found between experimental and control groups.

C. Conditions for immunization were identical to those described in section A above.

Immunogen	No of lung colonies/mouse (No. of colonies with diameter >1 mm)				
NeuAcGM3	13(8)	20(11)	21(7)	22(7)	13(5)
NeuAcGM3 lactone	9(4)	4(3)	6(4)	8(4)	6(1)
control	19(10)	10(4)	16(8)	8(3)	7(4)

Discussion

Natural occurrence of GM3 lactone in B16 melanoma cells was detected by rapid processing extraction followed by TLC immunostaining with MoAb M2590, which has much higher affinity with GM3 lactone than with native GM3. The presence of multiple lactone bands indicated complexity of structure, albeit the major one could be the same as described by Yu et al. (4) (see Figure 3). The structure could have a large, stable hydrophobic domain providing better immunogenicity than native GM3. The presence of GM3 lactone was further confirmed by detection of [^{3}H]-labelled gangliosidol after reductive cleavage applied directly to native cells.

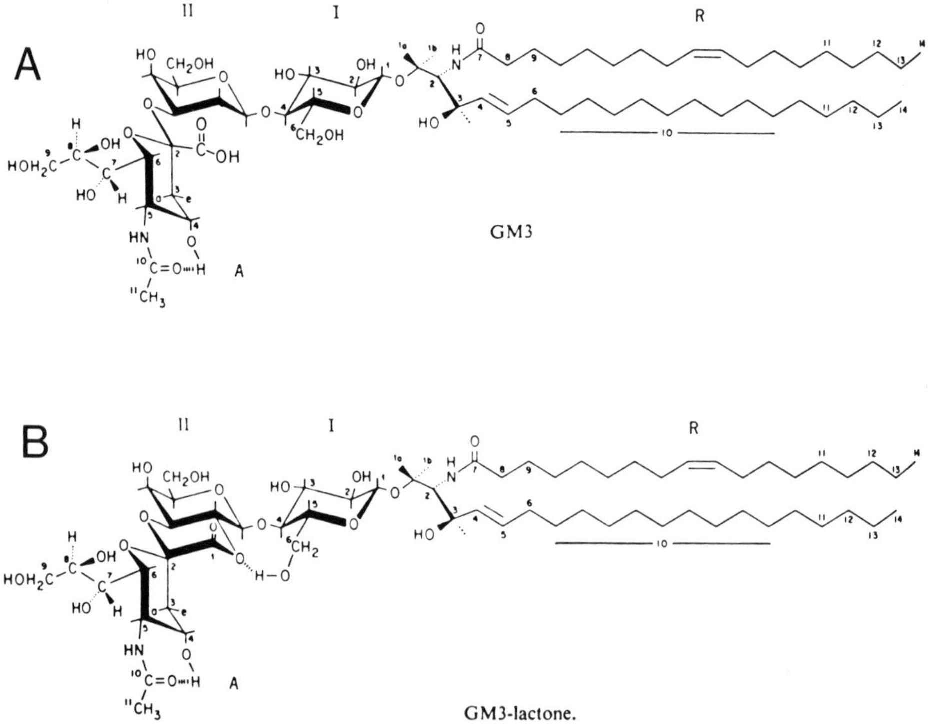

Figure 3. Structure of NeuAcGM3 (A) and its lactone (B), according to Yu et al. (4).

Data from a series of preliminary experiments as described above clearly indicate that GM3 lactone is strongly immunogenic in mice, producing enhanced B16 melanoma growth in intensively lactone-immunized mice (8x intravenous injection of 2 µg GM3 lactone with 50 µg *S. minnesotae*). In striking contrast, weaker immunization (i.e., 2x intravenous injection of the same dosage of NeuAcGM3 lactone, but not other types of GM3) results in clear reduction of metastatic B16 deposits to the lungs. This finding was confirmed by separate experiments by two independent investigators (Drs. T. Dohi and H. Inufusa). The immunological basis of such *in vivo* effect remains to be studied. It might be an antibody-dependent cytotoxic effect, complement-dependent effect, or induced cytotoxic killer T cell effect. Interestingly, stronger immunization with an extended period of time enhanced, rather than suppressed, tumor growth. This phenomenon may provide a clue for investigation of an important mechanism leading to suppression of tumor growth by lactones. A series of human tumor-associated ganglioside antigens in many common human cancers has been discovered, including fucoganglioside antigen ($III^3FucV^3FucVI^3NeuAcnLc_6$), which is highly expressed in lung, gastrointestinal and colonic adenocarcinoma (10, 11). This particular fucoganglioside can be readily converted to two types of lactone, although their structures have not been identified. Preliminary studies on such fucoganglioside lactones indicate that they have higher immunogenicity than native fucogangliosides. Thus, the approach involving immunization with ganglioside lactones could provide a useful, perhaps general, method to enhance the immunogenicity of tumor-assiciated lactones for preparation of tumor vaccines. However, it is important to note that immune responses in mice and humans are entirely different, and that the results of our studies with mice may not be directly adaptable to humans. Therefore, careful intensive study will be necessary before lactone preparations can be developed as effective vaccines against human cancers.

References

1. Taniguchi, M., Wakabayashi, S. Shared antigenic determinant expressed on various mammalian melanoma cells. Jap. J. Cancer Res. 75, 418–426, 1984.
2. Hirabayashi, Y., Hanaoka, A., Matsumoto, M., Matsubara, T., Tagawa, M., Wakabayashi, S., Taniguchi, M. Syngeneic monoclonal antibody against melanoma antigen with interspecies cross-reactivity recognizes GM3, a prominent ganglioside of B16 melanoma. J. Biol. Chem. 260, 13328–13333, 1985.
3. Nores, G. A., Dohi, T., Taniguchi, M., Hakomori, S. Density-dependent recognition of cell surface GM3 by a certain anti-melanoma antibody, and GM3 lactone as a possible immunogen: Requirements for tumor-associated antigen and immunogen. J. Immunol. 139, 3171–3176, 1987.
4. Yu, R. K., Koerner, T. A.W., Ando, S., Yohe, H. C., Prestegard, J. H. High-resolution proton NMR studies of gangliosides: III. Elucidation of the structure of ganglioside GM3 lactone. J. Biochem. (Tokyo) 98, 1367–1373, 1985.
5. Gross, S. K., Williams, M. A., McCluer, R. H. Alkali-labile, sodium borohydride-reducible ganglioside sialic acid residues in brain. J. Neurochem. 34, 1351–1361, 1980.
6. Riboni, L., Sonnino, S., Acquotti, D., Malesci, A., Ghidoni, R., Egge, H., Mingrino, S., Tettamanti, G. Natural occurrence of ganglioside lactones: Isolation and characterization of G_{Dib} inner ester from adult human brain. J. Biol. Chem. 261, 8514–8519, 1986.
7. MacDonald, D. L., Patt, L. M., Hakomori, S. Notes on improved procedures for the chemical modification and degradation of glycosphingolipids. J. Lipid Res. 21, 642–645, 1980.
8. Dohi, T., Nores, G. A., Hakomori, S. An IgG3 monoclonal antibody established after immunization with GM3 lactone: Immunochemical specificity and inhibition of melanoma cell growth in vitro and in vivo. Cancer Res. (in press).
9. Hakomori, S., Saito, T. Isolation and characterization of a glycosphingolipid having a new sialic acid. Biochemistry 8, 5082–5088, 1969.

10. Fukushi, Y., Nudelman, E., Levery, S. B., Rauvala, H., Hakomori, S. Novel fucolipids accumulating in human cancer: III. A hybridoma antibody (FH6) defining a human cancer-associated difucoganglioside (VI^{3}NeuAcV^{3}III^{3}Fuc$_2$nLc$_6$). J. Biol. Chem. 259, 10511–10517, 1984.
11. Fukushi, Y., Kannagi, R., Hakomori, S., Shepard, T., Kulander, B., Singer, J.W. Localization and distribution of difucoganglioside (VI^{3}NeuAcV^{3}III^{3}Fuc$_2$nLc$_6$) in normal and tumor tissues defined by its monoclonal antibody FH6. Cancer Res. 45, 3711–3717, 1985.

28. Role of Soluble GM3 Melanoma Antigen in Anti-tumor Immune Responses of Mice

Y. Harada, M. Sakatsume, and M. Taniguchi

Introduction

Recent accumulating evidence has indicated that gangliosides, glycosphingolipids with sialic acid, are secreted or shed into the local environment of cells as well as being present on the cell membrane and thus influencing the immune responses under certain conditions (1–13). In fact, their immunomodulatory effects, especially on cellular immune responses, have been demonstrated on two lines of evidence. First, several investigators have reported on antigen-nonspecific immunoregulatory effects of gangliosides, demonstrating that gangliosides at a relatively high concentration (more than 10 µg/ml) inhibit proliferative responses of T cells *in vitro* stimulated by mitogens, alloantigens or conventional protein antigens (4, 6–9). The suppression of T cell responses is not due to cell death, but to the inhibition of the influx of calcium into the T cells followed by stimulation by mitogen (10). It has also been demonstrated that gangliosides inhibit RNA synthesis as well as DNA synthesis (7). However, the precise inhibitory mechanisms still remain to be solved.

In addition to the above findings, antigen-specific T cell responses against gangliosides have also been reported (11–13). Bellamy et al. (11) have successfully established ganglioside-specific human T cell lines from cerebrospinal fluids of multiple sclerosis patients. The T cell lines have been shown to react with GM1, GD1a, GD1b or GQ1b gangliosides which are major components in human myelin and are believed to be potential candidates for the target antigen in multiple sclerosis. We have also demonstrated that cytotoxic T cells and suppressor T cells in antimelanoma immune responses in mice recognize GM3 gangliosides (12, 13). It is therefore, apparent that gangliosides possess the antigenicity to stimulate T cells and affect cellular immunity associated with certain disease status in an antigen specific as well as antigen nonspecific manner.

Recent developments in the monoclonal antibody technology have enabled us to characterize tumor antigens and various types of gangliosides as tumor associated antigens in many cases of tumors, such as cancers of pancreas, lung, stomach, colon, and melanomas and teratocarcinomas, etc. (reviewed in 14). In some cases, such as melanoma antigens, GM2 or GD2 gangliosides were demonstrated to have immunodominant epitopes for human immune systems, because the cell lines producing anti-GM2 or anti-GD2 monoclonal antibodies are successfully established by the Epstein-Barr virus transformation technique using peripheral lymphocytes of melanoma patients (15, 16).

Although gangliosides are ubiquitous in normal tissues and cells, they do work as antigens and are not tolerant in some disease status. Thus, the precise cellular and molecular mechanisms of immune responses to gangliosides are important in understanding the pathogenesis of diseases, including tumors.

In the present communication, we summarize our recent studies on specific immune responses against melanoma antigen composed of GM3 gangliosides as immunodominant epitopes in mice and propose a new concept of tumor antigens. We also discuss the biological role of GM3 gangliosides and anti-GM3 T cells in antimelanoma immune responses, especially in the escape mechanisms of melanoma cells from the immunological surveillance system.

Enhancement of Melanoma Growth in Mice

In our previous studies, we found that syngeneic cytotoxic T lymphocytes (CTL) raised in the *in vitro* primary culture system using B16 C57BL/6 mouse melanoma killed several human melanoma cell lines as well as mouse melanoma (17). This suggests that there exists cross-species melanoma antigen on the cell surface shared among at least mouse and human.

In order to analyze the cross-species melanoma antigen, we raised monoclonal anti-melanoma antibodies by fusion of P3U1 myeloma and C57BL/6 spleen cells hyper-immunized with syngeneic B16 melanoma cells. One of the anti-melanoma antibodies (M2590) was shown to have cross-species melanoma reactivity with mouse, human and hamster melanomas but did not react with various normal tissues (18). Thus, M2590 seems to recognize similar epitopes to those of anti-melanoma CTL.

Hirabayashi et al. have determined the primary structure of the cross-species epitope of melanoma antigen by methylation analysis, endoglycosidase treatment and fast atom bombardment spectrometry, and found it to be the GM3(NeuAc) ganglio-side (19). However, the GM3 with melanoma antigenicity does not have any particular structural difference in the primary sequence from normal ubiquitous GM3 ganglio-side. Even in a fatty acid composition of melanoma GM3, major ceramides consisted of C16:0, C22:0, C24:0, and C24:1, which are also most popular in normal GM3.

Further analysis at the cellular level has revealed that anti-melanoma CTL activity was blocked by the addition of M2590 anti-GM3 antibody in the effector phase of CTL

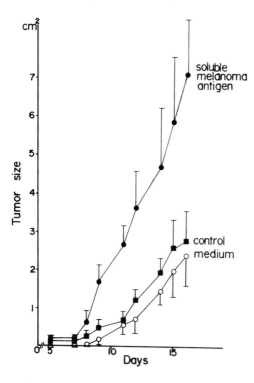

Figure 1. Enhancement of melanoma growth *in vivo* by injection of soluble melanoma antigen. C57BL/6 mice were intraperitoneally injected with soluble melanoma antigen (10^5 g supernate of B16 spent culture medium: amounts equivalent to 1.8 mg GM3/mouse) (●). As controls, fresh culture medium (○) and saline (■) were used. Simultaneously, mice were inoculated subcutaneously on the back with 10^6 B16 melanoma or EL-4 lymphoma cells. The size of tumor was measured at days indicated. The data were expressed as mean values of 10 experimental mice.

responses in a melanoma specific manner, indicating that the GM3 structure is indeed involved in the recognition and killing processes of anti-melanoma CTL (13).

The cross-species melanoma antigen detected by M2590 seemed to be shed or released from melanoma cells, because we detected the antigens reactive with M2590 as a soluble form in the culture supernatant of B16 melanoma cells ultracentrifuged at 10^5g. This soluble melanoma antigen was found to have the following decisive biological properties in anti-melanoma immune responses. First, the soluble antigen (equivalent to 0.03–0.1 µg GM3) effectively blocked anti-melanoma CTL activity in a melanoma specific manner in the effector phase of CTL responses. Second, the antigen selectively generated anti-melanoma suppressor T cells (Ts) that inhibited the generation of anti-melanoma CTL in the induction phase of CTL responses (Figure 1).

It is thus quite likely that the shedding molecule might modulate tumor formation *in vivo*, possibly by abrogating anti-melanoma CTL activity both in the induction and effector phases of CTL responses. To investigate *in vivo* effects of the soluble melanoma antigen, we injected it into mice simultaneously inoculated with 10^6 tumor cells on the back and measured the size of the tumor. In fact, three successive intraperitoneal injections of the soluble melanoma antigen (total amounts equivalent to 1.8 mg GM3/mouse) into tumor-bearing mice greatly enhanced melanoma growth but not EL-4 lymphoma growth (12). The results support our assumption that the soluble antigen selectively induces negative immune responses resulting in the enhancement of melanoma growth.

Similar findings have also been described by Ladisch et al. (5). They showed that intradermal injection of 1 pmol of purified gangliosides obtained from highly tumorigenic cells markedly increased tumorigenicity of potentially poorly tumorigenic cells *in vivo*. This might be due to a mechanism similar to the one previously described in our system.

Induction of Anti-melanoma Suppressor T Cells *in vitro*

In order to prove the above possibility that enhancement of melanoma growth by soluble tumor antigen is due to the induction of anti-melanoma Ts, we set up an *in vitro* culture system. C57BL/6 naive spleen cells were cultured with soluble antigen for several hours. The cells were then extensively washed and added to the anti-melanoma (B16) CTL induction system, in which C57BL/6 naive spleen cells were cultured with mitomycin-C treated syngeneic B16 melanoma cells for 4 days, and the cytotoxic activity was then assayed by the ^{51}Cr-release method.

Surprisingly, the cells incubated with the antigen for 12 h or 24 h almost completely suppressed the CTL responses to syngeneic melanoma cells. The suppression was specific for melanoma because the same cells did not inhibit anti-EL-4 lymphoma CTL or anti-allo CTL responses (12) (Figure 2).

Two types of T cells, CD4$^+$ and double negative I-J$^+$ T cells, are involved in this suppression. Treatment of anti-melanoma Ts either with anti-Thy 1, anti-CD4 or anti-

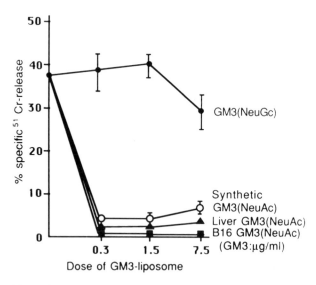

Figure 2. Induction of anti-melanoma Ts by GM3(NeuAc) but not by GM3(NeuGc) liposomes. Naive C57BL/6 spleen cells were cultured with various GM-liposomes (0.3 mg GM3/ml), such as GM3(NeuGc) (●), melanoma GM3(NeuAc) (■), normal GM3(NeuAc) (▲) and semi-synthetic GM3(NeuAc) (○), for 12 hr. They were then extensively washed and added to the *in vitro* primary anti-melanoma CTL induction system (suppressor/responder ratio of 1/4).

I-J but not anti-CD8 plus complement abrogated the Ts activity. When the cells treated with anti-CD4 and anti-I-J, either of which could not have any suppressor activity at all, were mixed two together, anti-melanoma Ts activity was, however, reconstituted (12). We have recently established several CD4[+] T cell clones with anti-melanoma Ts activity. When 1 x 10[4] cloned cells were added to the anti-melanoma CTL induction system at the beginning of the culture, anti-melanoma CTL responses were specifically diminished to the background level. On the other hand, no helper activity was observed for any numbers (10^2–10^5) of the cloned cells tested. These are, therefore, different from helper T cells (Th), despite their identical cell surface phenotypes to Th, and are one of the two types of T cells responsible for anti-melanoma suppression. It is necessary to establish I-J[+] double negative Thy-1[+] cell lines in order to understand cellular and molecular mechanisms of immune suppression against tumor-resistance.

Epitope for Anti-melanoma Ts

The epitope for anti-melanoma Ts was investigated. As GM3(NeuAc) ganglioside was found to be the immunogenic epitope for mouse syngeneic monoclonal antibody, such as M2590, thus to possess the melanoma antigenicity and to be detected in the soluble antigen, we assumed that the GM3 epitope might also have antigenicity for T cells. To test this possibility, anti-melanoma Ts was attempted to be induced by GM3 enriched fractions from the soluble melanoma antigen or by GM3 itself. Materials purified with an anti-GM3 column from soluble antigen, pronase treated soluble antigen and also GM3(NeuAc)-liposomes by itself successfully induced anti-melanoma Ts. On the other hand, GM3(NeuGc)-liposome did not induce any suppression of anti-melanoma Ts and also that induced by GM3(NeuAc)-liposome did not suppress anti-allo CTL or anti-EL-4 CTL responses (12). Thus, the described suppression were specific for melanoma. In addition, as phenotypes of anti-melanoma Ts induced by GM3(NeuAc)-liposome are the same as those induced by the soluble melanoma antigen, the epitope for melanoma Ts is GM3(NeuAc) and anti-melanoma Ts can distinguish two molecular species of GM3.

New Concept of Tumor Antigens

As previously described, at least the epitopes for anti-melanoma Ts and monoclonal anti-melanoma antibody (M2590) are demonstrated to be GM3(NeuAc), but their primary structure is the same as normal GM3. No structural difference has been detected at the level of the primary sequence. However, the reactivity of anti-melanoma antibody was selectively found on melanoma but not on normal cells with abundant GM3 expression, while the M2590 antibody did react with normal GM3 if it was bound on silica plate. The results suggest that the melanoma epitope is composed of the tertiary but not the primary structure.

In fact Nores et al. have found that M2590 antibody seems to recognize the density of GM3, because the antibody only reacts with high density (more than 8–12 mol %) but not with low density (less than 5 mol %) of GM3(NeuAc) (20). Similar phenomenon were also observed at the T cell level. Anti-melanoma Ts were only induced by GM3-liposome at a density of about 10–20 mol % whereas no Ts activity was obtained at a density of less than 10 mol %.

The above findings have raised a basic question on the concept of tumor antigen widely accepted at present which is believed and actually in some cases is found to have some structural differences on the primary sequence from normal components. It has also introduced a novel idea that the tertiary structure of gangliosides with normal primary sequence generates immunogenicity in some conditions. The mechanism that accounts for the generation of melanoma antigenicity of GM3 with normal primary sequence is still unclear. The experiments to solve this problem are now underway.

With respect to the structure of melanoma antigenic epitope related to GM3, Nores et al. (20) have demonstrated that the lactone form of GM3(GM3-lactone) was more immunogenic rather than GM3, and also that M2590 anti-melanoma GM3 antibody showed a high affinity (kd = 0.3 to 0.5 µg/ml) for GM3 lactone but a low affinity (kd = 6 to 15 µg/ml) for GM3. Therefore, the conformation of GM3 with melanoma antigenicity may have the tertiary structure similar to GM3 lactone; however, we do not know the detailed mechanisms of how the GM3 lactone-like conformation is generated by the high density of GM3.

Intriguing is the finding that anti-melanoma GM3 Ts repertoire seems to be very large in size and already exists in the naive or unprimed conditions, because only

12–24 h incubation of naive spleen cells with soluble melanoma antigen or GM3-lipo-some reproducibly induces anti-melanoma Ts, indicating that no clonal expansion of the functional repertoire is necessary in this Ts induction (12). This strongly suggests that the anti-GM3 Ts repertoire may be generated ontogenically during T cell develop-ment or by stimulation with GM3 on normal cells, possibly having a tertiary structure different from but cross-reactive with melanoma GM3.

It is thus quite likely that the anti-GM3 Ts play a role to maintain self(GM3) tolerance and melanoma GM3 secreted from melanoma cells stimulates this repertoire suppressing anti-self(GM3) and/or anti-melanoma CTL activity so that melanoma can escape from the immune system (Figure 3).

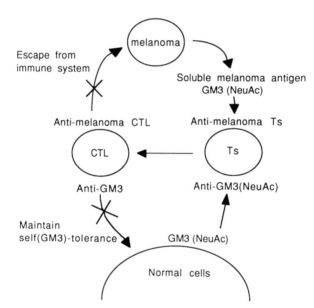

Figure 3. Role of anti-GM3 Ts in escape mechanisms of melanoma cells from immuno-logical surveillance.

Acknowledgement

This work was supported by Grants-in-Aid for Cancer Research and for Scientific Research on Priority Areas from the Ministry of Education, Science, and Culture, Japan, the Princess Takamatsu Cancer Foundation and the Uehara Memorial Founda-tion, Japan. We thank Ms. Chimi Saito for preparation of this manuscript.

References

1. Price, M. R., Baldwin, W.W. Shedding of tumor cell surface antigens. In: Dynamic Aspects of Cell Surface Organization, Ed.; Poste, G., Nicolson, G. Elsevier, Amsterdam 423–471, 1977.

2. Black, P. H. Shedding from the cell surface of normal and Cancer Cells. Adv. Cancer Res. 32, 75–199, 1980.

3. Kloppel, T. M., Keenan, T.W., Freeman, M. J., Morre, D. J. Glycolipid-bound sialic acid in serum: Increased levels in mice and humans bearing mammary carcinomas. Proc. Natl. Acad. Sci. USA 74, 3011–3013, 1977.

4. Ladisch, S., Gillard, B., Wong, C., Ulsh, L. Shedding and immunoregulatory activity of YAC-1 lymphoma cell gangliosides. Cancer Res. 43, 3808–3813, 1983.

5. Ladisch, S., Kitada, S., Hays, E. F. Gangliosides shed by tumor cells enhance tumor formation in mice. J. Clin. Invest. 79, 1879–1882, 1987.

6. Miller, H. C., Esselman, W. J. Modulation of the immune response by antigen-reactive lymphocytes after cultivation with gangliosides. J. Immunol. 115, 839–843, 1975.

7. Lengle, E. E., Krishnaraj, R., Kemp, R. G. Inhibition of the lectin-indued mitogenic response of thymocytes by glycolipids. Cancer Res. 39, 817–822, 1979.

8. Whisler, R. L., Yates, A. J. Regulation of lymphocyte responses by human gangliosides. J. Immunol. 125, 2106–2111, 1980.

9. Gonwa, T. A., Westrick, M. A., Macher, B. A. Inhibition of mitogen- and antigen-induced lymphocyte activation by human leukemia cell gangliosides. Cancer Res. 44, 3467–3470, 1984.

10. Krishnaraj, R., Lin, J., Kemp, R. Lectin- and ionophore-stimulated Ca^{2+} influx in murine lymphocytes: Inhibition by disialoganglioside. Cell Immunol. 78, 152–160, 1983.

11. Bellamy, A., Divison, A. N., Feldmann, M. Derivation of ganglioside-specific T cell lines of suppressor or helper phenotype from cerebrospinal fluid of multiple sclerosis patients. J. Neuroimmunol. 12, 107–120, 1986.

12. Takahashi, K., Ono, K., Hirabayashi, Y., Tanicuchi, M. Escape mechanisms of melanoma from immune system by soluble melanoma antigen. J. Immunol. 140, 3244–3248, 1988.

13. Ono, K., Hiraga, Y., Hirabayashi, Y., Taniguchi, M. Mouse melanoma antigen recognized by cytotoxic T lymphocytes with cross-species reactivity. Cancer Res. 48, 2730–2733, 1988.

14. Hakomori, S. Tumor-associated carbohydrate antigens. Ann. Rev. Immunol. 2, 103–126, 1984.

15. Irie, R. F., Sze, L. L., Saxton, R. E. Human antibody to OFA-I, a tumor antigen, produced *in vitro* by Epstein-Barr virus-transformed human B-lymphoid cell lines. Proc. Natl. Acad. Sci. USA 79, 5666–5670, 1982.

16. Tai, T., Paulson, J. C., Cahan, L. D., Irie, R. F. Ganglioside GM2 as a human tumor antigen (OFA-I-1). Proc. Natl. Acad. Sci. USA 80, 5392–5396, 1983.

17. Wakabayashi, S., Taniguchi, M., Tokuhisa, T., Tomioka, H., Okamoto, S. Cytotoxic T lymphocytes induced by syngeneic mouse melanoma cells recognize human melanomas. Nature 294, 748–750, 1981.

18. Taniguchi, M., Wakabayashi, S. Shared antigenic determinant expressed on various mammalian melanoma cells. Jpn. J. Cancer Res. (GANN) 75, 418–426, 1984.

19. Hirabayashi, Y., Hamaoka, A., Matsumoto, M., Matsubara, T., Tagawa, M., Wakabayashi, S., Taniguchi, M. Syngeneic monoclonal antibody against melanoma antigen with interspecies cross-reactivity recognizes GM3, a prominent ganglioside of B16 melanoma. J. Biol. Chem. 260, 13328–13333, 1985.

20. Nores, G. A., Dohi, T., Taniguchi, M., Hakomori, S. Density-dependent recognition of cell surface GM3 by a certain anti-melanoma antibody, and GM3 lactone as a possible immunogen: Requirements for tumor-associated antigen and immunogen. J. Immunol. 139, 3171–3176, 1987.

29. Immunization of Melanoma Patients with Purified Gangliosides

*P. O. Livingston, G. Ritter,
H. F. Oettgen, and L. J. Old*

Introduction

The gangliosides GM2, GD2, and GD3 are differentiation antigens that have been shown to function as effective targets for monoclonal antibody therapy of melanoma (1, 2, 3). We focused on GM2 in the initial studies because its distribution on various cell lines detected by an anti-GM2 Mmab (4) and on various tissues (detected by extraction and thin-layer chromatography) was quite restricted. The immunogenicity of these gangliosides has been explored in the mouse by analyzing the humoral immune response after vaccination. Vaccination with GM2 combined with Salmonella minnesota mutant R595 or BCG, but not with GM2 alone, results in frequent production of anti-GM2 IgM, especially after pre-treatment of the mice with low-dose cyclophosphamide (Cy) to decrease suppressor cell activity (5).

Immunogenicity of GM2 in Patients with Melanoma

Based on these findings in the mouse, we have treated patients with metastatic melanoma who are free of disease after surgery with a series of ganglioside vaccines and used ELISAs and immune thin layer chromatography (ITLC) with purified gangliosides to analyze the serological response (6). The results are summarized in Table 1.

Normal donors and untreated patients with melanoma rarely had a high titer antibody response (>1/80 by ELISA) against GM2. Vaccines containing GM2 alone did not induce antibody reponses, vaccines containing R595/GM2 induced occasional antibody responses, and vaccines containing BCG/GM2 induced high titer antibodies

Table 1. Serological response of humans to immunization with gangliosides.

	No. subjects	No. subjects producing high titer antibodies
Normal subjects, not vaccinated (GM2 antibodies)	44	1
Stage III melanoma patients vaccinated with GM2	48	0
Stage III melanoma patients vaccinated with:		
GM2 Alone	6	0
GM2 + R595	5	0
Cy + GM2 + R595	6	2
GM2 + BCG	5	3
Cy + GM2 + BCG	40	34
Cy + GD2 + BCG	12	0
Cy + GD3 + BCG	12	0

in most patients. Pretreatment with low-dose Cy (200 mg/M^2) increased the immuno-genicity of R595/GM2 and BCG/GM2 vaccines. The results of ELISA assays on GM2 for the initial six patients receiving the Cy-BCG/GM2 immunization are shown in Figure 1.

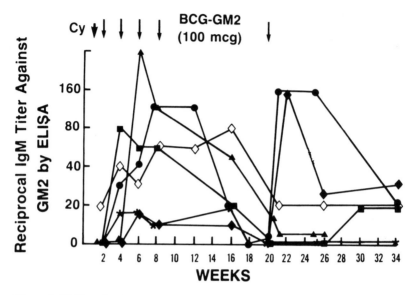

Figure 1. GM2 antibody response of stage III melanoma patients with purified GM2 ganglioside vaccines. Each curve represents the response of an individual patient. Arrows indicate time of Cy injection or vaccine injection.

All patients received a single dose of Cy and five immunizations with BCG/GM2 (indicated at the top). Each curve represents the course of GM2 antibody titers in an individual patient. Five patients produced high titer (1/80 or higher) antibody reactive with GM2. Overall, 34 of 40 patients immunized with Cy-BCG/GM2 have produced high titer IgM antibodies, and 8 of the initial 24 patients produced high titer IgG anti-bodies. The specificity of these antibodies was analyzed using ITLC and inhibition assays with a panel of gangliosides. Antibody reactivity was restricted to GM2 and N-glycolyl GM2. The suggestion, based on retrospective analysis, that production of GM2 antibodies is associated with delayed recurrence of melanoma (see Figure 2) is now being tested in a prospective randomized trial.

Relative Immunogenicity of GM2, GD2, and GD3 in the Mouse and in Patients with Melanoma

The heterogeneity of ganglioside expression by melanomas makes induction of an immune response against several melanoma gangliosides in a polyvalent vaccine appealing. Toward this end we have conducted preclinical and clinical vaccination

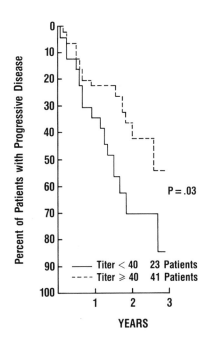

Figure 2. Correlation between GM2 antibody response after vaccination and time to melanoma progression.

trials with additional gangliosides. In contrast to the Cy-BCG/GM2 vaccines, Cy-BCG/GD2 or Cy-BCG/GD3 vaccines did not induce high-titer antibody responses in 12 patients immunized with each ganglioside (see Table 1). While GM2 is more immunogenic than GD3 in man, the reverse is true in the mouse (7), as shown in Table 2.

As we thought it possible that the immunogenicity of melanoma gangliosides was inversely related to their expression in normal tissues, we compared the immunogenicity of five gangliosides in man and in mouse (based on our results and the work of others) with their known expression in normal tissues (5). The results are summarized in Table 3.

Table 2. Serological response of the mouse to immunization with gangliosides.

	No. mice	No. mice producing high titer antibodies
Non-vaccinated normal mice (GM2 and GD3 antibodies)	10	0
Mice vaccinated with:		
R595 (GM2 and GD3 antibodies)	10	0
R595 + GM1	10	7
R595 + GM2	10	1
R595 + GM3	10	0
R595 + GD2	10	1
R595 + GD3	10	8

Table 3. Correlation of ganglioside immunogenicity with expression in normal (nonbrain) murine and human tissues.

Ganglioside	Tissue expression		Immunogenicity	
	Man	*Mouse*	*Man*	*Mouse*
GM1	weak	weak	strong	strong
GM2	weak	strong	strong	weak
GM3	strong	strong	weak	weak
GD2	unknown	unknown	intermed.	weak
GD3	intermed.	weak	weak	strong

No correlation was detected between ganglioside expression in normal brain and immunogenicity, consistent with the brain being an immunologically privileged site (8). However, the immunogenicity of most gangliosides correlated inversely with expression in normal non-brain human and murine tissues, supporting the view that variations between species in ganglioside expression in normal tissues may result in corresponding variations in ganglioside immunogenicity. Mice showed no toxicity from high titer antibodies induced against gangliosides expressed at low levels in normal tissues, suggesting that normal tissue ganglioside levels low enough to permit antibody induction by appropriate vaccination may not be high enough for the development of autoimmune disease. The levels of GM2, GD2, and GD3 expressed in melanoma cells ar at the least ten-fold higher than those in the major organs (excluding brain) that we reviewed (7, 9). We have recently initiated studies to determine whether this level of ganglioside expression on melanoma cells will permit immune rejection of melanoma in the mouse or delayed recurrence in melanoma patients.

Future Directions

Based on these findings, we have attempted to synthesize 9-O-acetyl GD3, another melanoma ganglioside with low expression in normal human tissues, and a series of congeners of GD3 which may induce antibodies reactive with GD3 more effectively than the parent molecule. Dr. Gerd Ritter will describe this aspect of our studies.

References

1. Houghton, A. N., Mintzer, D., Cordon-Cardo, C., Welt, S., Fliegel, B., Vadhan, S., Carswell, El., Melamed, M. R., Oettgen, H. F., and Old, L. J. Mouse monoclonal IgG3 antibody detecting GD3 ganglioside: a phase I trial in patients with malignant melanoma. Proc. Natl. Acad. Sci. USA 82, 1242, 1985.
2. Cheung, N.-K.V., Lazarus, H., Miraldi, F. D., Abramowsky, C. R., Kallick, S., Saarinen, U. M., Spitzer, T., Strandjord, S. E., Coccia, P. F., and Berger, N. A. Ganglioside GD2 specific monoclonal antibody 3F8: a phase I study in patients with neuroblastoma and malignant melanoma. J. Clin. Oncol. 5, 1430–1440, 1987.
3. Irie, R. F. and Morton, D. L. Regression of cutaneous metastatic melanoma by intralesional injection with human monoclonal antibody to ganglioside GD2. Proc. Natl. Acad. Sci. 83, 8694–8698, 1986.
4. Natoli, E. J. Jr., Livingston, P. O., Cordon-Cardo, C., Pukel, C. S., Lloyd, K. O., Wiegandt, H., Szalay, J., Oettgen, H. F., and Old, L. J. A murine monoclonal antibody detecting N-acetyl and N-glycolyl GM2: characterization of cell surface reactivity. Cancer Res. 46, 4116–4120, 1986.
5. Livingston, P. O., Jones Calves, M., and Natoli, E. J. Jr. Approaches to augmenting the immunogenicity of the ganglioside GM2 in mice: purified GM2 is superior to whole cells. J. Immunol. 138, 1524–1529, 1987.
6. Livingston, P. O., Natoli, E. J. Jr., Jones Calves, M., Stockert, E., Oettgen, H. F., and Old, L. J. Vaccines containing purified GM2 ganglioside elicit GM2 antibodies in melanoma patients. Proc. Natl. Acad. Sci. USA 84, 2911–2915, 1987.
7. Livingston, P. O., Ritter, G., and Jones Calves, M. Immunogenicity of the gangliosides GM1, GM2, GM3, GD2, and GD3 in the mouse. Cancer Res., in press, 1988.
8. Head, J. R. and Billingham, R. E. Immunologically privileged sites in transplantation immunology and oncology. Perspectives in Biology and Medicine 29, 115–131, 1985.
9. Tsuchida, T., Saxton, R. E., and Irie, R. F. Gangliosides of human melanoma: GM2 and tumorigenicity. J. Natl. Cancer Inst. 78, 55–59, 1987.

30. Development of Melanoma Vaccines: Gangliosides as Immunogens

G. Ritter, P. O. Livingston,
E. Boosfeld, H. Wiegandt, R. K. Yu,
H. F. Oettgen, and L. J. Old

Indroduction

In studies investigating the humoral immune response against gangliosides in patients with malignant melanoma after immunization with ganglioside vaccines, it has been shown that GM2 is consistently immunogenic, whereas GD2 elicits antibody responses only occasionally and GD3 is not immunogenic (1–3). The lack of immunogenicity of GD3 is disappointing because it is the most common cell surface ganglioside of human melanomas (4) and because treatment with the mouse IgG3 monoclonal antibody R24, which recognized GD3, has induced tumor regression in a small number of patients with melanoma (5). We have therefore attempted to increase the immunogenicity of GD3 vaccines by modifying the GD3 molecule. GD3 lactones, amides, methyl esters and gangliosidols were synthesized, and their reactivity with monoclonal antibodies recognizing GD3 was determined. In addition to GD3 itself, human melanomas express 9-O-acetyl GD3 (6, 7). As nothing is known about its immunogenicity, we have prepared a series of O-acetylated GD3 derivatives for use in future studies.

Material and Methods

Glycolipids and chemicals: GM3, GM2, GM1, and GD3 gangliosides were obtained from Fidia Research Laboratories (Abano Terme, Italy); neutral glycosphingolipids were prepared from human spleen in our laboratory by published procedures (8). High performance thin layer chromatography (HPTLC) silica gel plates were obtained from E. Merck (Darmstadt, FRG); preparative (21.4 x 250 mm) and semi-preparative (10 x 250 mm) aminopropyl and C18 high pressure liquid chromatography (HPLC) columns were obtained from Rainin Instruments Co. (Ridgefield, NJ); analytical (3.9 x 300 mm) aminopropyl HPLC-column and Sep-Pak C18-cartridges were obtained from Waters Associates (Milford, MA); DEAE-Sephadex A 25, Sodium-borohydride, 4-chloro-1-naphthol and N-acetyl-imidazole were obtained from Sigma Chemical Co. (St. Louis, MO).

Enzymes: Endoglycoceramidase was kindly provided by Dr. Makoto Ito from the Mitsubishi-Kasei Institute of Life Science (Tokyo, Japan); *V. cholerae* sialidase (E.C. 3.2.1.18) was obtained from Calbiochem-Behring Corporation (La Jolla, CA).

Monoclonal antibodies (mAbs): mAbs rabbit anti-mouse conjugated with horseradish peroxidase was obtained from Dako Corporation (Santa Barbara, CA); mAb D1.1 was kindly provided by Dr. David A. Cheresh (Scripps-Clinic, La Jolla, CA, ref. 6); mAb ME 311 was provided by Dr. Jan Thurin (The Wistar Institute, Philadelphia, PA, ref. 7) and Jones antibody was provided by Dr. Andrew S. Blum (Rockefeller University, New York, NY, ref. 9). mAbs R24, C5, and K9 were generated in our laboratory (10).

GD3 derivatives: Lactones were prepared by treating GD3 with glacial acetic acid as described (11). Amides were obtained by aminolysis of GD3 lactones (12). Gangliosidols were obtained by reduction of GD3 lactones with sodium borohydride (13) and methyl esters were prepared by treating GD3 with iodomethane (14). Purity of these derivatives was confirmed by HPTLC. O-acetylation of GD3 was performed with N-acetyl-imidazole (15).

HPTLC: TLC-analysis was performed on HPTLC silica gel plates. Gangliosides and ganglioside derivatives were run in solvent system chloroform/methanol/0.2 % aqueous $CaCl_2$ 60:35:8 (v/v), neutral glycosphingolipids in chloroform/methanol/water 65:25:4 (v/v), ceramides in chloroform/methanol 95:5 (v/v) (16), and oligosaccharides in ethanol/n-butanol/pyridine/water/glacial acetic acid 100:10:30:3 (v/v) (17). Gangliosides, ganglioside derivatives, and oligosaccharides were visualized by spraying with orcinol/H_2SO_4 or resorcinol/HCl, neutral glycosphingolipids by staining with orcinol/H_2SO_4, and ceramides by treatment with iodine vapor and Coomassie Blue stain (18). Two dimensional TLC with or without intermediate base treatment was performed as described (12).

ITLC: Immunostaining of gangliosides and ganglioside derivatives with mAbs after separation on HPTLC silica gel glass plates was performed by a modification of the method of Magnani (19) as described (20). For analysis of the reactivity of GD3 derivatives with anti-GD3 antibodies, TLC-plates were covered with mAbs R24, C5 or K9 for 4 h or over night at room temperature, or over night at 4 °C.

HPLC: Analytical and preparative separation of individual O-acetyl GD3 derivatives were performed by HPLC (Waters 501 system) using aminopropyl columns and acetonitrile/phosphate buffer gradients (21) followed by desalting on C18 columns.

Enzyme hydrolysis: O-acetyl GD3 derivatives were treated with *V. chloreae* sialidase (22), neutral cleavage products were separated by DEAE-Sephadex chromatography (23, 24) and analyzed by TLC before and after treatment with 0.05 M NaOH in methanol for 1 h at 37 °C. Endoglycoceramidase treatment of O-acetyl GD3 derivatives was performed as described (16). Oligosaccharides and ceramides were analyzed by TLC before and after treatment with NaOH. Susceptability of O-acetyl GD3 derivatives to cleavage by serum esterase activity was analyzed as follows: 20 μg GD3 or GD3 derivatives were incubated in of 50 μl of fresh human serum or in PBS containing 2 % BSA for 24 h at 37 °C. The glycolipids were re-extracted with chloroform/methanol/water 10:10:1 (v/v), purified by Sep-Pak C18 chromatography (25) and analyzed by TLC and ITLC with mAbs R24 and D1.1. Determination of GD3-lactone stability: 50 μg GD3-lactones were incubated in 100 μl HCl in water at pH 4.0, 5.0, 6.0, 7.0, and 8.0 at 4 °C, 24 °C, and at 37 °C. Aliquots were taken after 1, 5, 24, 48, and 120 h and analyzed by TLC. After staining with orcinol/H_2SO_4 relative amounts of reconverted GD3 were determined by densitometry using a Shimadzu dual wavelength TLC scanner (model CS 930) at 440 nm.

Results

Preparation of GD3 lactones, amides, gangliosidols, and methyl esters. Ganglioside GD3 was chemically modified to construct derivatives that might be more immuno-

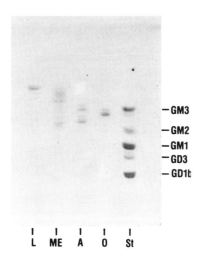

-GM3
-GM2
-GM1
-GD3
-GD1b

L   ME   A   0   St

Figure 1. TLC-analysis of GD3 derivatives. L, lactones; ME, methylester; A, amides; O, gangliosidols; St, reference gangliosides; HPTLC silica gel plate; running solvent: chloroform/methanol/0.2 % aqueous CaCl2 60:35:8 v/v; spray reagent: resorcinol/HCl.

genic than GD3 itself. The derivatives were characterized by TLC (Figure 1).

Two major products were obtained by treatment of GD3 with glacial acetic acid. Their TLC-patterns corresponded to those of GD3-lactone I and GD3-lactone II as described (26). After mild base treatment both derivatives co-migrated with the parent GD3. Following separation on DEAE-Sephadex according to charge, product I was eluted in the monosialo fraction, whereas product II was found in the neutral fraction.

GD3-lactones were used as starting material for the synthesis of GD3-amides and GD3-gangliosidols. After aminolysis two major products migrating as double bands could be detected on TLC, designated as GD3-amide I and II, respectively. In contrast to GD3-lactones, the amides had the same running mobilities in a 2-D TLC analysis, after being kept in a chamber saturated with ammonia between the two runs. Two bands with similiar Rf-values were detected after GD3 was reduced to gangliosidols. The major band was slightly slower than GM3 (gangliosidol I), whereas the minor band comigrated with GM3 (gangliosidol II). When stained with resorcinol reagent, both developed an atypical orange-yellowish color that has been described by others (27). TLC-analysis of the methyl ester fraction obtained after treatment of GD3 with iodomethane, revealed at least 3 alkalisensitive bands, referred as methyl ester I, II, and III, with increasing speed of migration. All methyl esters migrated faster than the parent GD3. The modified GD3 derivatives were free of GD3 or other detectable contaminants as determined by TLC.

Immune reactivity of these GD3 derivatives with established anti-GD3 mAbs R24, C5, and K9 was investigated by ITLC. Results are shown in Table 1. None of the GD3 derivatives reacted with anti-GD3 antibodies when incubated at 4 °C over night or at room temperature for 4 h, except methyl ester I which reacted with mAbs R24 and K9 after over night incubation at 4 °C. However, both lactones showed reactivity when incubated with GD3 antibodies at room temperature over night.

To determine whether this was in fact a reaction with the lactones or rather with break down products of the labile lactone structure, we tested lactone stability under various conditions of pH, temperature and incubation time by TLC. The results are

Table 1. Immune reactivity of GD3 derivatives with anti-GD3 monoclonal antibodies as determined by ITLC. Incubation times were over night at 4 °C and 4 h and over night at 25 °C, respectively; mAb dilutions: K9, C5 and R24 20 µg/ml; HRP-rabbit-anti-mouse 1:200.

Derivate	anti-GD3 MABS					
	K9		C5		R24	
	4 °C	25 °C	4 °C	25 °C	4 °C	25 °C
GD3	+	+	+	+	+	+
GD3-methyl-ester-I	+	−[a]	−	−[a]	+	−[a]
GD3-methyl-ester-II & III	−	−	−	−	−	−
GD3-amide-I	−	−	−	−	−	−
GD3-amide-II	−	−	−	−	−	−
GD3-ol-I	−	−	−	−	−	−
GD3-ol-II	−	−	−	−	−	−
GD3-L-I	−	−[a]	−	−[a]	−	−[a]
GD3-L-II	−	−[a]	−	−[a]	−	−[a]

*determined by ITLC; incubation times were overnight at 4 °C and 4 h at 25°, respectively.
[a]positive after overnight incubation.

shown in Figure 2. After incubation at 4 °C only traces of reconverted GD3 were detected, whereas at room temperature, and particularly at 37 °C, pH and time dependent lactone degradation to GD3 could be observed.

Preparation of O-acetylated GD3 derivatives. We converted GD3 to O-acetyl forms of GD3 by the method of Haverkamp et al. (15), using N-acetyl-imidazole in pyridine as a mild acetylation reagent. The process of acetylation was monitored by HPTLC (Figure 3). Four major bands were obtained, with only little GD3 remaining. The fractions were isolated by preparative HPLC (Figure 4). Fractions F1, F2, and F3 were rechromatographed to high purity, desalted by reversed phase chromatography, and characterized by TLC-analysis. TLC migration before and after base treatment is shown in Figure 5. Before base treatment, F1 migrated between GM1 and GD3, F2 ran slightly faster than GM1, and the two major bands of F3 migrated between GM2 and GM3. All fractions were sensitive to base treatment and were reconverted to a product co-migrating with GD3. Immune reactivity of the fractions with anti-ganglioside monoclonal antibodies was investigated by ITLC (Table 2). GD3 and F1 showed reactivity only with anti-GD3 antibodies, whereas F2 and F3 reacted with monoclonal antibodies against 9-O-acetyl GD3 as well as GD3. The reactivity with antibodies against 9-O-acetyl GD3 was lost after base treatment.

Further information about the localization of the acetyl groups was obtained by TLC-analysis of oligosaccharides and ceramides after treatment with endoglycoceramidase. Ceramides and base treated ceramides derived from O-acetylated GD3 comigrated with ceramide from native GD3, indicating that the acetylation site was not

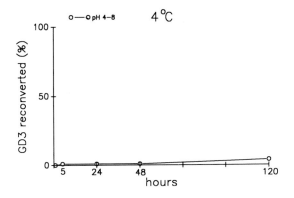

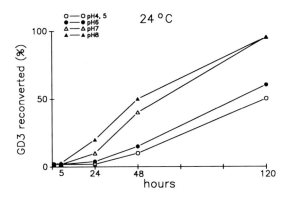

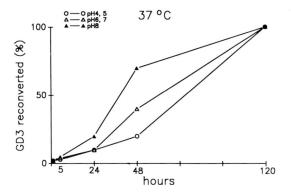

Figure 2. Conversion of GD3-lactones to GD3. 50 µg lactones were incubated in 100 µl of HCl in water at pH 4.0, 5.0, 6.0, 7.0, and 8.0 at 4 °C, 24 °C and at 37 °C. Aliquots were taken after 1, 5, 24, 48, and 120 hours and analyzed by TLC. relative amounts of reconverted GD3 was determined by densitometry as described in material and methods.

on the ceramide moiety. Oligosaccharides, however, showed different mobility, with a migration pattern similiar to that of their parent gangliosides. After base treatment they co-migrated with GD3-oligosaccharide.

TLC-analysis after treatment with *V. cholerae* sialidase revealed that the hydrolysis product derived from F1 migrated between ceramidemonohexoside and ceramidedi-

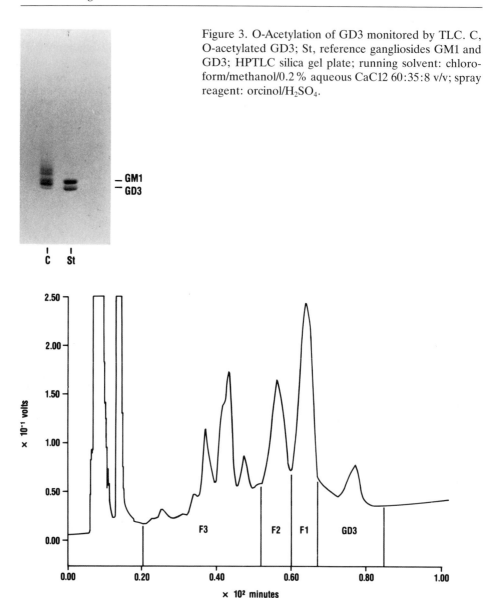

Figure 3. O-Acetylation of GD3 monitored by TLC. C, O-acetylated GD3; St, reference gangliosides GM1 and GD3; HPTLC silica gel plate; running solvent: chloroform/methanol/0.2 % aqueous CaC12 60:35:8 v/v; spray reagent: orcinol/H$_2$SO$_4$.

Figure 4. Separation of O-acetyl-GD3 derivatives by preparative HPLC. NH2-column (21.4 x 250 mm); buffer 1: acetonitrile/5 mM phosphate 83:17 v/v; pH 5.6; buffer 2: acetonitrile/20 mM phosphate 1:1 v/v; pH 5.6 programmed as follows: 30 min isocratic buffer 1/buffer 2 90:10 v/v; 90 min with a linear gradient from buffer 1/buffer 2 90:10 v/v to buffer 1/buffer 2 50:50 v/v; 30 min isocratic buffer 1/buffer 2 50:50 v/v; flow rate 9 ml/min; eluting gangliosides were monitored at 205 nm in a flow-through detector. F1–3 representing isolated fractions.

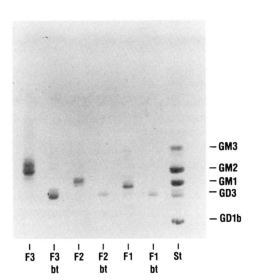

Figure 5. TLC-analysis of isolated O-acetyl-GD3 derivatives F1, F2, and F3 before and after base treatment. bt referring to base treated fraction; HPTLC silica gel plate; running solvent: chloroform/methanol/0.2 % aqueous CaC12 60:35:8 v/v; spray reagent: orcinol/H_2SO_4.

hexoside, that most of F2 co-migrated with ceramidedihexoside derived from GD3, and that the hydrolysis products of F3 co-migrated with ceramidedihexoside and the F1 hydrolysis product. Only bands co-migrating with ceramidedihexoside could be detected after base treatment (data not shown). A more detailed analysis of fractions F1, F2, and F3 including fast atom bombardment mass spectrometry and nuclear magnetic resonance is in progress.

As immunization of melanoma patients with these O-acetylated GD3 derivatives is envisaged, it seemed important to determine whether they are resistant or susceptible to cleavage by serum esterases. After *in vitro* exposure to fresh human serum for 24 h at 37 °C, followed by re-extraction and TLC-separation, the O-acetylated GD3 derivatives were recovered unchanged.

Table 2. Immune reactivity of O-acetyl-GD3 derivatives F1, F2 and F3 with anti-ganglioside monoclonal antibodies as determined by ITLC. mAbs were incubated at 4 °C overnight; mab dilutions: K9, C5 and R24 20 µg/ml; D1.1. 1:500; Jones antibody 1:200; ME 311 supernatant 1:5; HRP-rabbit-anti-mouse 1:200.

	MABS					
	anti-9-0-AcGD3			anti-GD3		
Derivative	D.1.1[1]	ME 311[2]	Jones[3]	R24[4]	C5[4]	K9[4]
GD3	−	−	−	+	+	+
F1	−	−	−	+	+	+
F2	+	+	+	+	+	+
F3	+	+	+	+	+	+

[1]Cheresh et al. 1984; [2]Thurin et al. 1985; [3]Blum et al. 1987; [4]Dippold et al. 1980, *tested by ITLC.

Discussion

GD3, the most common ganglioside of human melanoma, has been an effective target for passive immunization with the mouse monoclonal antibody R24, which has been shown to induce regression of melanoma metastases (5). However, using GD3-containing vaccines for active immunization, an immune response against GD3 is not induced in man, although it has been shown that ganglioside GM2 was consistantly immunogenic (1) and GD2 could occasionally elicited a specific immune response (3).

Recently, Nores et al. (13) observed in the mouse, where GM3 is non-immunogenic, that an immune response against GM3 could be induced when a modified GM3 molecule, GM3 in its lactonized form, was used as immunogen instead of native GM3. Also, immunization of rabbits with GM1 methylester resulted in polyclonal sera cross-reactive with GM1, whereas GM1 gangliosidol and GM1-N-methylamide elicited high titer immune responses which did not crossreact with parent GM1. Anti-GM1-N-methylamide sera reacted with other derivatives such as GM1 methylester or GM1 gangliosidol (14, 28). Reactivity of mouse monoclonal anti-GD2 antibodies with GD2 lactone (29), and mouse monoclonal anti-GM3 antibody M2590 with GM3 lactone (13) and C7-NeuAc-GM3 have been shown (28). We have modified the GD3 molecule in attempts to overcome its poor immunogenicity in man and have synthesized GD3 methylester, amides, gangliosidols, and lactones. We plan to investigate the potency of these derivatives to induce an immune response crossreactive with GD3 in patients with malignant melanomas. Analysis of the crossreactivities of these derivatives with established anti-GD3 monoclonal antibodies by ITLC revealed reactivity of antibodies R24 and K9 only with the lower migrating band of the GD3 methylester fraction. However, performing ITLC under harsher conditions, i.e. incubating the monoclonal antibodies on the plate overnight at room temperature, resulted in staining of two bands on the position of GD3 lactone I and II, respectively. This reactivity was considered to be due to degradation of GD3 lactone to GD3, since investigation of GD3 lactone stability showed a considerable degree of conversion of GD3 lactone to GD3 after overnight incubation at room temperature, while only traces of GD3 could be detected after incubation at 4 °C.

We have also studied the O-acetylation of GD3. In man, expression of 9-O-acetyl-GD3 seems to be strongly restricted to malignant melanoma, as it is not expressed on the cell surface of normal human tissues (7, 30). Recently, O-acetyl-GD3 was also found to be a major constituent in malignant melanoma of the fish genus *Xiphophorus,* but not in benign melanoma or in normal skin. As this species is phylogenetically distant from man, this result suggests a special role for these melanoma-associated GD3 derivatives (31). Not much is known about the immunogenicity of O-acetyl-GD3 derivatives in man, although autoantibodies reactive with O-acetyl-GD3 have been detected in some sera from patients with malignant melanoma (32). We have performed chemical O-acetylation of GD3 to produce these derivatives for use as possible candidates for melanoma vaccine construction. Various derivatives derived from these conversions were isolated by preparative HPLC and characterized in terms of TLC migration, susceptability to base treatment and reactivity with anti-ganglioside monoclonal antibodies. ITLC-analysis of O-acetylated GD3 derivatives with mouse monoclonal antibodies D1.1, ME 311 and Jones antibody, which were all described to recognize 9-O-acetyl-GD3 (6, 7, 9), revealed reactivity of these antibodies with a wide range of different O-acetylated GD3 derivatives. This reactivity was lost after base treatment. Although all base-sensitive derivatives have different mobilities after separation by TLC, showing that they differ in the number and position of their intersugar linkages, they seem to contain a common epitope recognized by these antibodies.

Furthermore, anti-GD3 monoclonal antibodies R24, K9, and C5 were observed to be reactive with the O-acetyl-GD3 derivatives. This might be interpreted to indicate that O-acetylation of GD3 does not affect the binding site of the anti-GD3 monoclonal antibodies used in this assay. However, it can not be excluded that this reactivity was with traces of GD3 formed by reconversion during incubation, even though no GD3 could be detected in experiments investigating the stability of O-acetyl-GD3 under comparable conditions. Hypothesizing that this crossreactivity is real, O-acetyl-GD3 might then be considered to be capable of inducing an immune response not only against itself but also against GD3. Studies investigating the immunogenicity of all of these GD3 derivatives in the mouse and in patients with malignant melanoma are underway, as are attempts at elucidating the fine structure of these compounds. These studies will tell us whether these derivatives induce an immune response in humans against GD3 and whether they are candidates for vaccine construction.

Summary

In studies aimed at inducing antibody production against gangliosides in patients with malignant melanoma by immunization with ganglioside vaccines, we found that GM2 is often immunogenic whereas GD2 elicits antibody production only rarely and GD3 is generally non immunogenic. GD3 is of particular interest because it is the predominant cell surface ganglioside of human melanomas, and because it has been an effective target for therapy with monoclonal antibody R24. We are attempting, therefore, to increase the immunogenicity of GD3 by chemical modification of the molecule. The following derivatives have been prepared: GD3 lactone, GD3 gangliosidol, GD3 amide, and GD3 methylester. The immunoreactivity of these GD3 derivatives with anti-GD3 monoclonal antibodies was confirmed by immuno thin layer chromatography. Another modification we have been exploring is O-acetylation. 9-O-acetyl-GD3 occurs naturally in human melanomas but its immunogenicity is not yet known. We have prepared a series of O-acetylated GD3 derivatives, purified them by HPLC and characterized them in terms of TLC-migration, susceptibility to base and enzyme actions and immunoreactivity with monoclonal antibodies. In preparation for *in vivo* studies we have determined the stability of some of the GD3 derivatives in serum. Studies of their immunogenicity in the mouse and in patients with melanoma are now underway.

References

1. Livingston, P. O., E. J. Natoli, Jr., M. Jones Calves, E. Stockert, H. F. Oettgen, and L. J. Old. Vaccines containing purified GM2 ganglioside elicit GM2 antibodies in melanoma patients. Proc. Natl. Acad. Sci. USA 84, 2911–2915, 1987.
2. Tai, T., L. D. Cahan, T. Tsuchida, R. E. Saxton, R. F. Irie, and D. L. Morton. Immunogenicity of melanoma-assiciated gangliosides in cancer patients. Int. J. Cancer 35, 607, 1985.
3. Livingston, P. O., E. Kaelin, C. M. Pinsky, H. F. Oettgen, and L. J. Old. IV. Serological response in stage II melanoma patients receiving allogeneic melanoma cell vaccines. Cancer 56, 2194, 1985.
4. Tsuchida, T., R. E. Saxton, and R. F. Irie. Gangliosides of human melanoma: GM2 and tumorigenicity. J. Natl. Cancer Inst. 78, 55, 1987.
5. Houghton, A. N., D. Mintzer, C. Cordon-Cardo, S. Welt, B. Fliegel, S. Vadhan, E. Carswell, M. R. Melamed, H. F. Oettgen, and L. J. Old. Mouse monoclonal IgG3 antibody detecting GD3 ganglioside: a phase I trial in patients with malignant melanoma. Proc. Natl. Acad. Sci. USA 82, 1242, 1985.
6. Cheresh, D. A., A. P. Varki, N. M. Varki, W. B. Stallcup, J. M. Levine, and R. A. Reisfeld. A monoclonal antibody recognizes an O-acetylated sialic acid in a human melanoma-associated ganglioside. J. Biol. Chem. 259, 7453, 1984.
7. Thurin, J., M. Herlyn, O. Hindsgaul, N. Stromberg, K. Karlsson, D. Elder, Z. Steplewski, and H. Koprowski. Proton NMR and fast atom bombardment mass spectrometry analysis of the melanoma-associated ganglioside 9-O-acetyl-GD3. J. Biol. Chem. 260, 14556, 1985.
8. Momoi, T. and H. Wiegandt. Separation and micro-detection of oligosaccharides of glycosphingolipids by high performance cellulose thin-layer chromatography-autoradiofluorography. Hoppe-Seyler's Z. Physiol. Chem. 361, 1201–1210, 1980.
9. Blum, A. S. and C. J. Barnstable. O-acetylation of a cell-surface carbohydrate creates discrete molecular patterns during neural development. Proc. Natl. Acad. Sci. USA 84, 8716, 1987.
10. Dippold, W. G., K. O. Lloyd, L. T. Li, H. Ikeda, H. F. Oettgen, and L. J. Old. Cell surface antigens of human malignant melanoma: definition of six antigenic systems with monoclonal antibodies. Proc. Natl. Acad. Sci. USA 77, 6114, 1980.
11. Yu, R. K., T. A. W. Koerner, S. Ando, H. C. Yohe, and J. H. Prestegard. High-resolution proton NMR studies of gangliosides. III. Elucidation of the structure of GM3 lactone. J. Biochem. 98, 1367, 1985.
12. Sonnino, S., R. Ghidoni, V. Chigorno, M. Masserini, and G. Tettamanti. Recognition by two-dimensional thin-layer chromatography and densitometric quantification of alkalilabile gangliosides from the brain of different animals. Anal. Biochem. 128, 104, 1983.
13. Nores, G. A., T. Dohi, M. Taniguchi, and S.-I. Hakomori. Density-dependent recognition of cell surface GM3 by a certain anti-melanoma antibody, and GM3 lactone as a possible immunogen: requirements for tumor-associated antigen and immunogen. J. Immunol. 139, 3171, 1987.
14. Handa, S. and K. Nakamura. Modification of sialic acid carboxyl group of ganglioside. J. Biochem. 95, 1323, 1984.
15. Haverkamp, J., R. Schauer, M. Wember, J. P. Kamerling, and J. F. G. Vligenthart. Synthesis of 9-O-acetyl- and 4,9-di-O-acetyl derivatives of the methyl ester of N-acetyl--D-neuraminic acid methylglycoside. Hoppe-Seyler's Z. Physiol. Chem. 356, 1575, 1975.
16. Ito, M. and T. Yamagata. A novel glycosphingolipid-degrading enzyme cleaves of the linkage between the oligosaccharide and ceramide of neutral and acidic glycosphingolipids. J. Biol. Chem. 262, 14278, 1986.

17. Veh, R.W., J.-C. Michalski, A. P. Corfield, M. Sander-Wewer, D. Gies, and R. Schauer. New chromatographic system for the rapid analysis and preparation of colostrum sialooligo-saccharides. J. Chromatogr. 212, 313, 1981.

18. Nakamura, K. and S. Handa. Coomassie brilliant blue staining of lipids on thin-layer plates. Anal. Biochem. 142, 406, 1984.

19. Magnani, J. L., D. F. Smith, and V. Ginsburg. Detection of gangliosides that bind cholera toxin: direct binding of ^{125}I-labelled toxin to thin-layer chromatograms. Anal. Biochem. 109, 399, 1980.

20. Ritter, G., W. Krause, R. Geyer, S. Stirm, and H. Wiegandt. Glycosphingolipid composition of human semen. Arch. Biochem. Biophys. 257, 370, 1987.

21. Gazzotti, G., S. Sonnino, and R. Ghidoni. Normal-phase high-performance liquid chroma-tographic separsation of non-derivatized ganglioside mixtures. J. Chromatogr. 348, 371, 1985.

22. Schauer, R. Characterization of sialic acids. In: V. Ginsburg (ed.), Methods in enzymology, Vol. L., part C, 64, 1978.

23. Ledeen, R.W., R. K. Yu, and L. F. Eng. Gangliosides of human myelin sialogalactosylcera-mide as a major component. J. Neurochem. 21, 829, 1973.

24. Iwamori, M. and Y. Nagai. A new approach to the resolution of individual gangliosides by ganglioside mapping. Biochem. Biophys. Acta. 528, 257, 1978.

25. Kubo, H. and M. Hoshi. Elimination of silica gel from gangliosides by using a reversed-phase column after preparative thinlayer chromatography. J. Lipid Res. 26, 638, 1985.

26. Ando, S. and R. K. Yu manusc. submitted.

27. MacDonald, D. L., L. M. Patt, and S.-I. Hakomori. Notes on improved procedures for the chemical modification and degradation of glycosphingolipids. J. Lipid Res. 21, 642, 1980.

28. Nakamura, K. and S. Handa. Biochemical properties of N-methylamides of sialic acids in gangliosides. J. Biochem. 99, 219, 1986.

29. Tai, T., I. Kawashima, N. Tada, and S. Ikegami. Different reactivities of monoclonal anti-bodies to ganglioside lactones. Biochim. Biophys. Acta. 958, 134, 1988.

30. Cheresh, D. A., R. A. Reisfeld, and A. J. Varki. O-acetylation of disialoganglioside GD3 by human melanomas cells creates a unique antigenetic epitope. Science 225, 844, 1984.

31. Felding-Habermann, B., A. Anders, W. G. Dippold, W. B. Stallcup, and H. Wiegandt. Melanoma-associated gangliosides in the fish genus xiphophorus. Cancer Res. 48, 3454, 1988.

32. Ravindranaths, M. H., J. C. Paulson, and R. F. Irie. Human melanoma antigen O-ace-tylated ganglioside GD3 is recognized by cancer antennarius lectin. J. Biol. Chem. 263, 2079, 1988.

31. Epitopes on Gangliosides GD2 and its Lactones: Markers for Gliomas and Neuroblastomas

K. Bosslet, H. D. Mennel, F. Rodden,
B. L. Bauer, F. Wagner,
H. H. Sedlacek, and H. Wiegandt

Abstract

Monoclonal antibodies (MAbs) BW 625 and BW 704 of IgG3, K-isotype, bound to immunochemically indistinguishable epitopes on ganglioside $II^3(NeuAc)_2$-GgOse$_3$-Cer. Despite this fact the MAbs showed a differential binding pattern on human glioma cell lines.

Furthermore, either MAb is able to mediate the antibody dependent cellular cytotoxicity reaction (ADCC) and the human complement dependent cytotoxicity reaction (CDC) with epitope expressing tumor cells. All cryopreserved tissue specimen from gliomas and neuroblastomas were immunohistochemically stained, whereas the small round cell tumors of childhood, melanomas and small cell lung carcinomas were essentially negative.

Positive staining of normal cryopreserved tissues was restricted to amyelinic axons, Hassal's bodies and some connective tissue fibers in thymus and the tegumentary epithelium of skin. The high selectivity of MAb BW 704 for gliomas and neuroblastomas, the lack of cross-reactivity with major tissues and the strong ADCC and CDC potential argue for the use of MAb BW 704 in immunotherapy of neuroblastomas and gliomas.

Introduction

Since the first description of hybridoma technology (Köhler and Milstein 1975) a variety of MAbs binding to tumor associated glycoprotein antigens (TAAs) were generated. Nowadays some of these MAbs binding to protein or carbohydrate epitopes on these TAAs represent tumor markers which are already used in routine histopathology (Gatter et al. 1983, Klöppel and Caselitz 1987), in treatment control and in the immunoscintigraphic localization of carcinomas and inflammatory processes (Mach et al. 1983, Seybold et al. 1988, Joseph et al. 1987).

In contrast, the clinical role of MAbs binding to carbohydrate moieties of gangliosides (Klenk 1942) is not yet established despite a few reports suggesting an application as tumor markers (Ladisch and Wu 1985) or as immunotherapeutic agents (Houghton et al. 1985).

The present report deals with MAbs binding to epitopes located on ganglioside $II^3(NeuAc)_2$-GgOse$_3$-Cer (short notations GD2 or GTri$_2$) isolated and characterized by Klenk (1968). Using immunochemical methods we characterized the MAbs BW 625 or BW 704 defined on GD2. Differences in the accessibility of the MAb defined epitopes on glioma cell lines as well as the Mabs' immunological properties will be presented as well. Finally, the distribution of the MAb BW 704 defined epitope on cryopreserved human neurogenic tumors and normal tissues will be described.

Material and Methods

Cell lines. The melanoma cell lines M 21, SKMel 28 and the neuroblastoma cell line SKNAS were kindly supplied by Dr. R. Reisfeld, Scripps Clinic, La Jolla, California. The T 98 human glioblastoma cell line was obtained from the ATCC (no. CRL 1690), the DETA colon carcinom was a gift from Dr. Vetterlein, Austrian Cancer Research Institute, Vienna.

Gliomas number 241, 302, 550, 543, 302, 553, and neurilemmoma 344, obtained from Drs. Tonn and Schönmayr, Department of Neurosurgery, University of Gießen, FRG, represent short term primary cell cultures derived from fresh surgical brain tumor material. All cell lines or primary cell cultures were passaged using routine cell culture conditions (Bosslet et al. 1986).

Immuno-thin-layer chromatography (ITLC). The ITLC method was based on the original methodological work of Magnani et al. (1982). Chromatography was performed using aluminium silica gel 60 HPTLC plates (Merck, Darmstadt, FGR). After chromatography in chloroform/methanol/0.2 % $CaCl_2$ water (50/40/10) gangliosides were immunostained using the corresponding MAbs followed by the avidin biotin peroxidase complex (ABC) method as suggested by Harpin et al. 1985.

Purified ganglioside GD2 was digested with 5 units/ml of Vibrio cholerae Neuraminidase (VCN) for 24 hrs in PBS, pH 7.0 VCN was removed by addition of 2 parts of 99.9 % ethanol and incubation overnight at -20° C. After centrifugation the VCN pellet was washed in chloroform/methanol (2/1), the chloroform/methanol and ethanol supernatants were evaporated and solubilized in chloroform/methanol/water (10/10/1). Samples were analyzed using the ITLC technique as outlined above.

Lactonisation of ganglioside GD2. Two procedures were used to generate GD2-lactones: 1 mg of purified ganglioside GD2 free acid was dissolved in 1 ml glacial acetic acid and stirred for 3 hrs at R.T. as described by Yu et al. (1985) (procedure 1) or treated for 1 h in 1 ml of formic acid/acetamid/water mixture (50/150/80 v/v), pH 1.9, as described by Wiegandt (1973) (procedure 2). Thereafter the samples were lyophilized, dissolved in chloroform/methanol/0.2 % $CaCl_2$ in H_2O (50/40/10) and 10 µg aliquots were chromatographed and immunostained using the ITLC method.

Alkali treatment of ganglioside lactones. Ganglioside lactones generated according to procedure 1 or 2 (see preceding chapter) were treated for 2 hrs at 37° C with 0.05 N NaOH in methanol (Tai et al. 1988). After evaporation samples were dissolved in chloroform/methanol/water (10/10/1 v/v) and chromatographed.

Induction and screening of monoclonal antibodies (MAbs). MAb BW 704 was induced by 4x i.p. injection of 10^7 M21 human melanoma cells, each in Balb/c mice in 1 week intervals. Immunized splenocytes were fused with the SP2-O Ag 14 murine myeloma cell line (Shulman et al. 1978) 3 days after the last immunization.

MAb BW 625 was induced in an identical manner as described for MAb BW 704, except alternating injections of M21 or SkMel 28 cells in 1 week intervals. The specificity of the MAbs was evaluated on cell lines using an indirect immunofluorescence assay in Terasaki plates (Brown et al. 1977). The alkaline phosphatase anti alkaline phosphatase method (APAAP) (Cordell et al. 1984) was applied to evaluate the MAbs' specificity on human cryopreserved tissues. Binding to human peripheral blood cells and thrombocytes was evaluated using cytofluorometric analysis (Reinherz et al. 1979).

MAb R24, binding to gangliosidide $II^3(NeuAc)_2$-Lac-Cer (short notations: GD3 or G_{Lac2}), a gift from Dr. Dippold, University of Mainz, FGR (Dippold et al. 1985) as well as MAbs BW 495 and BW 181 (Boslet et al. 1986, Bosslet et al. 1984) served as isotype matched, idiotype mismatched internal experimental controls.

Isotyping of MAbs. The double diffusion technique in agarose according to Ouchterlony (1948) was used for the isotyping of MAbs.

Derivation of intracranial tumors and brain tissues. MAb BW 704 was tested in 36 human intracranial tumors. Ten of them were malignant gliomas (WHO III–IV) six were differentiated gliomas (WHO I–II) eleven were meningiomas, four neurinomas, three pituitary adenomas and one metastasis. Furthermore different parts from human brain were tested in the same way. These parts comprised cerebral cortex (parietal, occipital, frontal and temporal), hippocampus, basal ganglia and cerebellum. Tumor biopsies were treated immediately after operation, whilst normal brain was removed 8 hours after death.

Tumors were immediately deep frozen in isopentan cooled in liquid nitrogen. Corresponding parts of the tumors were used for histological, immunohistochemical, cytological and electron-microscopic analysis. Furthermore, parts of the tumors were explanted in vitro and subjected to different diagnostic methods, including marker immunohistochemistry and proliferation kinetic analysis. Results of this investigations were published elsewhere (Mennel et al. 1988).

Parts of normal brain were equally deep frozen. After that, tumor biopsies and normal brain were cut in a cryomicrotome and used for antigen antibody reactions. The visualization of the reaction products was performed using the APAAP method. In all biopsies, antibody reactions using MAb BW 704 were performed; in addition HE and cresylviolett staining and controls were investigated.

Antibody-dependent cell-mediated cytotoxicity (ADCC) and complement-mediated cytolysis (CDC). The capacity of MAbs BW 625 and BW 704 to perform human K-cell-mediated tumor cells lysis and human complement mediated lysis was evaluated according to the procedure described by Schulz et al. (1983). Briefly, ^{51}Cr labelled tumor target cells were incubated for 4 hrs with peripheral blood mononuclear cells at various effector to target cell ratios (ADCC) or for 2 hrs with human complement (CDC).

Specific lysis in % was evaluated using the formula:

$$\frac{\text{exp. counts} - \text{low control counts}}{\text{high control counts} - \text{low control counts}} \times 100$$

Results

Immunochemical charcterization of the MAb BW 625 or BW 704 defined epitopes on ganglioside GD2. Bovine brain gangliosides were used as standards to define the ganglioside bearing the epitopes detected by MAb BW 625 or BW 704. The ITLC analysis depicted in Figure 1 showed that both MAbs detected a single ganglioside band running at a position corresponding to GD2 (compare the bovine brain resorcinol standards lane A with bovine brain ITLC lanes B and D). The absence of other even only slightly stained bands argues against cross-reactivity of both MAbs with other bovine brain gangliosides (see lanes B and D).

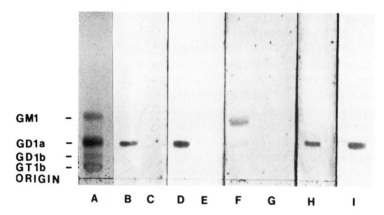

Figure 1a. HPTLC analysis of bovine brain gangliosides (see Materials and Methods).

A: bovine brain ganglioside standards stained with resorcinol, lanes B - I represent the same gangliosides immunostained with MAb BE 625, MAb BW 704 or MAb R24
B: Immunostaining with MAb BW 625 without VCN pretreatment
C: Immunostaining with MAb BW 625 after pretreatment with 5 U VCN/ml
D: Treatment like B, immunostaining with MAb BW 704
E: Treatment like C, immunostaining with MAb BW 704
F: Treatment like B, immunostaining with MAb R24
G: Treatment like C, immunostaining with MAb R24
H: Immunostaining of purified GD2 with MAb BW 625
I: Immunostaining of purified GD2 with MAb BW 704

Isolated and purified GD2 was equally well stained using both MAbs. Pretreatment of brain gangliosides with 5U VCN/ml resulted in a loss of binding of both MAbs to GD2. A similar loss of binding of GD3 to MAb R24 was observed when the ganglioside GD3 (Dippold et al. 1985) had been pretreated with VCN (see Figure 1a).

Taken together, MAbs BW 625 and BW 704 detect a VCN-sensitive epitope on the ganglioside GD2 that is not expressed on other bovine brain gangliosides including GD3, GM3, GM2, GM1, GT1a, GT1b, GD1b, GD1a, and GM4. As suggested by this immunochemical analysis the epitopes on GD2 recognized by both MAbs seem to be identical.

In order to further characterize the MAb BW 625 or BW 704 defined epitopes on ganglioside GD2 lactones were generated using two different methods (see Materials and Methods). Both MAbs showed reactivity with the lactonized GD2 ganglioside (see Figure 1b).

Ganglioside GD2, GD2-lactone 1 and 2, as produced by procedure 1, as well as GD2 and GD2-lactone 1, as produced by procedure 2, were stained to a similar extent by either antibody. After mild alkaline treatment of GD2-lactones, a procedure generating the original ganglioside GD2, only the ganglioside GD2 could be immunostained suggesting that the quickly migrating bands are no degradation products of GD2, but its lactones expressing the MAb defined epitopes.

Binding studies on neurogenic tumor derived primary or permanent cell lines. The binding of MAbs BW 625 and BW 704 to neurogenic tumor cell lines was evaluated

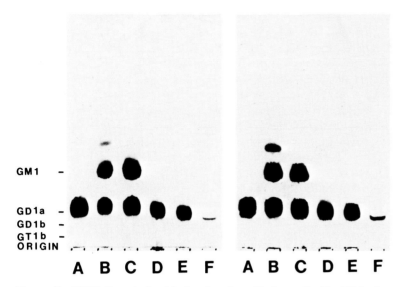

Figure 1b. HPTLC analysis of isolated and purified ganglioside GD2 after various chemical treatments. The left plate represents gangliosides immunostained using MAb BW 625, the right plate depicts identically treated gangliosides immunostained with MAb BW 704.

A: purified ganglioside GD2

B: purified ganglioside GD2 pretreated according to procedure 1 (see Materials and Methods) showing ganglioside GD2, GD2-lactone 1 and 2

C: purified ganglioside GD2 pretreated according to procedure 2 showing ganglioside GD2 and GD2-lactone 1

D: purified ganglioside GD2 pretreated according to procedure 1 (see Materials and Methods) followed by mild alkaline treatment

E: purified ganglioside GD2 pretreated according to procedure 2 (see material and methods) followed by mild alkaline treatment

F: bovine brain gangliosides immunostained with the anti GD2 MAbs

Table 1. Differential membrane immunofluorescence* of cell lines or primary cultures from neurogenic tumors by MABs BW 625 and BW 704.

MAb	Target structure	Gliomas						Neurilemmoma	Melanoma
		241	302	550	543	302	553	344	M21
BW 704	GD2	++	+	++	+ sc	+	+	+	+
BW 625	GD2	(+)	−	−	−	−	+	−	+
R24	GD3	(+)	+	+	+	+	−	(+)	+
BW 495	200 kDa GP	−	−	−	−	−	−	−	−
BW 181	mycoplasma	−	−	−	−	−	−	−	−

*In the Terasaki-IIF assay fluorescence intensity was evaluated:
++ = strong membrane fluorescence, + = significant membrane fluorescence,
−/(+) = no significant membrane fluorescence.
sc = single cells.

using an immunofluorescence assay performed with living adherent cells in Terasaki plates (Brown et al. 1977). A summary of a representative experiment is given in Table 1. MAb BW 704 bound to all neurogenic tumor cell lines tested (row 1), whereas MAb BW 625 bound to two neurogenic tumor cell lines out of the same panel only (row 2). As controls MAb R24 (specific for ganglioside GD3) binding to the majority of neurogenic tumor cell lines (row 3) as well as MAb 495 (specific for human epithelium) and MAb BW 181 (specific for mycoplasma hyorhinis), both negative on neuroectoderm derived tumors, were used (rows 4 and 5). In summary, the data from Table 1 indicate that the binding specificity of the two anti GD2 MAbs BW 625 and BW 704 is totally different despite the fact that both bound to immunochemically indistinguishable epitopes selective for GD2. MAb BW 704 bound to all cell lines tested in contrast to MAb BW 625 which bound to a minority only. The lack of binding of MAb BW 495 argues against the epithelial nature of the cell lines, because this MAb binds to epithelially derived tumors only (Bosslet et al. 1986). The lack of fluorescence staining obtained with the anti mycoplasma MAb BW 181, indicates that the cell lines investigated were not contaminated with mycoplasma hyorhinis. The finding argues against artifactual modifications of the cellular membranes leading to unexpected changes in the accessibility of membrane associated epitopes.

Immunological properties of MAbs BW 625 and BW 704. After having observed differences in the specificity of the anti GD2 MAbs BW 704 and BW 625 on neurogenic tumor derived primary cell lines we investigated the MAbs' potential to perform a) human complement mediated cytolysis (CMC) and b) the antibody-dependent cell-mediated cytotoxicity (ADCC) against human tumor cell targets.

The binding specificity of MAbs BW 704 and BW 625 as evaluated using the Terasaki IIF assay to a glioma, melanoma, neuroblastoma, and colon carcinoma cell line as well as their capacity to mediate tumor cell cytolysis via human complement is presented in Table 2a, b. Only those target cells were efficiently lysed to which the MAbs bound to a significant extent (compare rows 1, 2, 3 in Table 2a with rows 1, 2, 3 in Table 2b).

MAb BW 704 was the reagent mediating the strongest complement cytolytic activity as well as the broadest specificity on the cell lines tested (compare row 1, Table 2b with rows 2, 3, and 4).

Table 2a. Indirect immunofluorescence* using living glioma, melanoma, neuroblastoma and colon carcinoma target cells.

MAb	Target structure	Isotype	T98	M21	SKNAS	DE-TA
BW 704	GD2	IgG3	++	++	++	—
BW 625	GD2	IgG3	—	++	(+)	—
R24	GD3	IgG3	—	+	+	—
BW 495	200 kDa GP	IgG3	—	—	—	++
BW 181	mycoplasma	IgG3	—	—	—	—

* In the Terasaki-IIF assay fluorescence intensity was evaluated:
++ = strong membrane fluorescence, + = significant membrane fluorescence,
—/(+) = no significant membrane fluorescence.

Table 2b. Human complement* dependent cytolysis using glioma, melanoma, neuroblastoma and colon carcinoma target cells.

MAb	Target structure	Isotype	% specific lysis** with target cells			
			T98	M21	SKNAS	DE-TA
BW 704	GD2	IgG3	50	58	39	2
BW 625	GD2	IgG3	7	40	6	4
R24	GD3	IgG3	6	28	35	0
BW 495	200 kD GP	IgG3	4	3	4	46
BW 181	mycoplasma	IgG3	6	2	1	4

*complement dilution 1:2
**2 hrs ^{51}Cr RA

The same panel of MAbs was investigated to mediate the ADCC with human peripheral blood mononuclear cells as effector cells. Data from a representative experiment are presented in Table 3, indicating that from all MAbs of IgG3 isotype tested MAb BW 704 mediated the strongest cytolytic potential with the GD2 expressing M21 melanoma cell line. The GD2 negative DETA colon carcinoma cell line was not significantly lysed by the anti GD2 reagents combined with the effector cells but was lysed by MAb BW 495 detecting an epithelial tumor associated 200 kDa glycoprotein (row 4, Table 3).

In summary, MAb BW 704 of IgG3 isotype and selective for ganglioside GD2 was able to perform human CDC and ADCC with those targets expressing the MAb BW 704 defined epitope. MAb BW 625 of IgG3 isotype and selective for GD2 as well only bound to a minority of those cell lines bound by MAb BW 704 and mediated CDC and ADCC to a smaller extent.

Distribution of the MAb BW 704 defined epitope on cryopreserved human tissues. In the previous sections it could be shown that the MAb BW 704 defined VCN-sensitive epitope on GD2 was expressed on all neurogenic tumor cell lines tested whereas the MAb BW 625 defined epitope on GD2 was expressed on a minority of the neurogenic tumor cell lines investigated. Therefore, the following labour-intensive analysis per-

Table 3. ADCC* using melanoma and colon carcinoma target cells.

MAb	Target structure	Isotype	% specific lysis** with target cells	
			M21	DE-TA
BW 704	GD2	IgG3	38	4
BW 625	GD2	IgG3	24	5
R24	GD3	IgG3	33	2
BW 495	200 kDa GP	IgG3	4	36
BW 181	mycoplasma	IgG3	2	1

*Human peripheral blood effector: target ratio = 50:1
**4 hrs CRA

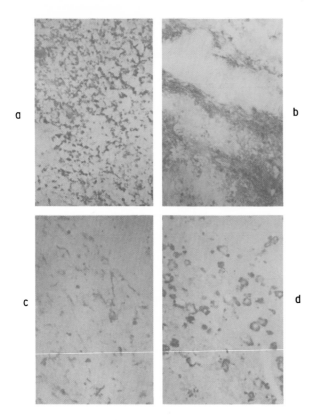

Figure 2. Photograph of a cryosection immunostained using MAb BW 704 combined with the APAAP technique.

2a: astrocytic cells diffusely stained with coarse processes and without staining of nuclei in an anaplastic astrocytoma III. Magnification 250x

2b: dense perivascular staining of glial processes in a glioma multiforme. The vessel with endothelium and connective tissue is not stained. Magnification 125x

2c: single glia cells and their processes in a cork-screw like form in a malignant polymorphic mixed glioma III. Magnification 250x

2d: strong cytoplasmic staining without a nuclear staining of "gemästet" astrocytes in a polymorphic astrocytoma III. Magnification 250x

formed on a broad panel of human normal tissues and tumors was restricted to the epitope detected by MAb BW 704. Immunohistochemical investigations with human neurogenic tumors and normal human brain are presented in Figure 2 and 3.

Positive staining was observed with gliomas, meningiomas and neurilemmomas. In normal human brain, astrocytes and presumably amyelinic axons of specific sites were positively stained. A summary of the reactivity of all intracranial tumors tested is given in Table 4.

The well differentiated gliomas (WHO I–II) were stained more strongly than the dedifferentiated gliomas (WHO III–IV), but all investigated gliomas showed a significant cytoplasmic and membranous staining (16/16). The 11 evaluated meningiomas as

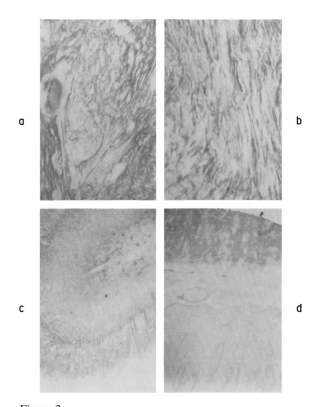

Figure 3.
3a: Strong membranous staining in an endotheliamatous meningioma. Magnification 250x
3b: Strong membranous staining in a neurilemmoma corresponding the cell architecture of the Antoni-A-formation. Magnification 250x
3c: Cortex with a medullary bundle (right corner at the top) in autoptic human brain. The center of the medullary bundle is not stained but in the branchings a weak staining can be seen. The branched axons form two ring shaped concentric condensation zones probably corresponding to the Baillarger stripes. These are penetrated by radially radiating positively stained amyelinic neurites. Magnification 50x
3d: Putamen from an autoptic human brain. A significant staining of fiber-producing astrocytes subventricularly can be seen. A weak staining at the periphery of medullary bundles can be observed whereas the central areas, the medulla, is not stained. Magnification 50x

well as the 4 neurilemmomas showed a strong membranous staining. In contrast, no binding to pituitary gland adenomas (0/5) or to a colonic cancer metastasis (0/1) was observed.

After having evaluated the expression of the MAb BW 704 defined epitope on intracranial tumors we investigated its expression on neuroblastomas, ganglioneuroblastomas, ganglioneurinomas and compared it with the expression on small round cell tumors of childhood.

Data from several experiments are summarized in Table 5 and show that the investigated small round cell tumors of childhood were negative whereas the neuroblasto-

Table 4. Specificity of MAB BW 704 on cryopreserved intracranial tumors as evaluated using the APAAP-technique.

Tumor type	Number of tumors positive	/	tested
well differentiated gliomas, grade I–II	6	/	6
malignant gliomas, grade III–IV	10	/	10
meningiomas	11	/	11
neurilemmomas	4	/	4
pituitary gland adenomas	0	/	5
carcinoma metastases	0	/	1

mas, ganglioneuroblastomas, and ganglioneurinomas were strongly positive. Only a few single cells in T-lymphomas were stained. These data indicate that MAb BW 704 could be used for the differential diagnosis of neuroblastomas and small round cell tumors of childhood.

Two further types of neuroectoderm derived tumours, melanomas and small cell lung carcinomas (SCLC) as well as unrelated carcinomas were investigated for the expression of the MAb BW 704 defined epitope. The data from these investigations are summarized in Table 6. Out of 10 melanomas investigated 4 showed a weak and heterogeneous staining. Two out of 11 SCLCs contained some slightly immunoreactive

Table 5. Specificity of MAB BW 704 on cryopreserved neuroblastomas and small round cell tumors of childhood as evaluated using the APAAP-technique.

	Number of tumors positive	/	tested
Neuroblastomas			
*grading I	5	/	5
grading II	10	/	10
grading III	6	/	6
ganglioneuroblastomas	3	/	3
ganglioneurinomas	3**	/	3
nephroblastomas	0	/	3
Ewing sarcomas	0	/	2
rhabdomyosarcomas	0	/	1
T-lymphomas	2***	/	5

  * grading according to Hughes
 ** ganglions +, Schwann's cells −
*** a few single cells positive

Table 6. Specificity of MAB BW 704 on cryopreserved melanoma, solo and unrelated carcinomas.

	Number of tumors positive	/	tested
Melanomas	4*	/	10
SCLC	2*	/	11
colon carcinomas	0	/	3
breast carcinomas	0	/	3
non SCLC:			
adeno carcinomas	0	/	3
squamous lung carcinomas	0	/	3
large cell carcinomas	0	/	3

* weak and heterogeneous staining of a few tumor cells.

Table 7. Specificity of MAB BW 704 on cryopreserved normal human tissues.

Tissue type	*Tissue components positive*	/	*negative*
brain	medullary sheath in cortex		white medulla
	medullary bundles in striatum = non-medullated axons		
peripheral nerves	non-medullated nerve		medullated nerve
peripheral blood cells			lymphocytes, monocytes, granulocytes, erythrocytes, thrombocytes }*
lymphoid organs	Hassal' bodies and connective tissue fibers in thymus		bone marrow spleen lymph nodes
	tonsillary epithelium		
hormone producing glands	a few connective tissues fibers in adrenal		pituitary gland parotid thyroid
other organs	tegumentary epithelium of skin		colon, stomach, pancreas, liver, lung, kidney, breast, testes, bladder

* cytofluorometric analysis

cells. No staining was obtained with colon, breast, and the three types of non small cell lung carcinomas.

After the evaluation of neuroectoderm derived tumours and unrelated carcinomas the expression of the MAb's BW 704 defined epitope was investigated on normal human tissues (Table 7). The white medulla of human brain was not stained, whereas the medullary sheath in the cortex and the medullary bundles in striatum were stained probably due to a reaction with the non-medullated axons. In peripheral nerve tissue medullated nerves did not react, whereas the non-medullated nerves showed a significant staining.

From the investigated lymphoid tissues only Hassal's bodies and connective tissue fibers in the thymus as well as the tonsillary epithelium expressed the MAb BW 704 defined epitope. Furthermore, a few connective tissue fibers in adrenal gland were stained, whereas all other hormone producing glands were essentially negative.

Furthermore, the tegumentary epithelium of the skin expressed the epitope. No staining was detected in organs like colon, stomach, pancreas, liver, lung, kidney, breast, testis, and bladder.

In summary, the MAb BW 704 defined ganglioside GD2 associated epitope was strongly expressed on brain tumors like astrocytomas, glioblastomas, meningiomas, neurilemmomas as well as on neuroblastomas, ganglioneurinomas, and ganglioneuroblastomas. A weak and heterogeneous expression was detected on some of the neuroectoderm derived small cell lung carcinomas and melanomas. Unrelated carcinomas were essentially negative. No staining was observed in most major human organs, except the non-medullated axons in brain and nerve, the tegumentary epithelium in skin, the connective tissue fibers in adrenal as well as Hassal's bodies and tonsillary epithelium.

Discussion

In this study it was demonstratet that the MAbs BW 625 and BW 704 bind to VCN-sensitive epitopes on ganglioside GD2 and its 2 lactones as revealed by immunochemical analysis (Figures 1a, b).

No binding to other brain gangliosides was observed. This high selectivity for GD2 discriminates MAbs BW 625 or BW 704 of IgG3 isotype immunochemically from the early murine IgM (Schulz et al. 1984) or human IgM (Katano et al. 1984) anti GD2 MAbs that were reported to show slight cross-reactivities with GD3 and GD1b.

A further consequence of the high selectivity of MAbs BW 625 and BW 704 for GD2 is probably a different tissue specificity compared with MAbs 126 (Schulz et al. 1984), 3F8 (Cheung et al. 1985) or the al series (Tai et al. 1988). Some of these anti GD2 MAbs (MAbs 126 or 3F8) bind strongly to melanomas or SCLC tumors which are only marginally or not at all stained by MAb BW 704 (see Table 6). Furtheron some normal tissues like skin melanocytes, benign nevi and supporting stroma and muscle of blood vessels were stained by MAb 126 but were not reactive with MAb BW 704 (see Table 7). These differences in tissue specificity argue for different epitopes detected by MAb BW 126 and MAb BW 704.

The fine specificity analysis on cryopreserved human tumors and normal tissues performed with the most sensitive APAAP technique revealed that the targets for MAb BW 704 were astrocytomas, glioblastomas, meningiomas, neurilemmomas, and neuroblastomas (Tables 4 and 5). The normal tissues expressing the MAb BW 704 defined epitope were some probably amyelinic axons in brain and peripheral nerve as well as the Hassal's bodies in thymus and the tegumentary epithelium in skin.

The most interesting observation of this study was the difference in the specificity of MAbs BW 625 and BW 704 on glioma cell lines (Table 1). Despite the fact that both MAbs bound to ganglioside GD2, its two lactones and not to VCN treated GD2 they showed a totally different binding specificity as outlined above. This observation argues for different epitopes on GD2 detected by MAbs BW 625 and BW 704, although the detailed immunochemical analysis did not reveal any differences.

These data clearly point out that the characterization of antigens, even though of low molecular weight (i.e. gangliosides), do not necessarily describe the fine specificity of MAbs binding to them. Phenomena like crypticity or accessibility on the membrane as well as conformational changes occurring during isolation of antigens must be considered. The biological characteristics of MAb BW 624 and BW 704 to perform the CDC and ADCC reaction with epitope positive tumor target cells argue for their potential in immunotherapy of neuroblastoma and brain tumors. Furthermore, the encouraging results obtained with MAb 3F8 (Cheung et al. 1987) in a phase I clinical study with neuroblastoma argue for the use, especially of MAb BW 704 in a similar clinical regimen.

Acknowledgements

The skilful technical assistance of H. Schmidt, N. Döring, B. Kranz, and G. Nikkhah as well as the excellent typing work of S. Lehnert is greatly appreciated.

References

1. Bosslet, K., Lüben, G., Stark, M., and Sedlacek, H. H. Molecular characteristics of two lung carcinoma cell line associated membrane antigens. Behring Inst. Mitt. 74, 27–34, 1984.
2. Bosslet, K., Kanzy, E. J., Lüben, G., and Sedlacek, H. H. A homogeneously expressed pancarcinoma epitope. Abstract: 5th NCI/EEORTC Symposium on New Drugs in Cancer Therapy, Amsterdam, Oct. 23–24, 1986.
3. Brown, J. P., Klitzman, J. M., Hellström, K. E. A microassay for antibody binding to tumor cell surface antigens using ^{125}I-labelled protein A from Staphylococcus aureus. J. Immunol. Methods 15, 57–66, 1977.
4. Cheung, N. K.V., Saarinen, U. M., Neely, J. E., Landmeier, B., Donovan, D., Coccia, P. F. Monoclonal antibodies to a glycolipid antigen on human neuroblastoma cells. Cancer Res. 45, 2642–2649, 1985.
5. Cheung, N. K.V., Lazarus, H., Miraldi, F. D., Abramowsky, C. R., Kallick, S., Saarinen, U. M., Spitzer, T., Strandjord, S. E., Coccia, P. F., and Berger, N. A. Ganglioside GD2 specific monoclonal antibody 3F8: A phase I study in patients with neuroblastoma and malignant melanoma. J. Clin. Oncol. 5, 1430–1440, 1987.

6. Cordell, J. L., Falini, B., Erber, W. N., Gash, A. K., Abdulaziz, Z., MacDonald, S., Pulford, K. A. F., Stein, H., and Mason, D. Y. Immunoenzymatic labelling of monoclonal antibodies using immune complexes of alkaline phosphatase and monoclonal antialkaline phosphatase. J. Histochem. Cytochem. 32, 219–229, 1984.

7. Dippold, W. G., Dienes, H. P., Knuth, A., Meyer zum Büschenfelde, K. H. Immunohistochemical localization of ganglioside GD3 in human malignant melanoma, epithelial tumors and normal tissues. Cancer Res. 45, 3699–3705, 1985.

8. Gatter, K. C., Cordell, J. L., Fami, B., Ghosh, A. K., Heryet, A., Nash, J. R. G., Pulford, K. A., Moir, J., Erber, W. N., Stein, H., and Mason, D. Y. Monoclonal antibodies in diagnostic pathology: Techniques and applications. J. Biol. Response Mod. 2, 369–395, 1983.

9. Hacker, W. G., Springall, D. R., Van Noorden, S., Bishop, A. E., Grimelius, L., and Polak, J. M. The immunogold-silver staining method. A powerful tool in histopathology. Virchows Arch. Pathol. Anat. 406, 449–461, 1985.

10. Harpin, M. L., Coulon-Morelec, M. J., Yeni, P., Danon, F., Baumann, N. Direct sensitive immunocharacterization of gangliosides on plastic thin layer plates using the peroxidase staining. J. Immunol. Methods 78, 135–141, 1985.

11. Houghton, A. N., Mintzer, D., Cordon-Cardo, C., Welt, S., Fliegel, B., Vadhan, S., Carswell, E., Melamed, M. R., Oettgen, H. F., and Old, L. J. Mouse monoclonal antibody detecting GD3 ganglioside: A phase I trial in patients with malignant melanoma. Proc. Natl. Acad. Sci. USA 82, 1242–1246, 1985.

12. Joseph, K., Höffken, H., Damann, V. In vivo labelling of granulocytes using ^{99m}Tc-labelled monoclonal antibodies: First clinical results. Nuc. Compact. 18, 223–229, 1987.

13. Katano, M., Saxton, R. E., Irie, R. F. Human monoclonal antibody to tumor-associated ganglioside GD2. J. Clin. Lab. Immunol. 15, 119–126, 1984.

14. Klenk, E. Über die Ganglioside, eine neue Gruppe von zuckerhaltigen Gehirn-Lipoiden. Hoppe-Seyler's Z. Physiol. Chem. 235, 24–36, 1942.

15. Klenk, E. Über eine Komponente des Gemisches der Gehirnganglioside, die durch Neuraminidaseeinwirkung in das T-Sachs Gangliosid übergeht. Hoppe-Seyler's Z. Physiol. Chem. 349, 288–292, 1968.

16. Klöppel, G. and Caselitz, J. Epithelial tumor markers: Oncofetal antigens (carcinoembryonic antigen, alpha fetoprotein) and epithelial membrane antigen. Current Topics in Pathology 77, 103–132, 1987.

17. Köhler, G. and Milstein, C. Continuous cultures of fused cells secreting antibody of predefined specificity. Nature 256, 495–497, 1975.

18. Ladisch, S. and Wu, Z. L. Detection of a tumor-associated ganglioside in plasma of patients with neuroblastoma. The Lancet II, 136–138, 1985.

19. Mach, J. P., Chatal, J. F., Lumbroso, J. D., Buchegger, T., Forni, M., Ritschard, J., Berche, Ch., Douillard, J.Y., Carrel, S., Herlyn, M., Steplewski, Z., and Koprowski, H. Tumor localization in patients by radiolabelled monoclonal antibodies against colon carcinoma. Cancer Res. 43, 5593–5600, 1983.

20. Magnani, J. L., Brockhaus, M., Smith, D. F., Ginsburg, V. A monosialoganglioside is a monoclonal antibody-defined antigen of colon carcinoma. Science 212, 55–56, 1982.

21. Mennel, H. D., Zinngrebe, J., Berweiler-Nippert, U., Lorenz, H. Meningiomas: Histogenesis and classification. A comparative morphological study. Zentralbl. allg. Phathol. pathol. Anat. 134, 27–40, 1988.

22. Ouchterlony, O. Antigen antibody reactions in gels. Arkiv Kemi Mineral. Geol. 26B, 1–3, 1948.

23. Reinherz, E. L., Kung, P. C., Goldstein, G., Schlossman, S. F. Separation of functional subsets of human T cells by a monoclonal antibody. Proc. Natl. Acad. Sci. USA 76, 4061–4065, 1979.

24. Schulz, G., Bumol, T. F., Reisfeld, R. A. Monoclonal antibody directed effector cells selectively lyse human melanoma cells in vitro and in vivo. Proc. Natl. Acad. Sci. USA 80, 5407–5411, 1983.
25. Schulz, G., Cheresh, D. A., Varki, N. M., Yu, A., Staffileno, L.V., and Reisfeld, R. A. Detection of ganglioside GD2 in tumor tissues and sera of neuroblastoma patients. Cancer Res. 44, 5914–5920, 1984.
26. Seybold, K., Locher, T. J., Coosemans, C., Andres, R.Y., Schubiger, A. P., and Bläuenstein, P. Immunoscintigraphic localization of inflammatory lesions: Clinical experience. Eur. J. Nucl. Med. 13, 587–593, 1988.
27. Shulman, M., Wilde, C. D., Köhler, G. A better cell line for making hybridomas secreting specific antibodies. Nature 276, 269–270, 1978.
28. Tai, T., Kawashima, I., Tada, N., and Ikegami, S. Different reactivities of monoclonal antibodies to ganglioside lactones. Biochim. Biophys. Acta 958, 134–138, 1988.
29. Wiegandt, H. Gangliosides of extraneural organs. Ztschr. Physiol. Chemie 354, 104–1056, 1973.
30. Yu, R. K., Koerner, T. A., Ando, S., Yohe, H. C., Trestegard, J. H. High resolution photon NMR studies of gangliosides. Elucidation of the structure of ganglioside GM3 lactone. J. Biochemistry, Tokyo 98, 1367–1370, 1985.

32. Determination of the Secondary Structures of Glycosphingolipids by NMR Spectroscopy

R. K. Yu

Summary

The primary and secondary structures of glycosphingolipids (GSLs) can be elucidated by high-field proton NMR spectroscopy and a number of 1-D and 2-D techniques. Using 2-D *J*-correlated spectroscopy which establishes scalar couplings of protons, the monosaccharide composition, anomeric configuration and aglycon structures of a GSL can be established. 2-D nuclear Overhauser effect (NOE) spectroscopy then establishes through-space intra- and inter-residue couplings of cross-relaxing protons. We have found that each anomeric proton is involved in NOE couplings with inter- and intra-residue protons; the latter can be used, in conjunction with Hard-Sphere Exo-Anomeric or AMBER potential energy calculations, to elucidate the preferred conformation of an oligosaccharide. We have found that the oligosaccharide residue of globoside exists in a unique "L-shaped" conformation which could be stabilized by hydrogen bonds and van der Waals interactions. Its terminal residue, however, is potentially flexible. Since GSLs are known to have a receptor role and are implicated in cell-cell recognition, enzyme-substrate interaction and antigen-antibody interaction, the determination of their conformation should be useful in understanding their biological functions.

It is well known that the carbohydrate portion of a glycosphingolipid is recognition, enzyme substrate interaction, antigen-antibody interaction, and other molecular events that may involve recognition processes. These events are necessarily governed not only by the primary structure but also by the secondary structure (solution conformation of the oligosaccharide moieties. The conformation for individual glycosidic bonds is governed by torsional angles $\varnothing$ and ψ as shown in Figure 1. $\varnothing$ is the torsional angle defined by the anomeric proton, anomeric carbon, glycosidic oxygen, and aglyconic carbon, and ψ is the torsional angle defined by the anomeric carbon, glycosidic oxygen, aglyconic carbon and aglyconic proton. Clockwise rotations viewed from the anomeric end are considered as positive. Thus, in disaccharide $\varnothing = O$ when H-1 and the aglyconic carbon are eclipsed, and $\psi = O$ when the anomeric carbon and the aglyconic proton are eclipsed. Information concerning the $\varnothing$ and ψ dihedral angles can be obtained experimentally from the three-bond coupling constants between ^{13}C and ^{1}H atoms in the glycosidic linkage, or the two-bond coupling constants between anomeric carbon and aglyconic carbon (1). However, these experiments are the relatively different to do because of the low nature abundance of the ^{13}C atom. On the other hand, the conformational preference of a glycosidic linkage can be obtained by energy

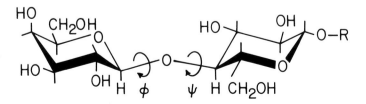

Figure 1. Dihedral torsional angles $\varnothing$ and ψ for a glycosidic linkage.

calculation programs such as the Hard Sphere Exo-Anomeric (HSEA) program devise by Lemieux and his associates (2). The program predicts that the $\emptyset$ and ψ angles about a glycosidic linkage to be essentially constant, typically $\emptyset = \pm 60° \pm 15°$ and $\psi = 0° \pm 30°$ (3), and non-zero differential chemical shifts of some of the protons are attributable to their electrostatic interaction with the oxygen atoms of the new sugar ring substituents. While the HSEA energy calculation has predicted conformations of a variety of oligosaccharides with certain degrees of certainty (2, 4, 5), it ignores energy terms which are important in determining the conformational properties. These terms include specific remote group effects, solvent effects, and H-bonding. In principle, one can improve the precision of the conformational analysis by the addition of a distance constraint in the form of pseudoenergy (6, 7). For example, under the dihedral angle constraints discussed above, the transglycosidic proton distance typically falls within 3Å. Since the cross-relaxation rate of protons (NOE) is inversely proportional to the distance of the proton pair to the sixth power, one can determine the distance by 1D- and 2D-NOESY experiments. By combining the potential energy calculations, which predict a set of energetically similar conformers, with distance constraint data in the form of pseudoenergy, it is possible to select the preferred "conformation" of an oligosaccharide. This principle has recently been applied to the analysis of the globotetraosyl head group of globoside, whose structure is shown in Figure 2.

Since the intra-residue 1,3- and 1,5-diaxial proton distance is fixed at 2.5Å, they serve as convenient internal reference to calculate inter-residue proton distances *(r)* employing NOESY. Table 1 lists the distance constraint data for globoside. These distances constraint data are converted into pseudoenergies based on the equation $Eab = W[ABS(rab^{-6} - roab^{-6}) - roab^{-6}]$, in which $roab$ is the distance between two protons determined on the basis of NOE experiments, rab is the distance between two protons at any stage of calculation, and W is a weighing factor. Such a function has a minimum of $rab = roab$ with the depth of the minimum proportional to $roab$. Energies become more positive to either side of the minimum with a rab^{-6} dependence. Thus, energies correctly mimic the precision of the NOE data at various distances.

Construction of models of the glycosidic linkages of globoside with data from Table 3 in conjunction with the allowed dihedral angles predicted by HSEA calculations (III,IV: $\emptyset = 40°$ to 60°, $\psi = -10°$ to $-50°$; II,III: $\emptyset = -40°$ to $-50°$; $= -10°$; I,II: $\emptyset =$

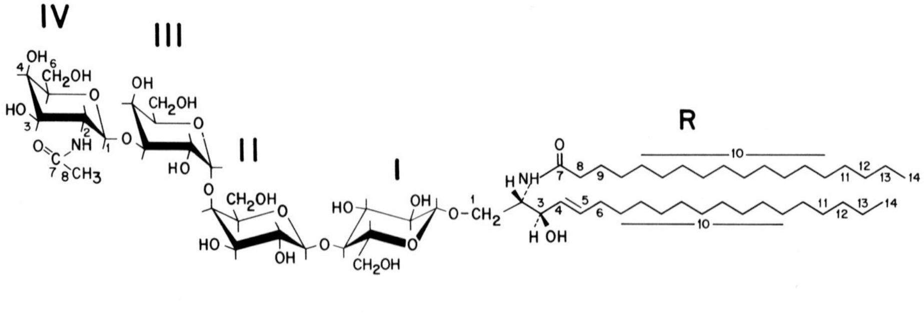

Figure 2. Structure of globoside.

Table 1. Interprotonic distance for globoside[a].

Proton Pair	r(250)[b]	r(1-dimensional)[c]
IV(1)-III(3)	2.3 ± 0.03	2.5
IV(1)-III(4)	2.9 ± 0.09	2.8
IV(1)-IV(3)[d]	2.5	2.5
IV(2)-IV(5)[d]	2.5	2.5
III(1)-II(4)	2.4 ± 0.03	2.5
III(1)-II(5)	3.5 ± 0.20	3.2
III(1)-II(6a)	2.6 ± 0.04	3.0
III(1)-II(6b)	2.6 ± 0.04	
III(1)-III(2)[d]	2.5	2.5
III(5)-III(3)[d]	2.5	
II(1)-I(4)	2.1 ± 0.02	
II(1)-I(6a)	2.8 ± 0.05	
II(1)-I(6b)	2.6 ± 0.03	
II(1)-II(5)[d]	2.5	

[a] Sample dissolved in DMSO-d$_6$, D$_2$O (98:2), distance expressed in Angstroms.
[b] Distances obtained using cross peak intensity data from NOESY experiments obtained with mixing time of 250 milliseconds.
[c] Distance obtained in one dimensional NOESY experiments, obtained through selective irradiation of a given anomeric resonance.
[d] Rigidly fixed proton pair used as a standard in computing interresidue distances.

20° to 60°, $\psi = 0°$ to $-10°$) reveal a one-state conformer to be that shown in Figure 3 (6, 8, 9).

While it is possible that such a conformation may be solvent dependent, several interesting features are apparent for this proposed structure: 1) an extended H-bond

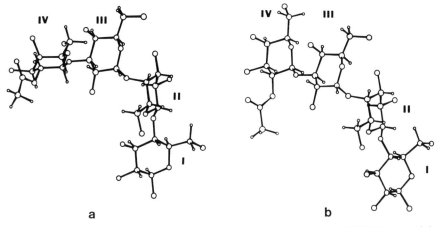

Figure 3. Molecular model of the globoside head group based on (a) HSEA potential energy calculations alone, and (b) HSEA calculations and distance constraint pseudoenergies through the use of the one-state conformer model. Hydroxyl protons are omitted since they are not considered in any of the calculations (Reproduced with permission from Reference 6).

network is optimized. Such extended H-bond networks could result in stabilizing secondary structures for oligosaccharides, as has been noted by Jeffery and Takagi (10); 2) a van der Waals interaction between the IV-2 acetamido methyl and the II-6 methylene may exist; 3) an overall "L-shape" for the oligosaccharide with a hydrophobic inner-side or "bay area" (containing the van der Waals interaction and extended H-bond network) and a hydrophilic outer-side (presenting all non-H-bonded hydroxyl groups) is apparent. Recent differential scanning calorimetry and lipid monolayer studies (11) have confirmed the existence of the L-shaped oligosaccharide conformation proposed above for globoside in acqueous solution.

Extension of the one-state model to a two-state model which takes into consideration of conformational averaging of two independent states further reveals that the terminal residue (βGalNAc) is relatively flexible (6, 7). It is tempting to speculate that this flexibility may account for the differential affinities of various globo-series glycosphingolipids to *E. coli* toxin (5). Additionally, the potentially flexible terminal residue could facilitate the displacement of globoside after its formation from globotriaosyceramide from the enzyme-substrate complex. Further studies are being carried out in relating the conformational information of glycolipids to their ligand binding property.

Acknowledgements

The author whises to acknowledge the collaborative efforts of Dr. J. H. Prestegard and Mr. J. N. Scarsdale during the course of this investigation. Financial Assistance was provided by USPHS grants NS-11853, NS-23012 and NS-26994.

References

1. Barker, R., Nunez, H. A., Rosevear, P. R., and Serianni, A. S. ^{13}C NMR analysis of complex carbohydrates, Methods Enzymol. 83, 58, 1982.
2. Lemieux, R. U., Bock, K., Delbaere, L. T. J., Koto, S., and Rao, V. S. The conformation of oligosaccharides related to the ABH and Lewis human blood group determinants. Can. J. Chem. 58, 631–653, 1980.
3. Thorgersen, H., Lemieux, R. U., Bock, K., and Meyer, B. Further justification for the *exo*-anomeric effect. Conformational analysis based on nuclear magnetic resonance spectroscopy of oligosaccharides. Can. J. Chem. 60, 44–57, 1982.
4. Bock, K., Arnurp, J., and Lonngren, J. The preferred conformation of oligosaccharides derived from the complex-type carbohydrate portions of glycoproteins. Eur. J. Biochem. 129, 171–178, 1982.
5. Bock, K., Breimer, M. E., Brignole, A., Hansson, G. C., Karlsson, K.-A., Larson, G., Leffler, H., Samuelsson, B. E., Strombert, N., Eden, C. S., and Thurin, J. Specificity of binding of a strain of uropathogenic Escherichia coli to Galα1-4Gal-containing glycosphingolipids. J. Biol. Chem. 260, 8545–8551, 1985.

6. Scarsdale, J. H., Yu, R. K., and Prestegard, J. H. Structural analysis of glycolipid head-group with one- and two-state NMR pseudo energy approaches. J. Am. Chem. Soc. 108, 6778–6784, 1986.

7. Scarsdale, J. N., Ren, P., Yu, R. K., and Prestegard, J. H. A molecular mechanistic-NMR pseudoenergy approach to the solution conformation of glycolipids. J. Computational Chem. 9, 133–147, 1988.

8. Yu, R. K., Koerner, T. A.W., Demou, P. C., Scarsdale, J. H., and Prestegard, J. H. Recent advances in structural analysis of gangliosides: primary and secondary structures. Adv. Exp. Med. Biol. 174, 87–102, 1984.

9. Yu, R. K., Koerner, T. A.W., Scarsdale, J. N., and Prestegard, J. H. Elucidation of glyco-lipid structure by proton nuclear magnetic resonance spectroscopy. Chem. Phys. Lipids 42, 27–48, 1986.

10. Jeffrey, G. A. and Takagi, S. Hydrogen-bond structure in carbohydrate crystals. Acc. Chem. Res. 11, 264–270, 1978.

11. Maggio, B., Ariga, T., and Yu, R. K. Molecular parameters and conformation of globoside and asialo-GM1. Arch. Biochem. Biophys. 241, 14–21, 1985.

33. Effects of Phorbol Esters, Dimethylsulfoxide, and Gangliosides on the Biosynthesis of Glycolipids by HL-60 Promyelocytic Leukemia Cells

X.-J. Xia, S. Ren, A. C. Sartorelli, and R. K. Yu

Summary

The relationship between glycosphingolipid synthesis and cellular growth and differentiation was investigated by measuring the incorporation of [^{14}C]-galactose into the glycolipids of HL-60 promyelocytic leukemia cells exposed to either 12-O-tetra-decanoylphorbol-13-acetate (TPA), dimethylsulfoxide (DMSO), GM3, GM1, or sulfatides*. All of these agents, except sulfatides, inhibited the growth of HL-60 cells and TPA, DMSO and GM3 induced their differentiation. Incorporation of [^{14}C]-galactose into trichloroacetic acid-precipitable material was increased in cells treated with TPA, GM3, or GM1, and decreased in cells exposed to DMSO or sulfatides. Radioactive glycosphingolipids were isolated in cells treated with the various agents to evaluate changes in ganglioside and neutral glycosphingolipid synthesis. Ganglioside synthesis, particularly GM3 formation, was increased in HL-60 leukemia cells grown in the presence of TPA, GM3, or GM1. In contrast, the formation of gangliosides was inhibited by the presence of DMSO, except for the synthesis of GM3, which was increased. Sulfatide treatment of HL-60 cells also decreased ganglioside biosynthesis. The incorporation of [^{14}C]-galactose into neutral glycosphingolipids was increased in cells treated with TPA, GM3, and GM1, and decreased in cells grown in the presence of DMSO or sulfatides. In cells treated with TPA, GM3, or GM1, the synthesis of GL2, a precursor of GM3, was significantly greater than that of control cells. This presumably accounts for the increased synthesis of GM3 in cells treated with the inducers of cellular differentiation. In addition, HL-60 cells grown either in the absence or the presence of TPA, DMSO, GM3, GM1, and sulfatides were found to synthesize glucosylceramide and small amounts of galactosylceramide. Galactosyl-ceramide synthesis was greater in cells treated with TPA than in cells treated with other agents. The findings indicate that glycosphingolipid metabolism is significantly modified in HL-60 leukemia cells induced to differentiate.

Introduction

Glycosphingolipids are located almost exclusively in the outer leaflet of plasma membranes (1). They have been shown to undergo characteristic changes in their composition and biosynthesis during cell differentiation and oncogenic transformation, and have been considered to be involved in cellular interactions and growth

---

* Abbreviations used: TPA, 12-O-tetradecanoylphorbol-13-acetate; DMSO, dimethylsulfoxide; Sulf, sulfatides; FBS, fetal bovine serum; TCA, trichloroacetic acid; PBS, phosphate buffered saline; BBG, bovine brain gangliosides; LacCer, lactosylceramide; PDGF, platelet-derived growth factor; EGF, epidermal growth factor. The ganglioside nomenclature is that of Svennerholm (23): GM3, NeuAcα2->3Galβ1->4Glcβ1->1Cer; GM1, Galβ1->3GalNacβ1->4 [NeuAcα2->3]Galβ1-4Glcβ1->1Cer; GD1a, NeuAcα2->3Galβ1->3HGalNAcβ1->[NeuAcα2->3]Galβ1->4Glcβ1->1Cer; GD1b, Galβ1->3GalNAcβ1->4 [NeuAcα2->8NeuAcα2->3]Galβ1->4Glcβ1->1Cer; GT1b, NeuAcα2->3Galβ1->3GalNAcβ1->4[NeuAcα2->8NeuAcα2->3]Galβ1->4Glcβ1->1Cer. GL1, monohexosylceramide; GL2, dihexosylceramide; GL3, trihexosylceramide; GL4, tetrahexosylceramide.

regulation (2). Differentiation associated differences in the profiles of neutral glyco-lipids (3, 4) and gangliosides (5–7) have been reported in leukemic cell lines of different degrees of maturity. Rosenfelder et al. (6) have demonstrated the incor-poration of [^{14}C]-labeled sugars into neutral glycosphingolipids of K562 and HL-60 leukemia cells. Buehler et al. (8) have performed comparative studies on the neutral glycosphingolipids synthesized by three human myeloid leukemias (K562, KG1, and HL-60). This study suggested that alterations occur in the biosynthesis of neutral glycosphingolipids and gangliosides during the differentiation of leukemic cells.

To gain further information on the effects of inducers of differentiation on the bio-synthesis of glycosphingolipids, we have evaluated synthesis of these molecules in HL-60 cells induced to differentiate by a variety of agents. TPA and GM3, which induced monocytic differentiation of HL-60 cells, markedly increased the extent of [^{14}C]-galactose incorporation into neutral glycolipids and gangliosides. DMSO, which induced granulocytic maturation of HL-60 cells, significantly inhibited [^{14}C]-galactose incorporation into neutral glycolipids and gangliosides, except for GM3. The findings suggest that the biosynthesis of glycosphingolipids, particularly GM3, is involved in the maturation of HL-60 leukemia cells.

Materials and Methods

Materials

DEAE-Sephadex A-25, Sephadex LH-20, TPA, and DMSO were purchased from Sigma Chemical Co. (St. Louis, MO). D-[1-^{14}C] galactose (Specific activity, 61 mCi/mmol) was obtained from Amersham (Arlington Heights, IL). Iatrobeads and HPTLC plates were purchased from Iatron Industries, Inc. (Tokyo, Japan) and E. Merck Co. (Darmstadt, West Germany), respectively. Gangliosides and sulfatide were isolated and purified from bovine and human brain by the method of Ledeen and Yu (9). Individual gangliosides and sulfatides were all demonstrated to be chromato-graphically pure on HPTLC plates. Kodak X-Omat AR film was from Eastman Kodak Company (Rochester, NY). All other reagents were of at least analytical grade.

Cell culture

HL-60 leukemia cells were grown in RPMI 1640 medium (Gibco, Grand Island, NY) supplemented with 10 % heat-inactivated fetal bovine serum (FBS, Gibco), 100 IU/ml of penicillin and 100 µg/ml of streptomycin at 37 °C in a humidified atmosphere of 95 % air-5 % CO_2. In experimental studies, cells were employed between passages 30 to 50 and seeded at a level of 4 to 7 x 10^5 cells/ml in RPMI 1640 medium containing 5 % FBS and either 10 nM TPA, 1.3 % DMSO, 100 µM GM3, 100 µM GM1, or 100 µM sulfatides.

Incorporation of [¹⁴C]-galactose into TCA-precipitable material

Twenty-five ml of HL-60 cell suspension was cultured with 18 uCi of D-[1-¹⁴C]galactose/flask for different periods of time in the absence or presence of TPA, DMSO, GM3, GM1, or sulfatides. An aliquot of the cell suspension was removed each day and transferred into a tube containing 1 ml of 25 % ice-cold TCA. After 10 min, the mixture was filtered (Millipore HA, 0.45 um) and the precipitate was washed with 5 ml of 5 % ice-cold TCA at least 4 times. The filters were placed in scintillation vials with 15 ml of scintillation fluid (Ecoscient, National Diagnostics, Inc., Manville, N.J.) and the radioactivity incorporated into the cells was determined using an LKB Rackbeta scintillation spectrometer.

Extraction and purification of glycosphingolipids

After incubation for 3 days in the absence or presence of various agents, cells were harvested and washed with PBS at least 3 times. After the addition of 0.2 to 0.4 ml of H_2O, cell pellets were sonicated for 3 min and the protein concentration determined by the method of Lowry et al. (10) using bovine serum albumin as the standard.

The sonicate containing 1 mg of protein (with 50 μg of BBG added as a carrier) was resuspended in 6 ml of chloroform:methanol (C:M, 1:1, v/v). The mixture was sonicated for 10 min, and the solvent was adjusted to a ratio of (C:M:Water of 30:60:8 v/v, solvent A) and further stirred overnight. After centrifugation, pellets were extracted with about 10 ml of solvent A and stirred overnight. The supernatants were combined and applied to a DEAE-Sephadex A-25 column (bed volume, 1.5 ml). The neutral glycolipid fraction was eluted with 15 ml of solvent A, and the acidic lipid fraction was eluted with 20 ml of C:M:0.8 M sodium acetate (30:60:8, v/v).

Analysis of [¹⁴C]-labeled gangliosides

The acidic lipid fraction was subjected to mild alkaline treatment (0.2 M NaOH in methanol at 37 °C for 2 hrs) to hydrolyze contaminating phospholipids, and then desalted by gel filtration on a Sephadex LH-20 column (bed volume, 20 ml). The recovered ganglioside fraction was separated on an HPTLC plate using C:M:aqueous 0.2 % $CaCl_2 \cdot 2H_2O$ (55:45:10, v/v) as the developing solvent system. Following chromatography, plates were air-dried and exposed to X-ray film for 5 to 8 days. Alternatively, plates were sprayed with resorcinol-HCl reagent (11) to locate gangliosides. The area corresponding to GM3 was removed by scraping the band from the plate, and transferred into a scintillation vial containing 0.1 ml of water and 15 ml of scintillation fluid. Vials were sonicated for 5 min and the radioactivities therein determined. Labeling of other gangliosides was measured as described for GM3.

Analysis of [¹⁴C]-labeled neutral glycosphingolipids

The neutral lipid fraction was treated with 0.2 M NaOH in methanol at 37 °C for 2 hrs to hydrolyze phospholipids, and then desalted by Folch partitioning (12). Neutral glycosphingolipids were separated on an HPTLC plate using C:M:Water (60:35:8, v/v) as the developing solvent. After chromatography, the plates were exposed to X-ray film for 5 to 8 days, and then sprayed with the orcinol-H_2SO_4 reagent (13). Labeling of GL1, GL2, and total neutral glycolipids by [^{14}C]-galactose was also determined in cells treated with various agents using a scintillation spectrometer, as described above.

Characterization of glucosyl and galactosylceramides on borate HPTLC plates

Borate HPTLC plates were prepared by spraying with 1 % $Na_2B_4O_7 \cdot 10H_2O$, drying at room temperature, and activation by heating at 95 °C for 2 hrs. Neutral glycosphin-golipids corresponding to 0.3 mg of cellular protein were applied to borate-HPTLC plates. The plates were developed using C:M:Water (60:35:8, v/v) as the developing solvent system. After plates were air-dried, they were exposed to X-ray film for ten days. The radioactivity of galactosyl- and glucosylceramides was determined as described previously.

Statistical evaluation

Results were compared by Student's t test and differences were considered statisti-cally significant when p values were less than 0.05.

Results

HL-60 leukemia cells were cultured in the presence of either TPA, DMSO, GM3, GM1, or sulfatides to measure the effects of these agents on cellular growth. All of the tested materials, except for sulfatides, inhibited cellular replication to varying degrees (Figure 1), with TPA being the most potent and GM3 and sulfatides the least inhibi-tory.

Incorporation of [^{14}C]-galactose into TCA-precipitable material was measured in HL-60 cells incubated for different periods of time in the presence or absence of TPA, DMSO, GM3, GM1, or sulfatides. The incorporation of [^{14}C]-galactose into cells treated with the various agents peaked on the second day (Figure 2). TPA, GM3, and GM1 enhanced the incorporation of [^{14}C]-galactose into the TCA-precipitable material of the cells, whereas DMSO inhibited incorporation and sulfatides had no effect.

The distribution of radioactivity in gangliosides was measured and the results are shown in Figure 3. The labelling of gangliosides by [^{14}C]-galactose was substantially modified by the presence of different agents in the culture medium. TPA, GM3, and GM1 enhanced the incorporation of [^{14}C]-galactose into gangliosides, while DMSO and sulfatides had an inhibitory effect (Figure 4). Examination of the GM3 fraction indicated that the synthesis of this ganglioside was enhanced when cells were treated with TPA, DMSO, GM3, or GM1 (Figure 5).

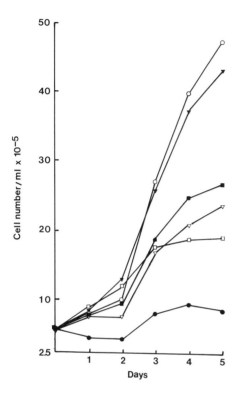

Figure 1. Effects of exogenously added TPA, DMSO, gangliosides and sulfatides on the growth of HL-60 leukemia cells.

HL-60 cells were grown in RPMI 1640 medium containing 5 % FBS in the absence of added agents (○) or in the presence of either 10 nM TPA (●), 1.3 % DMSO (□), 100 uM GM3 (■), 100 uM GM1 (▽), or 100 uM sulfatides (▼). The number of cells was determined using a Counter ZM particle counter at various times. Each value represents the mean ± S.E. of at least three separate determinations.

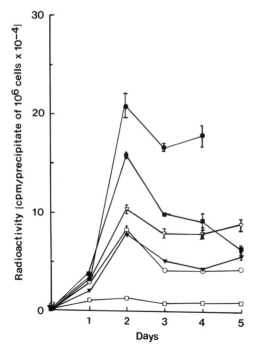

Figure 2. Effects of exogenously added TPA, DMSO, gangliosides and sulfatides on the incorporation of [^{14}C]-galactose into TCA-precipitable material of HL-60 cells.

The conditions were employed as for Figure 1. Control (○); 10 nM TPA (●); 1.3 % DMSO (□); 100 uM GM3 (■); 100 uM GM1 (▽); or 100 uM sulfatides (▼). Each value represents the mean ± S.E. of four separate experiments.

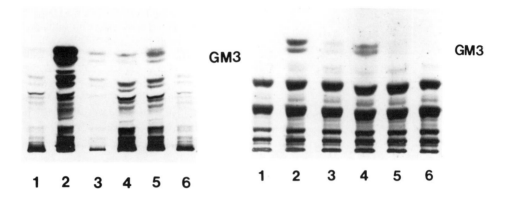

Figure 3. HPTLC chromatograms of [^{14}C]-labeled gangliosides from HL-60 cells exposed to [^{14}C]-galactose.
A. HPTLC autoradiograms; B. HPTLC chromatograms visualized by spraying with resorcinol-HCl reagent. 1. Control; 2. TPA; 3. DMSO; 4. GM3; 5. GM1; 6. sulfatides. The developing solvent system was chloroform:methanol:0.2% CaCl$_2$ · 2H$_2$O (50:45:10, v/v).

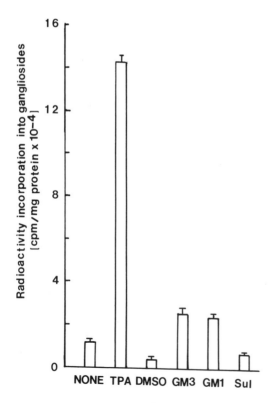

Figure 4. Effects of exogenously added TPA, DMSO, gangliosides and sulfatides on the synthesis of gangliosides.

After HPTLC chromatography of gangliosides labeled with [^{14}C]-galactose, the area corresponding to gangliosides was removed by scraping the silica from plates. Radioactivity was determined as described in "Materials and Methods". Sul:sulfides. Each value represents the mean ± S.E. of at least three separate experiments.

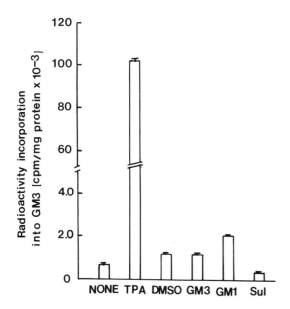

Figure 5. Effect of exogenously added TPA, DMSO, gangliosides and sulfatides on the synthesis of GM3.

After HPTLC chromatography of gangliosides labeled with [^{14}C]-galactose, the band corresponding to GM3 was removed from plates and radioactivity was determined as described in "Materials and Methods". Sul:sulfatides. Each value represents the mean ± S.E. of at least three separate experiments.

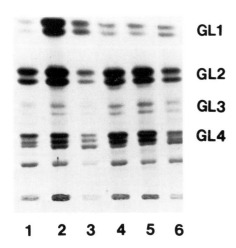

Figure 6. HPTLC autoradiograms of [^{14}C]-labeled neutral glycolipids from HL-60 cells to exposed [^{14}C]-galactose.

1. Control; 2. TPA; 3. DMSO; 4. GM3; 5. GM1; 6. sulfatides. HPTLC and autoradiography were performed as described in "Materials and Methods".

Neutral glycosphingolipids were analyzed using HPTLC followed by autoradiography (Figure 6). The total radioactivity of neutral glycosphingolipids of cells treated with TPA, GM3, and GM1 was higher than that of the control cells (Figure 7). However, treatment with DMSO or sulfatides decreased the biosynthesis of glycosphingolipids (Figure 7). The radioactivity of GL1 and GL2 in cells treated with various agents was also examined (Figure 8). TPA, DMSO, GM3, and GM1 increased the incorporation of [^{14}C]-galactose into GL1, while sulfatides had no effect. Labeling of GL2 was greater in cells treated with TPA, GM3, or GM1 than in the corresponding untreated control, but lower than in the control in HL-60 leukemia cells cultured in the presence of DMSO or sulfatides.

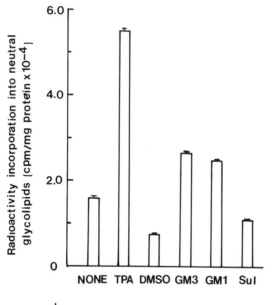

Figure 7. Effect of exogenously added TPA, DMSO, gangliosides and sulfatides on neutral glycolipid synthesis.

After HPTLC chromatography, the area corresponding to neutral glycolipids was removed by scraping from the plate and radioactivity was determined as described in "Materials and Methods". Each value represents the mean ± S.E. of at least three separate experiments.

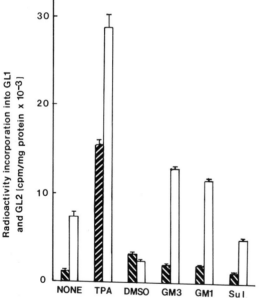

Figure 8. Effects of exogenously added TPA, DMSO, gangliosides and sulfatides on the synthesis of GL1 and GL2.

Radioactivity in GL1 and GL2 from [14C]-galactose was determined in bands corresponding to GL1 and GL2 after HPTLC separation. GL1, shaded bar; GL2, open bar. Each value represents the mean ± S.E. of at least three separate experiments.

Glucosyl- and galactosylceramides were characterized through their separation using borate HPTLC plate (Figure 9). The results indicated that HL-60 cells synthesized glucosylceramide, as reported by Buehler et al. (8). In addition, a small amount of galactosylceramide was also synthesized. TPA increased the labeling of both galactosyl- and glucosylceramides.

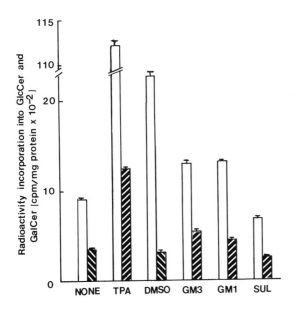

Figure 9. Effects of exogenously added TPA, DMSO, gangliosides and sulfatides on the synthesis of glucosyl- and galactosylceramides. Radioactivity in glucosyl- and galactosylceramides was determined in bands corresponding to gal- or glc-cer after HPTLC autoradiography on borate plates. Each value represents the mean ± S.E. of at least three separate experiments. Glc-Cer (□), Gal-Cer (■).

Discussion

In agreement with the reports of other laboratories (14, 15), we have found that TPA, DMSO, and GM3 inhibited the replication of HL-60 leukemia cells. Under the cell culture conditions employed in our experiments, GM1 also had an inhibitory effect; this observation is in contrast to the results of another group (14), which reported a stimulation of cell growth by this ganglioside. The reason for this difference is not known but may be related to differences in culture conditions.

TPA and GM3 induces the differentiation of HL-60 cells along the monocytic pathway (14, 17, 18), and DMSO initiates maturation along the granulocytic route (19). Since all of these agents stimulate GM3 synthesis, it has been suggested that an enrichment of membrane GM3 may be involved in the terminal differentiation process (2). GM3 and GM1 have been postulated to inhibit replication through cell-cell contact inhibition (2). In addition, the concentration-dependent binding of platelet-derived growth factor (PDGF) to certain cells has been reported to be altered by exogenous GM3 and GM1 (15, 16). Thus, ganglioside-dependent cellular growth inhibition may be caused by an altered affinity of this receptor to PDGF (15, 16). GM1 and GM3 inhibited PDGF-stimulated phosphorylation of tyrosine (17), suggesting that at the level of the membrane, GM1 and GM3 may modulate receptor function by affecting the degree of tyrosine phosphorylation, thereby altering affinity for growth factors.

We have found that differentiated HL-60 leukemia cells exhibit modifications glycolipid metabolism. Thus, the labeling of gangliosides, in particular GM3, and neutral glycolipids by [14C]-galactose was increased by the presence of TPA, GM3, or GM1. In addition, the incorporation [^{14}C]-galactose into GM3 was also increased significantly by DMSO. The increased labeling of glycosphingolipids suggests an increase in sialyl- and glycosyltransferase activities rather than a decrease in the rate of glycolipid degradation, since no significant change in sialidase activity was found during the monocytic differentiation of HL-60 cells (4). Nojiri et al. (20) reported that after treatment of HL-60 cells with the granulocytic differentiating agent DMSO for 3 days, sialidase activity was increased by 70 %. However, except for GM3, the labeling of gangliosides by galactose in cells treated with DMSO was decreased. This result may also reflect a change in the enzymatic activities involved in the metabolism of gangliosides, and this effect might be part of the reason for the low incorporation of galactose into total gangliosides in HL-60 cells exposed to DMSO.

Our results with neutral glycosphingolipids were generally similar to those reported by Momoi et al. (21) and Buehler et al. (8), except that we found that HL-60 cells also synthesized galactosylceramide. Their work (8, 21) with TLC analysis and TLC-autoradiography of neutral glycolipids from HL-60 cells demonstrated that the major neutral glycolipids cochromatographed with LacCer (GL2) and nLc4Cer (GL4). Compounds comigrating with monohexosylceramide and trihexosylceramide have been detected as minor components.

The mechanism by which glycosyltransferase activities are regulated in HL-60 cells remains unknown. However, we have previously found a parallel increase in sialyltransferase and protein kinase C activities when HL-60 cells were cultured in the presence of TPA, DMSO, or GM1 (22). The possibility exists that sialyl- and glycosyltransferase activities may be modified by phosphorylation by protein kinase C. The finding that HL-60 cells induced to differentiate into monocyte- and granulocyte-like forms show a significant increase in the labeling of GM3, together with the fact that the exogenous addition of GM3 inhibits the growth of these cells, support the concept that this ganglioside may participate in the termination of proliferation in mature cells by a cell-cell contact mechanism.

Acknowledgements: This research was supported in part by Grant CA-02817 from the National Cancer Institute and Grant NS-11853 from the National Institutes of Health.

References

1. Karlsson, K.-A. Aspects on structure and function of sphingolipids in cell surface membranes. In: Abrahamsson, S., Pascher, I. (eds): Structure of Biological Membranes. New York, Plenum, 1977, pp. 245–.
2. Hakomori, S.-I. Glycosphingolipids in cellular interactions, differentiation, and oncogenesis. Annu. Rev. Biochem. 50, 733–764, 1981.
3. Klock, J. C., Machers, B. A., and Lee, W. M. F. Complex carbohydrates as differentiation markers in malignant blood cells. Blood Cells. 7, 247–255, 1981.
4. Nojiri, H., Takaku, F., Tetsuka, T., Motoyoshi, K., Miura, Y., and Saito, M. Characteristic expression of glycosphingolipid profiles in the bipotential cell differentiation of human promyelocytic leukemia cell line HL-60. Blood, 64, 534–541, 1984.

5. Saito, M., Nojiri, H., and Yamada, M. Changes in phospholipid and ganglioside during differentiation of mouse myeloid leukemia cells. Biochem. Biophys. Res. Commun. 97, 452–462, 1980.

6. Rosenfelder, G., Ziegler, A., Wernet, P., and Braun, D. G. Ganglioside patterns: new biochemical markers for human hematopoietic cell lines. J. Natl. Cancer Inst. 68, 203–209, 1982.

7. Fukuda, M., Koeffler, H. P., and Minowada, J. Membrane differentiation in human myeloid cells: expression of unique profiles of cell surface glycoproteins in myeloid leukemic cell lines blocked at different stages of differentiation and maturation. Proc. Natl. Acad. Sci. USA 78, 6299–6303, 1981.

8. Buehler, J., Qwan, E., DeGregorio, M.W., and Macher, B. A. Biosynthesis of glycosphingolipids by human myeloid leukemia cells. Biochemistry, 24, 6978–6984, 1985.

9. Ledeen, R.W. and Yu, R. K. Gangliosides: structure, isolation, and analysis. Methods Enzymol. 83, 139–191, 1982.

10. Lowry, O. H., Rosebrough, M. J., Farr, A. L., and Randall, K. J. Protein measurement with the Folin phenol reagent. J. Biol. Chem. 193, 265–275, 1951.

11. Svennerholm, L. Quantitative estimation of sialic acid. II. A calorimetric resorcinol-hydrochloric acid method. Biochim. Biophys. Acta 24, 604–611, 1957.

12. Jordi, F., Lees, M., and Sloane-Stanley, G. H. A simple method for the isolation and purification of total lipids from animal tissues. J. Biol. Chem. 226, 497–509, 1957.

13. Sewell, A. C. An improved thin-layer chromatographic method for urinary oligosaccharide screening. Clin. Chim. Acta 92, 411–414, 1979.

14. Nojiri, H., Takaku, F., Terui, Y., Miura, Y., and Saito, M. Ganglioside GM3: an acidic membrane component that increases during macrophage-like cell differentiation can induce monocytic differentiation of human myeloid and monoloid leukemic cell lines HL-60 and U937. Proc. Natl. Acad Sci. USA 83, 782–786, 1986.

15. Bremer, E. G., Hakomori, S. I., Bowen-Pope, D. F., Raines, E., and Ross, R. Ganglioside-mediated modulation of cell growth, growth factor binding, and receptor phosphorylation. J. Biol. Chem. 259, 6818–6825, 1984.

16. Bremer, E. G., Schlessinger, J., and Hakomori, S. I. Ganglioside-mediated modulation of cell growth. Specific effects of GM3 on tyrosine phosphorylation of the epidermal growth factor receptor. J. Biol. Chem. 261, 2434–2440, 1986.

17. Rovera, G., O'Brien, T. G., and Diamond, L. Induction of differentiation in human promyelocytic leukemia cells by tumor promoters. Science, 204, 868–870, 1979.

18. Rovera, G., Santoli, D., and Damsky, C. Human promyelocytic leukemia cells in culture differentiate into macrophage-like cells when treated with a phorbol diester. Proc. Natl. Acad. Sci. USA 76, 2779–2783, 1979.

19. Collins, S. J., Ruscetti, F.W., Gallagher, R. E., and Gallo, R. C. Terminal differentiation of human promyelocytic leukemia cells induced by dimethyl sulfoxide and other polar compounds. Proc. Natl. Acad. Sci. USA 75, 2458–2462, 1978.

20. Nojiri, H., Takaku, F., Tetsuka, T., and Saito, M. Stimulation of sialidase activity during cell differentiation of human promyelocytic leukemia cell line HL-60. Biochem. Biophys. Res. Commun. 104, 1239–1246, 1982.

21. Momoi, T. and Yokota, J. Alterations of glycolipids of human leukemia cell line HL-60 during differentiation. J. Natl. Cancer Inst. 70, 229–236, 1983.

22. Xia, X. J., Gu, X. B., Sartorelli, A. C., and Yu, R. K. Effects of inducers of differentiation on protein kinase C and CMP-N-acetylneuraminic acid: lactosylceramide sialyltransferase activities of HL-60 leukemia cells J. Lipid Res. (in press)

23. Svennerholm, L. Chromatographic separation of human brain gangliosides. J. Neurochem. 10, 613–623, 1963.

34. Summary and Perspectives

S. Hakomori

Current trends in ganglioside and glycolipid research can be described in terms of several categories: (i) structural analysis, particularly focused on the conformation of the molecules; (ii) study of the functional roles of gangliosides and glycolipids in the regulation of cell growth and cellular interactions; and (iii) analysis of the antigenicity and immunogenicity of gangliosides and glycolipids expressed by cancer cells.

Structural analysis and the search for new molecular species of glycolipids remain important basic studies. An increasing diversity of molecular species have been recognized, and systematic assembly of this variety, as presented by Herbert Wiegandt, not only provides interesting linkages between phylogeny and ontogeny of the molecular species but also furnishes basic information on antigenic recognition sites. Studies directed more toward secondary and tertiary structure using NMR application, presented by Robert Yu and Jan Thurin, may define the exact three-dimensional configuration of epitopes that antibodies recognize. Such knowledge is increasingly important for efforts aimed at designing molecules of greater immunogenicity.

Studies directed at the functional role of gangliosides and glycolipids have developed in two directions: (a) gangliosides as receptors for ligands, and their role in cell-cell, cell-bacteria, and cell-virus interactions, an area somewhat outside the scope of this symposium, although of great importance in the immediate future, and (b) gangliosides as modulators of secondary signal transmission at the cell surface. There is growing evidence that receptor-associated kinases as well as C-kinase activities are inhibited or promoted by certain gangliosides, as presented by Yoshi Nagai, Robert Yu, and myself, and there will be increasing interest in this line of study as it relates to the broader field of signal transmission. A new aspect is the role of gangliosides in the regulation of calcium influx coupled with adenylcyclase activity, as discussed by Sarah Spiegel. Exciting future developments are to be expected, although the factors involved are highly complex.

Much interest in this symposium was focused on the role gangliosides and glycolipids play in determining tumor antigenicity and immunogenicity. Gangliosides and neutral glycolipids have been identified as tumor cell surface antigens with monoclonal antibodies in a large variety of tumors, particularly tumors of neuroectodermal origin such as melanoma and astrocytoma, colorectal and other gastrointestinal cancers, and lung cancer.

Glycolipids, including gangliosides, are also markers for lymphocytes, macrophages, and other immunocytes. They may be differentiation antigens of immunocytes and could act as modulators of the receptors for lymphokines. The presence of certain gangliosides on T cells, as discussed by Peter Mühlradt and Alan Houghton, may indicate such a possibility. The finding that gangliosides released from tumor cells may modulate the host's immune response, as discussed by Jacques Portoukalien and Stephan Ladish, provides important new information not only on immune regulation by gangliosides in general but also on the modification of immune regulation in the tumor-bearing host. More specifically, the studies reported by Masaru Taniguchi indicate that release of a GM3-protein complex from melanoma cells induces suppressor T cells and results in escape of the tumor from inhibition by the host's immune system. A similar mechanism may be operating with other glycolipid antigen-protein complexes in other tumor systems. An obvious need for future research is to evaluate the role each tumor ganglioside plays in modulating the host's immune response.

The most important knowledge gained by the application of monoclonal antibody technology to tumor immunology is the chemical definition of tumor antigens, many of which have now been identified as carbohydrate structures. Gangliosides are one such category. The epitopes recognized are defined with increasing precision, as discussed by Kenneth Lloyd, Ten Feizi, Takao Taki, Pamela Fredman, Wolfgang Dippold, Sandro Sonnino, Takashi Tai, Klaus Bosslet and their colleagues. However, attempts at passive immunization with monoclonal antibodies to gangliosides and active immunization with ganglioside vaccines have been limited so far to melanoma and neuroblastoma. Administration of an IgG3 mouse monoclonal antibody recognizing the ganglioside GD3 resulted in partial tumor regression in a small number of patients with melanoma, as demonstrated in the careful pioneering work of Alan Houghton, Herbert Oettgen, Lloyd Old, and their colleagues at Memorial Sloan-Kettering and Wolfgang Dippold in Mainz. Similar observations were made by Nai-Kong Cheung in patients with neuroblastoma, using an IgG3 mouse monoclonal antibody recognizing the ganglioside GD2. Further clinical application of antibodies directed to other glycolipid or carbohydrate antigens expressed by common cancers will obviously be important for future studies. The mechanisms activated by such antibodies that lead to suppression of tumor growth are probably multiple, and detailed study of the patients treated with these antibodies will be important so that factors that contribute to tumor regression or protect tumors from antibody-mediated inhibition can be defined.

Establishment of human monoclonal antibodies by the groups at Memorial Sloan-Kettering and UCLA will continue to be an important area of research for two reasons. First, one of the limitations of treatment with mouse monoclonal antibodies is the development of an anti-mouse Ig response. Second, human monoclonal antibody technology permits a detailed dissection of gangliosides and other glycolipids the human immune system can recognize. Reiko Irie emphasized that it will be necessary to develop a complete anti-ganglioside human monoclonal antibody library in order to be able to treat human melanoma effectively. Such an effort will certainly be important, and added motivation is provided by the UCLA group's apparent success in inducing regression of superficial cutaneous melanoma metastases by intralesional application of anti-GD2 and anti-GM2 ganglioside human IgM antibodies. Other uses of monoclonal antibodies such as administration of antibodies conjugated with cytotoxic drugs or toxins, or the development of anti-idiotype antibodies, have gained much interest in recent years; however, these approaches have not yet been used with ganglioside antibodies.

As Philip Livingston, Herbert Oettgen, and Lloyd Old and their associates at Memorial Sloan-Kettering have observed, purified gangliosides coated on BCG or other bacterial adjuvants can induce production of ganglioside antibodies in patients with malignant melanoma. Of the major melanoma gangliosides, GM2 was found to be most immunogenic. Whether antibody production against GM2 is associated with delayed recurrence of melanoma is now being tested in a prospective controlled study. GD3 and GD2, on the other hand, have been found to be poorly immunogenic in patients with melanoma, and approaches to increasing their immunogenicity are therefore needed. The presence of ganglioside lactones in mouse melanoma, and their stronger immunogenicity as compared with native gangliosides, suggest that ganglioside lactones or other derivatives are superior immunogens as demonstrated by Gustavo Nores and myself, and this approach has also been pursued by Gerd Ritter,

Philip Livingston, Herbert Oettgen, and Lloyd Old. Undoubtedly, this direction will be an important aspect of research in the immediate future. The approach could be used not only for ganglio-series antigens but also lacto- and globo-series tumor antigens.

An increasing number of glycolipids and gangliosides have been identified as tumor antigens with monoclonal antibodies in the past several years. Continuous efforts are justified to generate antibodies of high affinity, desired specificity, and favorable isotype. The use of such antibodies, or the use of purified ganglioside and glycolipid antigens for active immunization, represent important approaches to developing effective treatment for patients with cancers expressing these antigens. Knowledge of the role played by gangliosides in immune regulation and in cell proliferation and other manifestations of the malignant phenotype will be crucial in the development of the approach. I believe that the symposium played an important role in assessing the promise of the field and clarifying the issues we are facing.

Index